"Recognizing Celiac Disease is an excellent up to date and most comprehensive manual that is based on the The National Institutes of Health sponsored Consensus Development Conference of June 2004.

The work delivers an overview of celiac disease with a concise picture of the pathogenesis, clinical manifestations, diagnostic tools and treatment of celiac disease. Most of all it expands on the nutritional deficiencies and complications of this disease, emphasizing the dietary management of these patients.

This work will serve as an excellent reference to physicians, medical students, dietitians, patients and the general public as well."

> *- Kenneth R. Falchuk, MD, Associate Clinical Professor of Medicine*
> *Havard Medical School*
> *Beth Israel Deaconess Medical Center*

"Recognizing Celiac Disease provides medical personnel with a concise picture of the many clinical manifestations of how this disease can be expressed. Additionally, it discusses in-depth, the multitude of diagnostic techniques necessary to conduct a comprehensive differential diagnosis, along with the detailed treatment considerations. Specifically, the complexities of gluten free diet regimens are meticulously discussed.

Recognizing Celiac Disease is a comprehensive celiac disease reference that will serve as a manual for physicians and medical personnel that diagnose and treat this complex disease process."

> *- Wayne A. Satz, MD, FAAEM, Associate Professor, Emergency Medicine*
> *Vice Chairperson, Clinical Affairs*
> *Medical Director, Temple University Hospital Emergency Department*

"Recognizing Celiac Disease is a monumental work. Assembling this knowledge about celiac disease will help those who suffer from it and those who care for individuals who have suffered from it to understand the signs, the symptoms, and the triggers that cause it. This is must reading for any health professional who deals with this disease, and for individuals who suffer from it. The book will aid in both diagnosing and managing celiac disease. Cleo Libonati is to be congratulated for transforming her lived experience with Celiac Disease into a manual that helps others live with it effectively."

> *- Afaf I. Meleis, PhD, DrPS (hon), FAAN*
> *Professor of Nursing and Sociology*
> *Margaret Bond Simon Dean of Nursing*
> *School of Nursing, University of Pennsylvania*

"Recognizing Celiac Disease is well written, accessible and includes an exhaustive and very comprehensive list of symptoms. Although all of the symptoms listed have been described in association with celiac disease, the reader should also notice that not necessarily all of them are attributable directly to celiac disease as their cause.

The work successfully communicates the disease process, scope and multisystem nature of celiac disease as well as addressing treatment of nutritional deficiencies, associated disorders and the many complications of the condition.

Recognizing Celiac Disease uses documented medical research to show how seemingly unrelated symptoms in different body systems can stem from celiac disease.

Physicians who are not familiar with celiac disease should have this book on their shelves. They will find this reference a practical source of information and an important aid in making a prompt diagnosis and treating their patients.

The book is useful for prospective patients to determine whether their complaints are consistent with celiac disease. It is also an excellent patient resource for self management, especially in identifying ongoing and future health problems related to celiac disease and bringing them to the attention of their physician for proper treatment.

Recognizing Celiac Disease is a useful reference that will serve as a helpful tool for health care providers and anyone diagnosed with the disease."

- Stefano Guandalini, MD
Professor of Pediatrics, University of Chicago
Chief of Pediatric Gastroenterology, Hepatology and Nutrition
University of Chicago Children's Hospital
Founder and Medical Director, The University of Chicago Celiac Disease Center

"Recognizing Celiac Disease is an excellent up to date resource for health professionals. As a Registered Dietitian for a major grocery store retailer I need a quick and valid source of information about Celiac's at my fingertips. This is the most comprehensive source I've seen and it will surely help me to better guide my consumers towards appropriate food choices for their condition."

- Jacqueline Gomes, RD, MBA
Corporate Dietitian, Pathmark Stores, Inc.

Recognizing Celiac Disease

Signs, Symptoms, Associated Disorders & Complications

Cleo J. Libonati, RN, BSN
Foreword by David M. Capuzzi, MD, PhD

Gluten Free Works Publishing

Fort Washington, Pennsylvania

Published by:
Gluten Free Works Publishing
Fort Washington, PA 19034
USA
2007

This book is available online at www.glutenfreeworks.com.
To order contact: sales@glutenfreeworks.com
Gluten Free Works is a registered trademark of Gluten Free Works, Inc.

Cleo Libonati, RN, BSN
Edited by John Libonati, Jr.

Cover design & Book design: Joanna Libonati at Ascension Design, Ambler PA
            www.ascensiondesign.net
Cover: Healthy Villi of Small Intestine. Based on the image, "Cross Section of Normal Mucosa," used with permission of Deutsche Zöliakie-Gesellschaft, e.V. Filderhauptstraße 61, 70799 Stuttgart. (Part 1 Reference 21)

Printed in the United States of America

Publisher's Cataloging-in-Publication
Libonati, Cleo J.
    Recognizing celiac disease : signs, symptoms,
  associated disorders & complications / Cleo J. Libonati
  ; foreword by David M. Capuzzi.
    p. cm.
    Includes bibliographical references and index.
    LCCN 2006934429
    ISBN-13: 978-0-9788626-4-0
    ISBN-10: 0-9788626-4-3

    1. Celiac disease. 2. Intestines--Diseases.
  I. Title.

RC862.C44L53 2006   616.3'99
                    QBI06-600328

10 9 8 7 6 5 4 3

Contents

Part 2 Health Manifestations of Celiac Disease

ACKNOWLEDGMENTS

Sincere thanks to David M. Capuzzi, M.D., Ph.D., Professor, Thomas Jefferson University, Jefferson Medical College, Philadelphia, Pennsylvania, for his encouragement and suggestions.

We also thank the many dedicated clinicians and researchers whose work was crucial to the content development of this guide. We hope many others will access their work for a fuller understanding of this complex disorder.

We would like to thank Mary Schluckebier, Executive Director of CSA-USA, for her support.

To my special family of celiacs:

This work would neither have been undertaken nor completed without the diligent editing of my son, John, who worked with me side-by-side every day in the difficult research and crafting of this unique and complex reference.

Special thanks to my daughter, Joanna, for the design and layout of the truly handsome text you hold in your hands.

Finally, this book is dedicated to my husband, John, for his unswerving support, assistance and legal expertise.

Disclaimer:

The author gathered information from numerous sources and compiled that information into this book, which, in the author's opinion, represents some of the most up-to-date information currently available about celiac disease. While every effort has been made to provide the most accurate and up-dated information, the publisher and author cannot be responsible for any error, omission, or dated material and neither the publisher nor the author make any warranty, express or implied, in regard to the contents of this book.

The publisher and author do not guarantee that the methods and findings noted in this book will in fact identify or exclude a diagnosis of celiac disease, alleviate or exacerbate symptoms, or cause or cure the disease. This book serves only to educate readers about the disease and familiarize the reader with the existing body of research. Readers are encouraged to refer to the cited source for its full content and context.

This book does not purport to take the place of qualified medical advice and treatment. Thus, any application of the recommendations set forth in the following pages is at the reader's own risk. Please contact a doctor or other medical professional when appropriate.

Foreword

By David M. Capuzzi, MD, PhD

*Professor of Medicine, Biochemistry and Molecular Pharmacology, Jefferson Medical College
Director of the Cardiovascular Disease Prevention Center, Thomas Jefferson University Hospital*

Celiac disease is an immune-mediated disorder that stems from an inherited intolerance to dietary gluten that is a common protein found mainly in wheat, barley, rye, and oats. Until recently, celiac disease was considered to be an extremely rare condition in the United States. However, more recent findings suggest that celiac disease is far more prevalent, and that up to one percent of the U.S. population may be afflicted with this greatly under-recognized genetic disorder.

The active form of the disease develops when gluten and/or its breakdown products, detected as foreign invaders, trigger a specific immune inflammatory response in the mucosal cells that line the small intestine. The ensuing reaction causes structural and functional changes in the intestinal lining cells. These are characterized by chronic inflammation of the small intestinal mucosa that leads to flattening of the fingerlike intestinal villa, infiltration of the mucosal lining with lymphocytes, and breakage of the normally tight junctions that interconnect the lining cells. The intestinal lining then becomes hyper-permeable and leaky. As a result, a variety of clinical manifestations may develop either in childhood or later in life. These include bloating, abdominal discomfort and distention, pain and diarrhea. Mal-absorption of fluid, a variety of nutrients, vitamins and minerals may then result in weight loss, failure to thrive, and clinical evidence of multiple deficiency states. Somewhat surprisingly, a majority of individuals afflicted with celiac disease commonly fail to recognize a relationship between ingestion of gluten-containing products and the appearance of symptoms.

An undefined relationship appears to exist between celiac disease and a variety of other clinical conditions that include auto-immune thyroiditis, hypoparathyroidism, osteoporosis, dental disease, IgA nephropathy, an immune-mediated kidney disease, neuropsychiatric conditions, and in some cases, even intestinal lymphoma and carcinoma.

My own interest in celiac disease stems from my participation in a pilot project on the effects of gluten-derived peptides in an animal model system, during my doctoral training in Physiological Chemistry at the Johns Hopkins University School of Medicine. From this early experience, I developed a keen appreciation of the complexity of conducting experiments and of obtaining meaningful data in this area of investigation.

In the summer of 2004, a Consensus Development Conference was convened and conducted by an independent panel of experts in the field of celiac disease to discuss and assess the body of existing medical knowledge then available, and to identify directions for future research. This meeting was sponsored and co-sponsored by various institutes of the National Institutes of Health and by other relevant governmental agencies. A report of the proceedings of this panel and its recommendations was issued.

Recognizing Celiac Disease is a carefully composed, comprehensive, and detailed work on the multifaceted aspects of this condition. This text consolidates updated pertinent information drawn from a myriad of research studies, case reports, and updates on new diagnostic and therapeutic approaches in patients with celiac disease in this growing field of medicine. This text will serve as a useful resource to a wide range of healthcare investigators, afflicted patients and many others with an interest in or involvement with this condition.

Preface

In Italy, the time between when symptoms begin and the disease is diagnosed is usually only 2 to 3 weeks. In the United States, the time between the first symptoms and diagnosis averages about 10 years.[1]

This manual was created to increase the rate of successful medical diagnosis of celiac disease by improving recognition of typical and atypical signs and symptoms, associated disorders, and complications.

This work views celiac disease as a specific form of gluten sensitivity. Gluten sensitivity includes any and all problematic health responses to gluten in any body system.

Celiac disease predominantly affects the small intestine, but may affect other body systems. It displays itself as an immune-mediated disease of the lining of the small intestine, that is distinguished by certain types of changes to the structure of intestinal cells.[2]

Hundreds of signs, symptoms, associated disorders and complications in celiac disease may be associated with gluten exposure. Health problems result from any combination of causes, including the direct effect of gluten inside and/or outside the gastrointestinal tract, malabsorption of nutrients, and immune mechanisms.

- Gluten exposure triggers the active form of celiac disease. Active celiac disease causes damage to the intestines. Intestinal damage results in nutrient malabsorption. Nutrient malabsorption leads to a multitude of health problems. Therefore, gluten exposure can lead to any health problem resulting from a lack of any single nutrient or combination of nutrients.

- Gluten is a protein that causes loss of intestinal lining integrity (hyperpermeability). This lost integrity allows fragments of gluten to pass through the lining into the bloodstream. Once in the bloodstream, they are transported throughout the body, damaging cells and potentially provoking an immune response in any body system.

- Health disorders caused by gluten may lead to other disorders in a cascading effect.

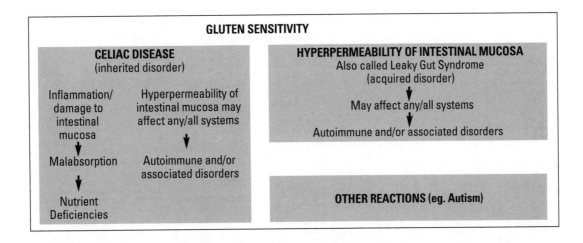

Introduction

Of 6,276 papers published on celiac disease in 30 years, only 48 had been published in the United States.[3]

    Celiac disease is the most common food sensitive enteropathy affecting Americans today. That said, clinical recognition of its full identity and range of manifestations remains seriously lacking in this country. To address these and other celiac disease-related issues, The National Institutes of Health (NIH) sponsored a Consensus Development Conference in June of 2004 and issued its Final Statement on August 9, 2004.

The Final NIH Consensus Statement issued August 9, 2004

- Celiac disease is an immune-mediated disorder with protean manifestations.

- Celiac disease is common, affecting 0.5 to 1.0 percent of the general population of the United States, but is greatly underdiagnosed.

- There are now specific and sensitive serologic tests available to aid in diagnosis that need to be more widely applied.

- The treatment of celiac disease remains a lifelong gluten-free diet, which results in remission for most individuals.

- The classic presentation of diarrhea and malabsorption is less common than previously thought. Atypical and silent presentations are increasing.

- Most individuals are being seen by primary care providers and a broad range of specialists. Therefore, heightened awareness of this disease is imperative.

- Education of physicians, registered dietitians, and other providers is needed. [4]

    This manual is based on the above NIH conclusions, past and current medical research, and the accumulated work of authorities on celiac disease and gluten sensitivity. It is comprised of two parts:

Part 1: Overview of Celiac Disease

- Describes gluten, taxonomy of gluten grains, sources of gluten-containing grains and common uses in food and safe alternatives in food preparation.
- Presents a concise picture of celiac disease, including background, description, pathophysiology, prevalence, manifestations, diagnosis, patient classification, management, and prognosis.
- Identifies the disruptive effects of celiac disease on both structure and function of the human digestive system.

Part 2: Health Manifestations of Celiac Disease

- Provides a comprehensive list of health manifestations noting relationship to celiac disease, prevalence, description, features, cause, and response to treatment with a gluten-free diet.

Part 1
Overview of Celiac Disease

CHAPTER 1
Gluten: The Environmental Trigger for Celiac Disease

CHAPTER 2
Celiac Disease

CHAPTER 3
Impact of Celiac Disease on the Digestive System

CHAPTER 1
Gluten: The Environmental Trigger for Celiac Disease

Description

Gluten is a formless storage protein in wheat, barley, rye and oat grains. Gluten is composed of smaller parts called peptides. These peptides are of two types: 1) water soluble peptides called glutenin, and 2) alcohol soluble peptides called prolamines.

The prolamines that trigger celiac disease reactions and related health disorders are gliadin in wheat, hordein in barley, secalin in rye, and avenin in oats. Avenin antibodies follow the same pattern as gliadin antibodies, but with a slightly lower magnitude.[5]

As shown in Figure 1.1 below, a grain of wheat, or seed, is composed of hull, bran, germ and endosperm. The hull seals and protects the embryonic plant from the environment. The bran is a layer of insoluble fiber that lies below the hull. The germ is a complete miniature living plant. The endosperm consists of stored nutrients and energy to be used by the germ upon germination. Gluten is combined with starch in the endosperm.

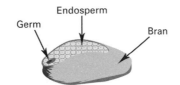

Figure 1.1 Anatomy of a Grain of Wheat

Wheat, barley, rye, and oats are related cultivated members of the grass family, which numbers about 6,000 grasses. In plant taxonomy, the name for wheat is triticum aestivum. Barley is hordeum vulgare. Rye is secale cereale. Oat is avena sativa. Figure 1.2 below illustrates their relationship in the Plant Kingdom.

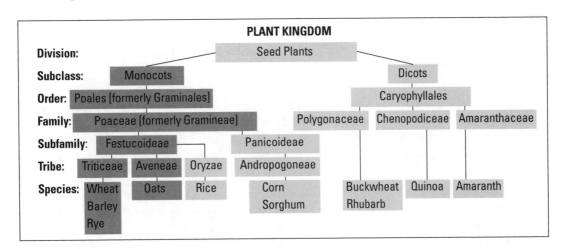

Figure 1.2 Plant Taxonomy Showing Relationship of Wheat, Barley, Rye, and Oats and Some Safe Grains and Plant Alternatives. Drawn by author with assistance of George Whiting, Associate Professor of Horticulture, Department of Landscape Architecture and Horticulture, Temple University, PA.

Sources of Gluten-Containing Grains

Although few in number, the gluten-containing grains, called toxic or unsafe grains, are widely used in food preparation. The excessively high use of unsafe grains in the Western diet makes avoiding consumption difficult.

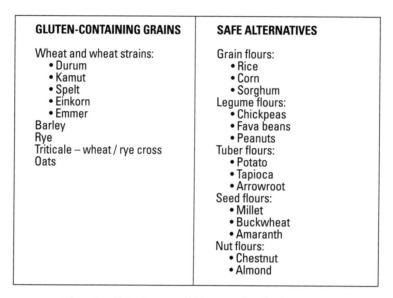

GLUTEN-CONTAINING GRAINS	SAFE ALTERNATIVES
Wheat and wheat strains: • Durum • Kamut • Spelt • Einkorn • Emmer Barley Rye Triticale – wheat / rye cross Oats	Grain flours: • Rice • Corn • Sorghum Legume flours: • Chickpeas • Fava beans • Peanuts Tuber flours: • Potato • Tapioca • Arrowroot Seed flours: • Millet • Buckwheat • Amaranth Nut flours: • Chestnut • Almond

Chart 1.1 Grain Sources of Gluten and Safe Alternatives.

Gluten-Containing Grains and Food

Wheat grain is milled into white flour, whole wheat flour, and coarse meal for a great number of uses. Gluten constitutes about 80% of the protein contained in wheat. It is by far the most common source of gluten, appearing in about 95% of processed foods. By law, wheat is the grain referred to whenever the name "flour" is used alone. Any other use of "flour" must identify the grain, such as rye flour or rice flour.

Over the centuries, wheat flour has been preferred in baking due to its unique elasticity and stickiness. These properties trap the air produced by yeast or raising agents, making dough and batter rise. Gluten holds other ingredients in suspension, allowing for a great variety of baked goods. At baking temperatures gluten coagulates, which maintains the shape of the product.

Flour and wheat starch are widely used as thickeners in condiments, sauces, gravies, soups, and casseroles. Flour is often used to bind or coat foods, such as meat before frying. Frozen potato products, French fries for example, can be dusted with flour at the manufacturing facility to prevent sticking. Bread crumbs are used in making or coating many dishes, including meatloaf, meatballs, sausage, patties, chicken and fish sticks.

The whole grain is used in cereals, bread, and cooked as a side dish such as couscous.

One hundred percent wheat gluten, called seitan, becomes firm to the bite and absorbs the surrounding broth and taste when cooked. It is substituted for meat by vegetarians. In other foods, such as bread and meat batters, gluten is added to increase the total protein content.

Barley grain is milled into coarsely ground meal and flour for use in baked goods, such as breads, rolls, and crackers. Soups, casseroles, and side dishes use the whole grain pearl barley or pot barley.

Barley is added to cold cereals like flakes, puffs, and granolas. It appears as malt or malt flavoring to provide flavor and coat cereals in order to keep them crisp. This practice contaminates "safe" grain cereals, such as corn flakes, corn puffs, rice flakes, and rice puffs.

Rye grain is milled into coarsely ground meal and rye flour. The flour is usually mixed with wheat for bread-making because the gluten in rye provides stickiness but lacks elasticity. Rye meal is used in cereal and muffins.

Oat grain is milled into flattened kernels and coarsely ground flour. The flour is mixed with wheat for bread and dough making. Oat bran is milled separately. Oats are widely used in granola, cereals, cookies, muffins, soups, and as a thickener.

Gluten-Containing Grains and Nutrition

The grains containing gluten are not necessary for good nutrition. Any nutritive benefit they have is cancelled by their damaging effect in a person with celiac disease.

Wheat, barley, rye, and oats can be replaced with other foods including safe grains, such as rice, corn, and sorghum. In addition, alternative flour is also made from ground nuts, vegetables like potatoes and tapioca, legumes that include beans, peas, lentils, and peanuts, and seeds such as buckwheat, amaranth, and millet. These safe foods have nourished people throughout history.

Chart 1.2 (page 6) lists a comparison of nutrients in wheat flour and gluten-free flours.

FLOURS 100 grams (about 1 cup)	Calories	Protein (g)	Fat (g)	Carbs (g)	Fiber (g)	Calcium (mg)	Iron (mg)	Magnesium (mg)	Phosphorus (mg)	Potassium (mg)	Sodium (mg)	Zinc (mg)	Copper (mg)	Manganese (mg)	Selenium (mg)	Thiamin (mg)	Riboflavin (mg)	Niacin (mg)	Pantothenic Acid (mg)	Vitamin B6 (mg)	Folic Acid (mg)	Vitamin B12	Vitamin E (mg)	Fatty Acid, Monounsaturated (g)	Fatty Acid, Polyunsaturated (g)
SOY FLOUR, FULL FAT	441	34.8	22	34	9.7	188	5.8	369	476	2041	12	3.6	2.2	2.1	7.5	0.4	0.9	3.3	3.28	1.2	227	227	2	4.82	12.3
PEANUT FLOUR, LOW FAT	428	33.8	22	31	16	130	4.7	48	508	1358	1	6	2	4.2	7.1	0.5	0.2	11	11.5	1.5	133	133	0	10.9	7
CHICKPEA FLOUR	387	22.4	6.7	58	11	45	4.9	166	318	846	64	2.8	0.9	1.6	8.3	0.5	0.1	1.8	1.76	0.6	437	437	0.8	1.5	2.98
AMARANTH FLOUR	374	14.5	6.5	66	15	153	7.6	266	455	366	21	3.2	0.8	2.3	0	0.1	0.2	1.3	1.28	1	49	49	0	1.43	2.89
RICE BRAN FLOUR	316	13.4	21	50	21	57	19	781	1677	1485	5	6	0.7	14	16	0	0.3	34	34	7.4	63	63	4.9	7.54	7.45
BUCKWHEAT FLOUR	343	13.3	3.4	72	10	18	2.2	231	347	460	1	2.4	1.1	1.3	8.3	0.3	0.4	2.8	7.02	1.2	30	30	0	1.04	1.03
QUINOA FLOUR	374	13.1	5.8	69	5.9	60	9.3	210	410	740	21	6	0.8	2.3	7	0.1	0.4	7	2.93	1	49	49	0.4	1.53	2.34
SORGHUM FLOUR	339	11.3	3.3	75		28	4.4	0	287	350	6	0	0	0		0.2	0.1	2.9	2.92	0	0	0	0	0.99	1.37
RICE FLOUR, BROWN	363	7.23	2.8	76	4.6	11	2	112	337	289	8	2.5	0.2	4	0	0.4	0.1	6.3	6.34	1.6	16	16	0	1	0.99
CORN FLOUR, WHOLE-GRAIN	361	6.93	3.9	77	13	7	2.4	93	272	315	5	1.7	0.2	0.5	15	0.2	0.1	1.9	1.9	0.7	25	25	0.4	1.01	1.75
RICE FLOUR, WHITE	366	5.95	1.4	80	2.4	10	0.4	35	98	76		0.8	0.1	1.2	15	0.1	0.1	2.6	2.59	0.7	0	4	0.1	0.44	0.37
WHEAT FLOUR, ALL-PURPOSE	364	10	1	76	2.7	15	1.2	22	108	107	2	0.7	0.7	0.7	34	0.1	0	1.3	0.4	0.4	0	0	0.3	0.1	0.4

Chart 1.2 Nutrient comparison of wheat and gluten-free flours compiled from USDA Nutrient Database.

Recognizing Celiac Disease Signs, Symptoms, Associated Disorders & Complications

CHAPTER 2
Celiac Disease

Celiac disease is the most commonly misdiagnosed, or missed diagnosis in medicine.[6]

BACKGROUND

The following history of celiac disease was provided by Celiac Sprue Association – USA:

> The earliest description of celiac disease was recorded in the second century A.D. In 1888 Samuel Gee published a monograph on celiac disease that "to regulate the food is the main part of treatment ... The allowance of farinaceous foods must be small ... but if the patient can be cured at all, it must be by means of diet."

> In the early 1900's a carbohydrate restricted diet was advocated where the only carbohydrates allowed were ripe bananas and rice. Then in the 1950's Dr. W. K. Dicke published work reporting that celiac children improved dramatically during World War II when wheat, rye and oat flour were scarce and therefore excluded from the diet. When these grains were reintroduced as a dietary mainstay after World War II the negative affect on celiac children was also noted. These observations were confirmed by other researchers who also demonstrated that "gluten" was the harmful component in wheat flour. Thus the gluten-free diet was born.

> In 2002, Shan et al. demonstrated that the gluten-free diet model was valid. These researchers identified a 33-mer peptide (a chain of amino acids) as the primary initiator of the inflammatory immune response to gluten in celiac disease. They also identified tissue transglutaminase as the major autoantigen in celiac disease. This identification resulted in a more sensitive and specific serum antibody test which can be used to screen for celiac disease or to track individual response to gluten exposure.

> Tissue transglutaminase was first identified by the late Dr. Elizabeth Ferguson of Glasgow, Scotland.

> Despite the advances in celiac disease, the inclusion of oats in a gluten-free diet remains controversial. Clinical studies suggest that some people with celiac disease tolerate uncontaminated oats. Other researchers have reported an inflammatory gastrointestinal immune response to oats. At this time there is no method to identify which people with celiac disease will tolerate uncontaminated oats and those who will not. The addition of oats is not a risk free choice for those on a gluten-free diet.[7]

Celiac Disease is the most common chronic intestinal disease in the world.[6]

DESCRIPTION

Celiac disease was traditionally defined as a gastrointestinal malabsorption disorder that presents early in childhood after the introduction of dietary gluten. It is now recognized that the clinical manifestations are highly variable, may present at any age, and involve multiple organ systems.[4]

Although also referred to as gluten sensitive enteropathy, non-tropical sprue or celiac sprue, celiac disease is the term most often utilized. The International Classification of Diseases (ICD) code for celiac disease is "579.0 Celiac Disease."

Celiac disease is an inherited lifelong intolerance to gluten, a protein found in the grains of wheat, barley, rye and oats. When ingested, gluten precipitates hyperpermeability and inflammation of the small intestinal lining, or mucosa, and damage to its structures and function. Damage to the mucosa interferes with nutrient absorption and triggers the formation of autoimmune antibodies.

Strict exclusion of gluten from the diet usually results in rapid healing of the mucosa, resolution or improvement of nutrient deficiencies, and the disappearance of many manifestations of celiac disease.

Celiac disease is a complex disorder with six components:

1. **Genetic.** It is inherited, meaning it runs in families.
2. **Chronic.** It never goes away. Damage worsens with continued gluten ingestion.
3. **Autoimmune.** The immune system attacks the body's own tissue.
4. **Digestive.** The digestive system is damaged, disrupting its ability to function.
5. **Malabsorption.** Nutrients are not properly absorbed by the damaged digestive system.
6. **Multi-system.** Every part of the body can be affected.

1. Genetic. People who have inherited genes for celiac disease have the "potential" to develop an autoimmune response triggered by gluten exposure. Potential means there can be no response without first eating food that is made with wheat, barley, rye, or oats. The gluten protein precipitates development of "active" celiac disease.

2. Chronic. Once developed, active celiac disease continues as long as gluten is consumed. Damage stops only when gluten-containing food is completely removed from the diet. Susceptibility to future harm from gluten remains because it is part of the genetic make-up.

3. Autoimmune. Celiac disease first affects the digestive tract. All health problems begin when partially digested sub units of gluten contact the surface of the small intestinal lining. A destructive, autoimmune response occurs in the small intestine at the site where gluten is being digested. Once the autoimmune reaction is triggered, inflammation and damage result.

4. Digestive. The body's interaction with toxic gluten prolamines produces a rapid inflammation of the small intestinal lining. The inflammation causes intestinal swelling and damage to the villi and crypts, resulting in progressive loss of the natural folds of the lining and the surface area available to absorb nutrients.

5. Malabsorptive. Loss of absorptive capacity results in malnutrition. Because damaged villi cannot properly digest, absorb or transfer the full amounts of nutrients into the bloodstream as required for health, deficiency in one or more nutrients follows. As a result, the body cannot work well and health problems develop.

6. Multi-system. Any part of the body can develop health problems. Manifestations result from one or a combination of causes, including the direct effect of gluten peptides inside and/or outside the gastrointestinal tract, nutritional deficiencies, and associated autoimmune mechanisms.

- Certain undigested peptides, called exorphins, adversely affect mental function due to their opioid effect, causing mental apathy, irritability, depression, anxiety, and other psychiatric disturbances.

- Undigested peptides, abnormally ciculating in the bloodstream, can directly harm any tissue on contact, causing disorders, such as non-alcoholic fatty liver disease and arthritis.

- Nutritional deficiencies can cause malfunctions in one or many parts of the body. For example, vitamin A deficiency leads to visual problems that begin as dry eyes but may end in blindness. Rough, scaly skin develops. Other problems caused by vitamin A deficiency include respiratory and urinary tract infections and reproductive failure.

- Associated autoimmune disorders and serious, disabling, or deadly complications can affect any body system.

Celiac disease is self-perpetuating in the continued presence of gluten.[8] Although under 10 mg of gliadin in wheat gluten a day seems to be tolerated by most celiacs, some individuals experience reactions to less than 5 mg per day. Dose dependent studies have shown that around 25 mg of gliadin produces symptoms and intestinal changes. 10 mg of gliadin equals 20 mg of gluten, which in turn equals 250 mg of wheat flour - less than 1/8 teaspoon.[9]

Considerable progress has been made in understanding celiac disease.[4]

PATHOPHYSIOLOGY

Contributing events that lead to the immune system response and intestinal damage characterizing celiac disease are thought to follow this sequence:

• Genetic predisposition allows for creation of antibodies.

• Exposure to gluten is the most important environmental factor in triggering celiac disease.[10]

• Gluten resists complete breakdown into harmless amino acids by normal digestive enzymes in all persons, whether or not they have celiac disease. Incomplete digestion yields undigested peptides.

• These undigested peptides relax intercellular tight junctions of the lining. The peptides then enter the submucosa. Tight junctions, the controlled spaces between cells lining the small intestines, serve as the main barrier to the passage of such large molecules.

• The enzyme, tissue tranglutaminase, deamidates, or alters, undigested peptides that have breached the tight junctions.

• HLA-DQ2 and/or HLA-DQ8, proteins present in the submucosa of affected individuals, bond to deamidated peptides to form molecular complexes that stimulate the immune system.

• These complexes trigger a potent inflammatory response by celiac disease-specific T lymphocytes. The ensuing inflammation damages the intestinal lining resulting in villous atrophy and crypt proliferation of varying degrees.

• Antibodies are produced against tissue transglutaminase, endomysium, reticulin, and gliadin.

Genes and the Role of HLA-DQ2 and HLA-DQ8

There is a strong genetic predisposition to celiac disease, with the major risk attributed to the specific genetic markers known as HLA-DQ2 and HLA-DQ8 that are present in affected individuals.[4] HLAs (human leukocyte antigen) are markers located on leukocytes that help them discriminate between host cells and foreign cells. Leukocytes are white blood cells that are quickly attracted to foreign cells and bind them for the purpose of destroying them.

HLA-DQ2 and HLA-DQ8 play an important part in the pathogenesis of celiac disease by binding to altered peptides derived from dietary gluten in wheat, barley, rye, and oats. Greater than 97 percent of celiac disease individuals have the DQ2 and/or DQ8 marker, compared to about 40 percent of the general population. Therefore, an individual negative for DQ2 or DQ8 is extremely unlikely to have celiac disease.[4] No difference in the clinical or pathological parameters of severity between HLA types was found.[11]

Protein Toxicity and the Role of Tissue Transglutaminase

The resistance of gluten prolamines to digestive enzymes is thought to be a key contributor to the pathogenesis of celiac disease by promoting the intestinal entrance of peptides able to trigger inflammation in at-risk individuals.[12] The toxic mechanism that ensues involves tissue transglutaminase, a ubiquitous intracellular enzyme. Tissue transglutaminase modifies proteins and peptides in the gut, by transamidation or deamidation of specific glutamine residues.

The interaction of tissue transglutaminase with long, undigested peptides of gliadin in wheat is the most studied. The peptides become toxic after tissue transglutaminase acts to deamidate, or break off, the rich glutamine residues present in gliadin to form glutamic acid. Glutamic acid is an amino acid that can be taken up by the enterocytes. Deamidation creates molecular compounds called epitopes, that are then seen as foreign by the host cell-mediated immune system.[13]

The deamidated peptide most studied is the 33-mer derived from alpha-gliadin in wheat gluten. The 33-mer is a peptide fragment of 33 residues (alpha2-gliadin 56-88) produced by normal gastrointestinal protein digestion. It contains six partly overlapping copies of three T cell epitopes and is a remarkably potent T cell stimulator after deamidation by tissue transglutaminase.[14]

In addition to findings on alpha-gliadin, analysis of one type of gamma-gliadin in wheat led to the identification of another 26-mer peptide that was also resistant to further gastric, pancreatic, and intestinal brush border degradation, and was a good substrate for transglutaminase. At least 60 disease-causing peptides that share the common characterisitics of the 33-mer and the 26-mer peptides have been identified.[15]

Intestinal Hyperpermeability and Breach of the Intestinal Barrier Defense System

Both gastric and small intestine permeability are disrupted in patients with celiac disease.[17] Gliadin is thought to initiate an autoimmune enteropathy by stimulating the innate immune response to increase intestinal permeability and by upregulating macrophage proinflammatory gene expression and cytokine production.[16]

Under normal circumstances, the interplay between immune cells and the contents of the intestines that would cause an immune response is prevented by a competent barrier defense system made up in large part by intercellular tight junctions, the controlled spaces between surface cells of the lining.[18]

Disruption of tight junctions leads to intestinal hyperpermeability (the so-called "leaky gut") that is implicated in the pathogenesis of celiac disease.

Only a single layer of epithelial cells, or enterocytes, separates the contents of the small intestine from immune cells in the underlying lamina propria and the internal environment of the body.[18] The lamina propria is the thin layer comprised of areolar connective tissue, blood vessels, and nerves that lies immediately beneath the surface epithelial cells.[19] A breach of this single layer of epithelial cells, by means of disrupted tight junctions, can expose immune cells in the lamina propria to a myriad of microorganisms and food antigens, leading to immune reactions.[18]

Zonulin is an intestinal protein that functions as a mediator of gut permeability. Gliadin induces zonulin release in enterocytes activated in part by opening of tight junctions. Zonulin release leads to a rapid increase in intestinal permeability that then allows gliadin to cross the intestinal barrier.[20]

Cell-Mediated Immune Response and Lymphocytosis

Cellular immunity seems to play the major role in the intestinal damage in celiac disease.[10]

An increase in the expression of HLA markers on cells in the surface layers of the intestinal mucosa is seen after 2 to 4 hours of exposure to gluten. Gluten peptides interact with the HLA molecules to activate an abnormal immune response, promoting a massing of killer lymphocytes.[10]

The intense inflammatory reaction that results as the killer immune cells amass to destroy the foreign substances produces villous flattening, characteristic of celiac disease.[13] The inflammatory response likely also affects the structural support and microcirculation of the villus, leading to collapse of the villus. The thickening of the crypt is not so much a response to loss of surface enterocytes but represents inflammation of the mucosa. This damage is most intense in the proximal small intestine and decreases toward the ileum.[10]

The extent of the damage to the intestine determines the malabsorptive consequences of the disease.[10] This largely explains the great number of possible symptoms, multi-system involvement, considerable variation among patients, and the variation of symptoms in the same individual at different times.

Humoral Response

Antibodies produced by the immune system in celiac disease involve immunoglobulin-A (IgA) and immunoglobulin-G (IgG). There is little or no immunoglobulin-E involvement. IgA and IgG are directed against a variety of antigens, including transglutaminase, endomysium, gliadin, and reticulin.[13] The antibodies are secreted into the intestinal lumen and are detected in circulating blood.[10]

The dynamics of the humoral response seem to parallel the cellular injury, although antibodies may arise before mucosal relapse and disappear before healing. Secreted antibodies against gliadin may be a vain attempt to exclude a harmful antigen, whereas antibodies to connective tissue (endomysium and reticulin) may target autoantigens in connective tissue (transglutaminase).[10]

Histopathology

The histopathology of celiac disease is a continuum from normal villous architecture with intraepithelial lymphocytosis, through partial villous atrophy to total villous atrophy.[11]

Villi are minute structures of the small intestinal lining that function to absorb nutrients from food. They wave in a pumping motion as the liquid mix of nutrients passes through them. Numbering in the millions, villi give the mucosa surface an appearance of velvet.

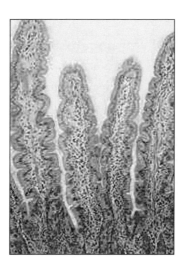

Figure 2.1 Cross Section of Normal Mucosa.[21] Used with permission Deutsche Zöliakie-Gesellschaft.

Progressive inflammation leads to collapse of villi and thickening of the crypts, resulting in loss of the ability to digest, absorb and transfer nutrients.

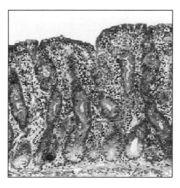

Figure 2.2 Cross Section of Mucosa of a Patient Suffering from Celiac Disease.[21] Used with permission Deutsche Zöliakie-Gesellschaft.

The intestinal surface can become flattened, losing both its folds and villi structures. The surface capacity to absorb nutrients can diminish from the size of a tennis court to the size of a table top.[1]

Importance of Distinquishing Non-Celiac Gluten Sensitivity Reactions

Gluten may be able to drive the immune system, even outside the gastrointestinal tract, to cause other diseases that we do not call celiac disease, but are still gluten-derived diseases.[29]

Celiac disease must be distinguished from non-celiac gluten sensitivity, which appears to affect many more people than celiac disease. Estimates run as high as 15% of the population. Non-celiac gluten sensitivity disorders do not involve the intestinal lesion that is characteristic of celiac disease, although they may involve other aspects including breach of the intestinal barrier and association with autoimmune diseases.

Increased intestinal permeability is a part of celiac disease, but it may also subject the non-celiac patient to gluten sensitivity reactions. Studies have revealed non-gastrointestinal manifestations with positive blood tests for anti-gliadin antibodies without evidence of celiac disease, indicating gluten entering the bloodstream via increased membrane permeability of the small intestine.[22] The cause may be bacterial flora, diet, psychological stress, oxidative stress, intense exercise, aging, drugs and toxins.[17]

Gluten, as a neuroactive compound derived from the intestinal lumen, can permeate either diseased or healthy mucosa, cross the blood-brain barrier and cause psychiatric, cognitive and behavioral disturbances.[23]

Factors other than gluten that disrupt tight intercellular junctions include the following:[17]

- Gastrointestinal infections from microbes such as rotavirus, parasites, pathogenic bacteria (Escherichia coli, Clostridium difficile toxins), and mycotoxins (toxins produced by fungi found in stored grain and dried fruit).

- Fats such as rancid fats, sodium caprate, (a medium-chain fat), and sucrose monester fatty acid, (a food-grade surfactant), induce significant disruption.

- Foods such as alcohol, lactose, caffeine, paprika, cayenne pepper, refined carbohydrates, some food preservatives and food additives.

- Medications such as oral antibiotics, NSAIDS such as aspirin and ibuprofin, corticosteroids, and oral contraceptives.

- Psychological stress

- Oxidative stress

- Excessive exercise

- Aging

Celiac Disease is 100 times more common than most things screened by doctors.[6]

PREVALENCE

Celiac disease is a common medical condition. Celiac disease was historically considered to affect just 1 in 5,000 persons in the United States. The assumption that celiac disease is a rare disease was a common error that led to the widespread failure to diagnose celiac disease.[24]

Advances in the understanding of the multi-system nature of celiac disease and the identification of sensitive serologic tests have led to the recognition that celiac disease is much more common than previously thought. United States population-based studies indicate the prevalence of celiac disease to be in the range of 0.5 to 1.0 percent. A study of Denver children under age 5 demonstrated a prevalence of 0.9 percent.[25] These findings suggest celiac disease affects up to 3,000,000 Americans.[4]

A study of 830 children initially enrolled as healthy newborns demonstrated a minimum prevalence of celiac disease of 1 per 69 newborns who completed the study. No child had anti-tissue transglutaminase immunoglobulins at the first visit at 1 to 1.5 years of age, but 9 children had anti-tissue transglutaminase immunoglobulins at the second visit at 2.5 years of age. One patient refused biopsy. Of the remaining 8, intestinal biopsy showed flat mucosa in 7, confirming the diagnosis of celiac disease. These statistics are similar to worldwide prevalence statistics that estimate celiac disease affects 1% of the human population.[26]

A systematic review of the prevalence of celiac disease in general Western populations and in populations at high risk for celiac disease revealed that the prevalence of celiac disease in patients suspected of having celiac disease varied depending on the reasons for suspecting celiac disease and whether the study was conducted at a referral center. In general, the prevalence ranged from 5% to 15%, but was as high as 50% in symptomatic patients evaluated in a hospital.[27]

The prevalence is higher still in high-risk groups. Clinicians in a variety of specialties should have a high index of suspicion for the diagnosis of celiac disease and, in particular, need to pay close attention to the identified high-risk groups.[27] First degree relatives of individuals with biopsy-proven celiac disease have villous atrophy on biopsy ranging from 4% and 12%. Second degree relatives also appear to have an increased prevalence, although this has been defined only by blood antibody tests.[4]

Certain populations with other disorders have an increased prevalence of celiac disease:

- 100% of persons with dermatitis herpetiformis.
- 20% of persons with collagenous colitis.
- 14.8% of persons with lymphocytic colitis.
- 14% of persons with anti-phospholipid syndrome.
- 3 to 8% of persons with type I diabetes mellitus.
- 5 to 12% of persons with Down syndrome.
- 7.9% of persons with Addison's disease.
- 5.7% of persons with cardiomyopathy.

A body of evidence shows that celiac disease is associated with protean manifestations outside the intestine, and neurological disorders are well recognized.[28]

MANIFESTATIONS

There is no typical presentation of manifestations.[10] More than 300 diverse signs, symptoms and related health conditions are known to indicate a person may have celiac disease. Each one may be the only manifestation of celiac disease.

Signs and symptoms may present following an environmental trigger such as high dose gluten challenge, gastrointestinal surgery, excessive physical, mental or emotional stress, pregnancy, and viral or bacterial infection.[10]

Most patients who get diagnosed exhibit the classic symptoms, such as diarrhea and anemia.[29]

However, it is very common for celiac disease to present with nongastrointestinal manifestations, sometimes with little or no gastrointestinal symptoms. About 60% of cases are now revealed by non-gastrointestinal manifestations where diagnosis is largely due to the use of blood tests.[30]

Patients with celiac disease have a larger burden of other diseases than the general public.[11] For example, untreated celiac disease increases the rate of cancers two to three times the average rate.[29]

Both nutritional and immune-related nongastrointestinal manifestations associated with celiac disease can increase in severity and outcome if the treatment plan does not include a gluten-free diet. In addition, the longer an individual with celiac disease is exposed to gluten, the higher the likelihood of other associated autoimmune disorders.[31] Some findings suggest that celiac disease itself is responsible for the high prevalence of other autoimmune diseases. Persistent stimulation by some proinflammatory cytokines could induce further processing of autoantigens and their presentation to T lymphocytes.[32]

Categorizing Manifestations

In view of the great number of health manifestations, it is helpful to categorize them by their relationship to celiac disease. A current system identifies manifestations as 1) classic signs and symptoms, 2) atypical signs and symptoms, 3) associated disorders, or 4) complications.[33]

1. Classic Signs and Symptoms refer to what have traditionally been considered to be the expected manifestations of celiac disease. Most patients with classic signs and symptoms present with anemia, weight loss, bloating, abdominal pain, steatorrhea, and diarrhea that can range from mild to massive. Classic signs and symptoms in children can also include lassitude, failure to thrive and a protruding abdomen.[4]

2. Atypical Signs and Symptoms refer to those signs and symptoms that are other than classic signs and symptoms. Examples include urinary tract infection, joint pain, weight gain, constipation, premenstrual syndrome, depression, headache, hypoparathyroidism, irritable bowel syndrome, kidney stones, and gastroesophageal reflux disease (GERD).

3. Associated Disorders refer to disorders that are caused by gluten exposure, related immune mechanisms and/or nutrient deficiencies. Examples include anxiety, insomnia, chronic fatigue syndrome, attention deficit/hyperactivity disorder, gall bladder dysfunction, Crohn's disease, hypertension, angina pectoris, cardiomyopathy, insulin dependent diabetes mellitus, Addison's disease, Grave's disease, alopecia, psoriasis, allergic rhinitis, and chromosome aberrations.

4. Complications refer to manifestations that develop with duration of celiac disease. Complications can effect physical, mental, and emotional derangement, disfigurement and pain. Examples include obesity, short duration of breast feeding, gastric ulcer, atherosclerosis, stroke, cataracts, pneumonia, osteoporosis, and various cancers.

To think early of the possibility of intolerance to gluten is to give the means of a very easy diagnosis.[34]

DIAGNOSING CELIAC DISEASE

The single most important step in diagnosing celiac disease is to recognize its myriad clinical features. No one test can definitively diagnose or exclude celiac disease in every individual. Just as there is a clinical spectrum of celiac disease, there is also a continuum of laboratory and histopathologic results.[4]

Serologic antibody studies are confirmed by endoscopy with small bowel biopsy. Other methods include ultrasound procedure, genetic testing, capsule endoscopy and gluten-free diet trial.

To be considered accurate, tests must have a high degree of sensitivity and specificity. Sensitivity is how likely the test will detect what is being looked for. Specificity is how likely what is being looked for determines that the patient has the disease.

> **All diagnostic tests must be performed while the patient is continuously eating a gluten-containing diet.**[4]
> In patients who have started a diet without any diagnostic test for more than 3 months serological tests may be inconclusive necessitating a gluten challenge. The periods of the gluten challenge and the amount of gluten necessary to provoke a serological response are individually different.[35]

1. History and Physical Examination

The investigating clinician must know and understand the manifestations of celiac disease and must be looking for symptoms consistent with celiac disease.

A detailed history of symptoms must be obtained. This history should include a comprehensive list of signs, symptoms, associated disorders and complications that the patient has experienced or is experiencing. A physical examination is then performed, seeking to reveal current celiac disease-related manifestations.

2. Serologic Antibody Screening (Blood Tests)

Blood tests are available to screen for celiac disease. Blood drawn from the patient is tested in an experienced laboratory for the presence of specific antibodies.

Tests performed by experienced laboratories are more reliable. Internal and external test controls are better established in experienced laboratories than in laboratories where the celiac disease serology panel is only one of the routine tests. More importantly, laboratories specializing in celiac serological testing have a larger number of positive and negative samples to validate their tests and they are able to set up more accurately the negative, intermediate and pathologic values.[35]

Based on very high sensitivities and specificities, the best available autoimmune antibody tests are the anti-human tissue transglutaminase antibody (tTG) test and the endomysial antibody (EMA) immunofluorescence tests. Both appear to have equivalent diagnostic accuracy.[4] The anti-gliadin antibody (AGA) test is less accurate for celiac disease, but accurate as an inexpensive test useful to screen for evidence of an immune reaction to gliadin.

Anti-Tissue Transglutaminase Antibody (tTG) Test. The tTG test sensitivity is 98% in adults and 96% in children. Specificity is between 95% and 99%. Since the analysis is performed by a computer, it is less costly than the EMA test. The best time to begin measuring tissue transglutaminase antibodies in children is age 2 to 3 years, as recommended in a recent prospective screening study for celiac disease.[26]

Endomysial Antibody (EMA) Test. The EMA test sensitivity is in excess of 90% with specificities over 95%. The test is more costly than the tTG because the actual lab work requires human evaluation.

Anti-Gliadin Antibody (AGA) Test. Antigliadin antibody tests have lower sensitivity (70 to 85%) and specificity (70 to 90%) for celiac disease. These tests are less specific in young children.[10]

Total Serum IgA Test. This test determines whether the individual has IgA antibody deficiency.

Antibody Test Results and Diagnosis: How They Work and What They Mean

- Positive Antibody Results.

  Raised IgA antibodies indicate short-term immune response, indicating ingestion of gluten 2-4 weeks preceding the test.

  Raised IgG antibodies demonstrate long-term immune response, indicating ingestion of gluten from three to six months, sometimes up to a year preceding the test.

- Negative Antibody Results.

  Blood tests that return negative results for both IgA and IgG antibodies would be considered negative, ***providing the patient has been regularly ingesting dietary gluten for the preceding three months.***[35]

continued next page

3. Endoscopy Procedure with Proximal Intestine Biopsies

Intestinal biopsy is the gold standard for diagnosis of celiac disease. Celiac disease is the most common disorder that a gastroenterologist would see.[29] Nevertheless, it has been demonstrated that the majority of patients with anemia, iron deficiency, weight loss, and diarrhea do not undergo small bowel biopsy at endoscopy. Endoscopy provides an opportunity to obtain tissue to diagnose celiac disease, thus biopsy should be strongly considered whenever endoscopy is performed.[37]

Biopsies of the proximal small bowel are indicated in individuals with positive celiac disease antibody test results except those with biopsy proven dermatitis herpetiformis.[4] Biopsies should also be performed on patients with negative antibody test results yet having symptoms consistent with celiac disease.

Endoscopic evaluation without biopsies is inadequate to confirm or exclude a diagnosis since endoscopic findings are not sufficiently sensitive for celiac disease. Multiple biopsies should be obtained because the tissue changes may be focal (patchy). Biopsies should be obtained from the second portion of the duodenum or beyond.[4]

Celiac disease can be associated with minimal mucosal changes. A patient may exhibit positive serology and seemingly normal histology, or tissue structure. However, damage to the absorptive villi may be submicroscopic. Submicroscopic damage would imply a reduction of intestinal absorption is already occurring, even in this latent stage of the disease. In these patients, more significant alterations of the villi may develop at a later date.[38]

The pathology report should specify the degree of crypt hyperplasia and villous atrophy as well as assess the number of intraepithelial lymphocytes.[4] A negative report may result from poor technique in obtaining the tissue to be biopsied or from inaccurate determination by the pathologist who examines it.[35]

Biopsy Results: What They Mean

Three distinct patterns of mucosal abnormalities have clinical relevance:

- Infiltration of the villous epithelium with lymphocytes and a normal villi and crypt architecture. This pattern is found in 40% of individuals with dermatitis herpetiformis and a portion of first degree relatives of celiacs who have no gastrointestinal symptomatology.

- A flat mucosa characterized by villous flattening and crypt elongation with inflammatory cells in the lamina propria, the connective tissue under the epithelium that contains blood vessels. This pattern is classically found in individuals with celiac disease who have gastrointestinal symptoms, but has also been reported in asymptomatic celiac relatives and individuals with dermatitis herpetiformis.

- A hypoplastic mucosa characterized by villous flattening and small crypts. This biopsy is found in the small group of patients with presumed severe celiac disease unresponsive to a gluten-free diet.

4. Additional Tests for Celiac Disease and Gluten Sensitivity

Ultrasound Procedure. Ultrasound is especially useful for exploring celiac disease in children because it does not require needle sticks or anesthesia. An ultrasound is performed to look for abnormal appearance of the small bowel wall. Compared to intestinal biopsy results, ultrasound identification of changes related to celiac disease has been found to have a sensitivity of 94% and a specificity of 88%.[39]

Genetic Testing – HLA Haplotypes. More than 97% of people with celiac disease share the same genetic HLA haplotype markers. These markers are HLA-DQ2 and HLA-DQ8. DQ2 and DQ8 have high sensitivity but poor specificity, indicating a low positive predictive value but a very high negative predictive value for celiac disease.

It is useful to test for the HLA-DQ2 and HLA-DQ8 genetic markers in the following patients:

1. Relatives of diagnosed patients with celiac disease and dermatitis herpetiformis.
2. Patients with negative blood tests that exhibit manifestations of celiac disease.
3. Patients with ambiguous biopsy results.
4. Patients who started a gluten-free diet before diagnostic testing.

HLA typing should not be used in the diagnosis of celiac disease in patients with type 1 diabetes mellitus because of the similarities of HLA types between patients with type 1 diabetes and those with celiac disease.[40]

Capsule Endoscopy Procedure. Capsule endoscopy is a useful test for obtaining continuous images of the entire digestive tract. It can be used as an additional test if biopsy results are inconclusive or as an alternative if patients cannot undergo endoscopy with biopsy. The patient swallows a pill-size capsule that contains a camera and miniature lights. The camera takes thousands of photographs of the inside of the entire digestive tract and transmits them to a computer that the patient wears throughout the day. The process is expensive, but highly accurate, noninvasive and easy to administer.

Gluten-Free Diet Trial. No test is 100% accurate. Serology tests and biopsies have returned negative on one occasion and positive on another or negative on one test and positive on a different type of test. If tests are negative, yet symptoms are still being experienced, then the patient should be put on a gluten restrictive diet. Remission of symptoms would indicate gluten sensitivity.

5. Definitive Diagnosis

Communication between the pathologist and the individual's physician is encouraged to help correlate the biopsy findings with laboratory results and clinical features. Second opinions on biopsy interpretation may be sought when biopsy results are discordant with serologic markers or clinical findings.

With concordant positive serology and biopsy results, a presumptive diagnosis of celiac disease can be made. Definitive diagnosis is confirmed when symptoms resolve subsequently with a gluten-free diet. A demonstration of normalized histology following a gluten-free diet is no longer required for a definitive diagnosis of celiac disease.[4]

When the diagnosis of celiac disease is uncertain because of indeterminate results, testing for certain genetic markers (HLA haplotypes) can stratify individuals to high or low risk for celiac disease. HLA haplotype testing provides high negative predictive value. Greater than 97 percent of celiac disease individuals have the HLA-DQ2 and/or HLA-DQ8 marker, compared to about 40 percent of the general population. An individual negative for DQ2 or DQ8 is unlikely to have celiac disease.

Patient preferences should be elicited in developing recommendations in the setting of a positive celiac disease serology and normal biopsy results. A single best approach cannot be prescribed. Choices include additional small bowel biopsies, periodic monitoring with celiac disease serology tests, or a trial of gluten-free diet.[4]

Failure to appreciate the variable clinical manifestations of celiac disease can lead to long delays between onset of symptoms and diagnosis.[2]

PATIENT CLASSIFICATION

There is an existing classification of patients with commonly accepted subphenotypes, or characteristics of celiac disease. Whether these subphenotypes are clinically useful remains to be determined. These include the following:

- **Classical Celiac Disease** is dominated by symptoms and secondary consequences of gastrointestinal malabsorption. The diagnosis is established by serological testing, biopsy evidence of villous atrophy, and improvement of symptoms on a gluten-free diet.

- **Celiac Disease with Atypical Symptoms** is characterized by few or no gastrointestinal symptoms. Nongastrointestinal manifestations predominate. Recent improvement of recognition of atypical features of celiac disease is responsible for much of the increased prevalence. As recognition improves further, atypical symptoms may become the most common presentations. As with classical celiac disease, the diagnosis is established by serologic testing, biopsy evidence of intestinal inflammation and villous atrophy, and improvement of symptoms on a gluten-free diet.

- **Silent Celiac Disease** refers to individuals who have no apparent symptoms but have a positive serologic test and villous atrophy on biopsy. These individuals are usually detected via screening of high-risk individuals, or detection of intestinal inflammation and villous atrophy through endoscopy and biopsy that was conducted for another medical reason.

- **Latent Celiac Disease** is defined by a positive serology but no inflammation and villous atrophy on biopsy. These individuals are asymptomatic, but later may develop symptoms and/or histologic changes.[4]

People with classic symptoms represent only the tip of the celiac iceberg. Below that tip are those with atypical, silent, and latent symptoms.[29] Figure 2.3 below illustrates the relationship between symptoms and intestinal damage in people who have positive antibody test results.

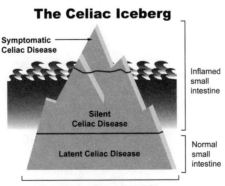

Figure 2.3: Illustration of the Celiac Iceberg.

Recognizing Celiac Disease Signs, Symptoms, Associated Disorders & Complications

It is early elimination of gluten which will make the various clinical manifestations disappear and so prevent the risk of evolution to a tumoral pathology.[34]

MANAGEMENT

The current management of celiac disease is a strict gluten-free diet for life.[4]

Treatment for celiac disease should begin only after a complete diagnostic evaluation including serology and biopsy.[4] The institution of a gluten-free diet should result in prompt and often dramatic improvement. Resolution of symptoms may take 3 to 6 months. Complete healing of the intestines may take longer in some individuals, especially the elderly. Recovery is more rapid and complete in children than in adults.[10]

The following are six key elements in the management of individuals affected by celiac disease as advanced by the NIH panel statement:

Consultation with a skilled dietitian.
Education about celiac disease.
Lifelong adherence to a gluten-free diet.
Identification and treatment of nutritional deficiencies and other manifestations.
Access to an advocacy group.
Continuous long-term follow-up by a multidisciplinary team.[4]

Consultation with a skilled dietitian

Gluten is so widely used that newly diagnosed patients need detailed lists of the foodstuffs to avoid, as well as a diet plan. Expert advice from a dietitian familiar with celiac disease is recommended. Properly kept food diaries can be instrumental in identifying gluten sources of accidental ingestion.

Education about celiac disease

Self-education is critically important. Learning about celiac disease and how to identify gluten-containing products is associated with improved self-management. Visual aids and Internet resources are helpful.

Lifelong adherence to a gluten-free diet

The management of celiac disease is a lifelong gluten-free diet. A gluten-free diet is defined as one that excludes wheat, rye, barley, and oats. Even small quantities of gluten are harmful, preventing remission or inducing relapse. Considering less than 5 mg of gliadin per day can cause symptoms in some people, eliminating gluten ingestion as completely as possible is prudent.

The strict definition of a gluten-free diet remains controversial due to the lack of an accurate method to detect gluten in food products and the lack of scientific evidence for what constitutes a safe amount of gluten ingestion.[4]

Identification and treatment of nutritional deficiencies and other manifestations

Health care providers should consider and treat nutritional deficiencies including vitamin, mineral, protein, carbohydrate and essential fatty acids. At diagnosis, obtain baseline serology of vitamins A, D, E, K, B_{12} and folate and minerals iron, calcium and phosphorus.[4] Mild cases may not require supplementation. Severe cases may require comprehensive nutritional replacement.

Access to an advocacy group

Participation in an advocacy group is an effective means of promoting adherence to a gluten-free diet and may provide emotional and social support.[4] There are hundreds of celiac disease support groups in the United States.

Continuous long-term follow up by a multidisciplinary team

Following initial diagnosis and treatment, individuals should return for periodic visits with the physician and dietitian to assess symptoms and dietary adherence, and monitor for complications. In children, this includes evaluation of growth and development. During these visits, health care providers can reinforce the benefits of adhering to a strict gluten-free diet for life.[4]

Repeat serologic testing may be used to assess response to treatment but that this may be used to assess improvement is unproven. These tests may take a prolonged time (up to 1 year) to normalize, especially in adults, and may not correlate with improved histology. Persistent elevated serological levels may suggest lack of adherence to a gluten-free diet or unintended gluten ingestion.[4]

Individuals eating so-called "gluten free" oats (not contaminated with wheat, rye or barley), require follow-up to detect clinical intolerance to oat gluten stemming from avenin-reactive T lymphocyte activity.

Intestinal permeability assessment by way of sugar absorption tests may be used for evaluating the severity of illness and is a good marker of response to gluten-free diet for follow-up in patients with celiac disease.[17] Hydrogen breath testing may also be used to monitor sugar digestion and follow-up.

Individuals who do not respond to a gluten-free diet require reevaluation. No established approach exists to screen for complications of celiac disease.

The damage should be reversible in most cases.[9]

PROGNOSIS

The personal cost of celiac disease can be great. Symptoms can cause discomfort ranging from inconvenience to deep personal distress that can leave the patient debilitated and unable to properly participate in life and work. Both benign and malignant complications of celiac disease occur, but can be avoided by early diagnosis and compliance with a gluten-free diet.[10]

A person with untreated celiac disease is more likely to die prematurely than the normal population, but a person with celiac disease following a strict gluten-free diet is likely to live five years longer than the average population.[6]

Clinical outcome depends on duration of exposure to gluten. The longer gluten is consumed, the more the body is damaged and the greater the likelihood of health disorders and complications developing. Early recognition of celiac disease manifestations is crucial for optimum prognosis.

Intestinal permeability improves within two months of starting a gluten-free diet. Measurable intestinal biopsy improvement requires ingestion of a gluten-free diet for at least three to six months. Complete recovery can take up to five years or more. Even then, recovery can remain incomplete.[41]

Despite a good clinical response, abnormal endoscopic and histological appearances persist in the majority of patients. In a study of 39 people who had clinically responded to a gluten-free diet that they had maintained for a mean of 8.5 years, endoscopic appearance was normal in 23%, reduced duodenal folds present in 46%, scalloping of folds 33%, mucosal fissures in 44% and nodularity in 33%. There was more than one abnormality in 46%. Histology, or cell structure, was normal in only 21%. The remainder had villous atrophy (69% partial, 10% total).[42]

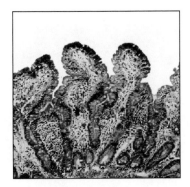

Figure 2.4 Recovering Villi.[43] Reprinted with permission from BCMJ 2001:43:7:392

Lack of adherence to strict gluten-free diet is the main reason for poorly controlled disease in adults. Baseline education significantly predicts dietary compliance and intestinal damage at follow-up.[44]

Refractory Sprue and Cryptic Intestinal T-Cell Lymphoma

Refractory sprue is a diagnosis of exclusion. In poorly responsive patients, diagnosis of refractory sprue can be established after exclusion of a limited number of conditions.[45] Refractory sprue is a severe complication of celiac disease characterized by persistence of symptoms and intestinal inflammation despite gluten-free diet.[10] It is marked by intractable diarrhea, villous atrophy, constant fatigue, and wasting malnutrition. Refractory sprue may occur after a positive initial response to gluten-free diet or without any evidence of preexisting celiac disease.[45]

The presence of an aberrant clonal intraepithelial T-cell population has led to the designation of refractory sprue as a cryptic intestinal T-cell lymphoma. In a subgroup of patients with enteropathy-associated T-cell lymphoma (EATL) there is progressive deterioration of a refractory form of celiac disease. EATL derives from a clonal proliferation of intraepithelial lymphocytes.[46] The prognosis is poor, although some patients respond to corticosteroids and immunosuppressive agents.[45]

Future Medical Therapy

Oral enzyme therapy is under intense investigation by researchers. An enzyme called prolyl-endopeptidase (PEP) has been shown to digest gliadin peptides into harmless parts.

Laboratory studies of intestinal biopsy specimens from patients with active celiac disease demonstrated that after prolonged exposure to high concentrations of PEP, the amount of immune stimulatory gliadin peptides reaching immune system cells was decreased. These results established a basis whether such conditions are achievable in the body.[12,15]

CHAPTER 3
Impact of Celiac Disease on the Digestive System

The digestive system consists of many organs and parts. Each performs its own function while interacting in harmony with others every time we eat. These complex organs and parts turn the food we eat into specific components to fuel, build, maintain, repair, regulate, and protect our bodies.

Muscles, nerves, reflexes, enzymes, and hormones of the digestive tract all work together to change food into nutrients that can be absorbed into the bloodstream and lymph system. These two transport systems then carry fresh supplies of nutrients throughout our body to nourish every individual cell.

Celiac disease interferes with this basic function by way of inflammation and damage to tissues and structures of the small intestinal lining, the mucosa. Alteration in form and function of the mucosa results in malabsorption of nutrients.

Celiac disease causes many gastrointestinal health problems. It affects the harmony of organs by disrupting the action of muscles, nerves, reflexes, enzymes, and hormones. Structural and functional changes lead to problems such as difficulty swallowing, reflux, nausea, abdominal bloating, constipation and diarrhea.

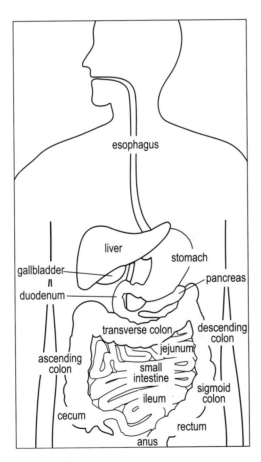

Figure 3.1: Organs of the Digestive System. Courtesy NIH.

HUNGER AND APPETITE

The brain monitors nutritional needs and employs a hunger mechanism to alert us when fresh food is needed. Hunger is mainly caused by the need for protein.

Hunger causes appetite, the desire for food. The tempting sight, smell, taste and expectation of food stimulate involuntary sensory nerves. By reflex action, these sensory nerves cause muscle and sensory activity in various digestive organs. Salivary glands in the mouth begin to secrete saliva as stomach glands and muscles become active.

Conditions Affecting Hunger and Appetite Associated with Celiac Disease.

- **Loss of appetite**, or anorexia, can result from just one nutrient deficiency or combinations of deficiencies. These nutrients include zinc, iron, magnesium, phosphorus, potassium, thiamine, vitamin B_{12}, and protein.*
- **Increased thirst** results from deficiencies of omega fatty acids and potassium.*

See Part 2: Categorized Manifestations of Celiac Disease for details.

ACTION OF THE MOUTH

Chewing food begins digestion. Food is made ready to swallow by the tearing and grinding action of the teeth and the chemical breakdown action of saliva. Saliva adapts to the type of food being chewed, dissolving substances and diluting materials that would be too concentrated for the stomach.

Saliva consists of mucin and salivary amylase. Mucin is a slippery carbohydrate-protein complex, which protects the lining of the mouth, lubricates the food for swallowing, neutralizes acids present in food and kills many bacteria that enter the mouth with food. Salivary amylase is a digestive enzyme that breaks down starch. Salivary amylase works best when the mouth is neutral or has a slightly alkaline Ph (not acidic).

Conditions and Diseases of the Mouth Associated with Celiac Disease.

- Painful mouth ulcers, both aphthous ulcers (canker sores) and non-aphthous ulcers.*
- Lowered saliva pH (acidic), predisposing to dental cavities and poor starch digestion.*
- Dental enamel defects.*
- Gingival inflammation, bleeding, and eventual tooth loss from infection resulting from deficiency of vitamin C.*

continued next page

- Cracking at the corners of the mouth, burning of the lips, mouth and tongue which appears magenta with hypertrophy or atrophy of papillae resulting from deficiency of riboflavin.*
- Pale, sore, and swollen tongue resulting from deficiency of iron.*
- Scarlet, swollen tongue with burning of the mouth resulting from deficiency of niacin.*
- Beefy red, smooth tongue with burning resulting from deficiency of vitamin B_{12}.*
- Oral inflammation resulting from deficiency of folic acid and vitamin B_6.*
- Increased susceptibility to infection resulting from deficiency of iron and vitamin A.*
- Impaired taste resulting from deficiency of zinc, vitamin B_{12}, and niacin.*

See Part 2 Health Manifestations of Celiac Disease for details.

ACTION OF THE PHARYNX AND LARYNX

Swallowing that is started by voluntary action in the mouth is completed by reflex through the pharynx. The pharynx is the area in the throat below the mouth in the larynx. The opening of the trachea, or glottis, is closed by the automatic action of the attached epiglottis leaning backward over it, to keep food from entering the lungs. Breathing is held by reflex to prevent choking.

Conditions and Diseases of the Pharynx and Larynx Associated with Celiac Disease.

- Burning of the throat resulting from deficiency of niacin.*
- Dysphagia, difficulty or the inability to swallow.*
- Cancer of the pharynx.*
- Post-cricoid carcinoma.*
- Laryngospasm resulting from deficiency of calcium, magnesium, vitamin D.*

See Part 2: Categorized Manifestations of Celiac Disease for details.

ACTION OF THE ESOPHAGUS

Located in the middle of the chest, the esophagus is a hollow muscular tube positioned behind the heart and lungs that generally follows the curvature of the spine. The average person's esophagus is approximately 10 inches (24 cm). In its resting state, the walls of the esophagus flatten front to back measuring almost one inch (about 2 cm) wide.

The esophagus performs swallowing through highly coordinated voluntary and involuntary muscle actions, called peristalsis, that quickly move the food into the stomach. These muscles move the food 2-3 cm per second. Liquids are able to rapidly pass into the stomach without peristalsis.

The thickened end of the esophagus works in concert with the lower esophageal sphincter (LES) to reliably pass food into the stomach. The LES is a strong muscle band surrounding the stomach opening. It relaxes to allow food into the stomach and closes to keep food from going back into the esophagus, preventing reflux.

Conditions and Diseases of the Esophagus Associated with Celiac Disease.
- Burning of the esophagus resulting from deficiency of niacin.*
- Dysphagia, difficulty or the inability to swallow.*
- Esophageal motor abnormalities.*
- Heartburn.*
- Gastroesophageal reflux disease (GERD).*
- Plummer-Vinson syndrome resulting from deficiency of iron.*
- Cancer of the esophagus.*
- Esophageal small cell carcinoma.*

See Part 2: Health Manifestations of Celiac Disease for details.

ACTION OF THE STOMACH

The stomach is a complex organ that is chemically monitored and controlled by the brain and nervous system. This form-changing muscular sack acts as a holding tank, mixing food until it is dissolved and broken down into a liquid state called chyme.

The shape and size of the stomach can vary considerably, depending on the position of the body and the amount of filling. When empty, the front and back of the stomach practically touch. A tough organ, the stomach can hold an entire meal because its wall is elastic and made of stretchable folds called rugae. It can stretch to hold nearly 2 liters of food and fluid.

Located in the upper abdomen, the stomach is composed of four specialized areas: cardia, fundus, body, and pylorus. Each is distinctly different in muscle and gland structure.

When food enters the cardia, it first falls to the pylorus initiating strong muscle contractions that push the food up toward the fundus. Muscle contractions of the main body portion follow, one after another, alternating with pyloric contractions. These powerful muscles churn the food and mix it with gastric juice, dissolving and breaking it down into liquid. The pylorus regulates this mixing of food and gastric juice for proper consistency before allowing it to pass into the small intestine.

Gastric juice is composed of a high concentration of hydrochloric acid and enzymes, pepsin and gastric lipase. Hydrochloric acid dissolves food tissues and kills most bacteria that are swallowed with food. Pepsin begins the digestion of proteins, working best in an acid environment. Gastric lipase is the enzyme that begins the digestion of fats.

Cells lining the stomach secrete about 3 liters of gastric juice from numerous, microscopic glands every day. The secretion of gastric juice is controlled by a hormone called gastrin. Stomach cells are replaced every three days due to the erosive effect of gastric juice.

Partially digested food can take 1½ hours to 6 hours before passing on to the small intestine, depending on the type and amount of food eaten. Rich food, raw food, and/or large quantities will substantially delay passage through the pylorus.

Conditions and Diseases of the Stomach Associated with Celiac Disease.
- Nausea and vomiting resulting from deficiency of magnesium, potassium, and niacin.*
- Indigestion resulting from deficiency of thiamin.*
- Delayed gastric emptying.*
- Low hydrochloric acid levels cause low pepsin output, resulting in poor protein digestion.*
- Gastric ulcer and ulcerations.*
- Gastritis, both lymphocytic and collagenous.*
- Increased permeability of gastric mucosa.*
- Increased susceptibility to H. Pylori Bacter infection, leading to ulcers.*

See Part 2: Health Manifestations of Celiac Disease for details.

ACTION OF THE SMALL INTESTINE

The liquid food mass, chyme, enters the small intestine where the work of digestion and absorption of proteins, carbohydrates, fats, vitamins, minerals, and bioflavanoids takes place.

The small intestine is a complex, hollow muscular tube comprised of three segments: the duodenum, jejunum, and ileum. It has an overall length of 22 feet (6.8 meters) and is the longest section of the digestive tract.

The inside lining of the small intestine is formed into tightly packed folds that overlay the muscle layer. This folding greatly increases the lining's surface area contacting the chyme. The folds are covered with multitudinous, tiny, hollow projections called villi. The barely visible villi (0.5 to 1.5 mm long) jut out into the passing chyme. By this formation, they provide significantly more surface area for absorbing nutrients than the folds alone can provide.

The total number of the jejunum and ileum villi is estimated at 4,000,000.

Enzymes that split the disaccharides, lactose, sucrose, and maltose, into simple sugars and small peptide chains into amino acids are produced by villi.

The walls of the villi are made up of microscopic absorptive cells that are continually exposed to digested nutrients moving along their surface. These cells do the actual work of absorbing nutrients. In addition, each of the absorptive cells has numerous microscopic projections called microvilli. The microvilli are collectively called the "brush border."

The prodigious numbers of microvilli dramatically increase absorption. Altogether, the folds, villi and microvilli in a healthy small intestine make up a huge surface area for absorbing nutrients that is calculated to equal the size of a tennis court.

Conditions and Diseases of the Small Intestine Associated with Celiac Disease.

- Malabsorption of nutrients including fat, protein, carbohydrate, minerals, and vitamins; worsened by folic acid deficiency.*
- Loss of membrane integrity of the gastrointestinal lining, thickening of epithelial cells and increased susceptibility to microbe invasion resulting from deficiency of vitamin A.*
- Sugar intolerance - lactose, sucrose, and maltose.*
- Abdominal distention resulting from gas, intestinal edema, and deficiency of niacin.*
- Abdominal pain resulting from inflammation, spasm, gas, and deficiencies of thiamin and vitamin B_{12}.*
- Steattorhea (foul-smelling, pale stool that floats) as a consequence of fat malabsorption.*
- Acute onset diarrhea.*
- Chronic diarrhea resulting from poorly absorbed nutrients and deficiencies of niacin and folic acid, and is made worse by zinc deficiency and potassium depletion.*
- Intermittent diarrhea and constipation resulting from deficiency of vitamin B_{12}.*
- Intestinal edema resulting from inflammation.*
- Increased intestinal permeability of small intestinal mucosa.*
- Increased susceptibility to Candida albicans mucosal infection.*
- Small bowel intussusception (telescoping bowel).*
- Colonic volvulus and ulcerative jejunoileitis.*
- Bovine beta casein enteropathy.*
- Development of food allergies.*
- Lymphocytosis.*
- Adenocarcinoma of small intestine.*
- Cryptic intestinal T-cell lymphoma (refractory sprue).*
- Enteropathy-associated T cell lymphoma (EATL).*

See Part 2: Health Manifestations of Celiac Disease for details.

THE DUODENUM

The duodenum is the first part of the small intestine, measuring 8 to 11 inches (20 to 28 cm). Muscular, vigorous, freely moveable, and capable of adapting its course according to the stomach contents, it is centrally located in the upper abdomen, touching parts of the pancreas, liver, gall bladder, right kidney, large intestine and stomach.

The duodenum continuously receives chyme from the stomach. Because the duodenum is naturally alkaline, the strong acid contents entering from the stomach stimulate the release of secretin, a hormone, from the duodenal wall. Secretin signals the release of bicarbonate, a natural antacid, from the adjacent pancreas. The strongly alkaline bicarbonate quickly neutralizes the acidic chyme.

Three juices act on the chyme. Duodenal juice secretes protein-splitting enzymes. Pancreatic juice digests starches, proteins and fats. Bile, produced by the liver and delivered by way of the gallbladder, emulsifies fat to render it into smaller particles.

Here is how complex carbohydrates, proteins and fats are digested in the duodenum:

1. Complex carbohydrates, primarily starch, must be broken down into simple sugars to be absorbed into the bloodstream.

   Pancreatic amylase, as part of pancreatic juice, finishes the digestion of starch begun by salivary amylase in the mouth. The resulting complex sugar, maltose, will later be broken down to simple glucose by the villi.

2. Proteins must be broken down into simple amino acids to be absorbed into the bloodstream.

   Four pancreatic enzymes, as part of pancreatic juice, finish the bulk of protein digestion that was begun by pepsin in the stomach. Trypsin and chymotrypsin break large chains of proteins into smaller amino acid chains, called peptides. Carboxypeptidase and aminopeptidase split off one amino acid at a time from the peptides. Amino acids can then be absorbed by villi.

3. Fats must be broken down into fatty acids and glycerol to enter the lymph system.

   Fat digestion, begun by gastric lipase in the stomach, is finished here. First, large fat globules are emulsified by bile. Then, the emulsified fat is acted on and digested by pancreatic lipase, another enzyme produced by the pancreas. Fatty acids and glycerol will be absorbed into the duodenal villi.

Other nutrients are also absorbed through the wall of the duodenum. Most vitamins and fluids are easily absorbed unchanged into the bloodstream, but mineral absorption is more complex.

Minerals absorbed in the duodenum include calcium, chloride, fluoride, sulfur, iron, copper, magnesium, and zinc. These larger minerals are soluble in stomach acid but not in the alkaline duodenal juice. To get across the absorbing cell wall of the small intestine and into the bloodstream, these minerals need to combine with a carrier, such as amino acids, sugars, and organic acids from food.

While small minerals such as fluoride are freely absorbed, metals must be carried across the cell wall by specific proteins to be absorbed.

Conditions and Diseases of the Duodenum Associated with Celiac Disease.

- Malabsorption of minerals including calcium, chloride, fluoride, sulfur, iron, copper, magnesium, and zinc.*
- Diminished active transport of calcium, magnesium, zinc, and other minerals across the gut and absorption resulting in part from deficiency of vitamin D.*
- Fat malabsorption binds minerals, causing loss in the feces and loose bowels or diarrhea.*
- Pancreatic insufficiency, resulting in fat malabsorption.*
- Scalloping of the duodenal folds.*
- Duodenal erosions and ulceration.*
- Postbulbar duodenal ulceration and stenosis.*

See Part 2: Health Manifestations of Celiac Disease for details.

THE JEJUNUM

The liquid chyme enters the jejunum, the second part of the small intestine. The jejunum continues the work of dismantling and preparing nutrients for entry into the body for its use.

The jejunum is about 8 feet (2.5 meters) in length with an average diameter measuring 1 ¼ to 1 ½ inches (3 to 3.5 cm). The jejunum lining forms tightly packed, circular folds on the inner muscle wall varying in height from 3 to 10 millimeters. Allowing for huge numbers of villi that cover them, the tiny folds maximize absorption area in a limited space and physically slow the passage of chyme for longer contact with the villi. Three carbohydrate-splitting enzymes, called disaccharidases, are imbedded in the microvilli cells. The vital task of these enzymes is to finish carbohydrate digestion by splitting them into simple sugars in the following way:

1. Lactase is located at the tips of the villi. This enzyme splits lactose, the complex sugar in milk, into galactose and glucose. These simple sugars easily pass into the blood vessels of the villi.

2. Sucrase, located further down the villi, splits sucrose into fructose and glucose, allowing these simple sugars to pass easily into the blood vessels of the villi.

3. Maltase, located near the base of the villi, splits maltose, the sugar that results from starch digestion, into glucose, which easily passes into the blood vessels of the villi.

Protein-splitting enzymes, called dipeptidases, are also located in the microvilli. Dipeptidases finish the digestion of protein by breaking down protein fragments, called dipeptides, into amino acids. Without these enzymes, proteins cannot be fully absorbed. Here is how it happens:

1. Dipeptidase enzymes are attached to the cell wall of the villi.
2. They split protein fragments into amino acid chains small enough to pass into the blood.
3. Absorptive cells draw the amino acid chains into the villi, while preventing large protein molecules from entering.

Other important nutrients that are absorbed in the jejunum include vitamin C, vitamin B_1, vitamin B_2, vitamin B_6, and folic acid.

Conditions and Diseases of the Jejunum Associated with Celiac Disease.

- Maldigestion and malabsorption of protein, carbohydrate, and fat.*
- Malabsorption of vitamin C, vitamin B_1, vitamin B_2, vitamin B_6, and folic acid.*
- Jejunal ulceration.*
- Edema.*
- Non-Hodgkin's lymphoma.*

See Part 2: Categorized Manifestations of Celiac Disease for details.

THE ILEUM

The last section of the small intestine is the ileum where final absorption of digested nutrients occurs. The ileum is about 13 feet long (4 meters), making it the longest segment of the small intestine. Its diameter is narrower than the jejunum, measuring an inch or less (2.5cm). The end of the ileum is closed by the ileocecal valve, which separates the small intestine from the colon.

The mucosa is composed of less tightly packed, circular folds covered by villi. The villi are more slender here and are fewer in number than in the jejunum. They produce the same enzymes and do the same work as the jejunal villi.

The work of the ileum ensures all the nutrients that can be absorbed are fully absorbed before leaving the small intestine. Nutrients that are digested and/or absorbed in the ileum include disaccharides, amino acids, vitamin A, vitamin D, vitamin E, vitamin K, and vitamin B_{12}.

Waste products leaving the small intestine pass through the ileocecal sphincter. This smooth muscle, circling the end of the ileum, controls the liquid mass as it enters the large intestine and prevents stool from reentering the ileum. The ileocecal sphincter responds to the gastrocecal reflex. This reflex acts to allow the ileum to empty its contents into the colon, making room for incoming new food. In this way, chyme in the upper regions of the small intestine moves down into the emptying ileum.

ACTION OF THE LARGE INTESTINE

The large intestine is the hollow, tube-shaped organ that provides for the breakdown of undigestible nutrients coming from the small intestine. In addition, the large quantity of fluid that has entered along the digestive tract is reabsorbed with sodium and potassium minerals. In the large intestine, the food mass waste is called feces or stool, changing from liquid to solid as it travels along by peristalsis. Stool takes 12 to 24 hours to reach the rectum.

The large intestine averages 4 to 6 feet in length, mainly consisting of the colon and rectum. The colon is segmented into four parts: ascending colon, transverse colon, descending colon, and sigmoid colon. The colon has the same mucus lining as the small intestine, but without villous structures. Cells that make up the lining are called colonocytes. There are no digestive enzymes secreted from these cells. Rather, digestion that takes place in the colon is largely for nourishment of the colon itself and is due to the important action of billions of beneficial bacteria, called flora. Intestinal flora thrive on arriving undigested nutrients coming from the small intestine. They break down complex molecules in food, that otherwise would be wasted, through a chemical reaction called fermentation. For example, this fermentation is the only way nutrients can be obtained from cellulose. Smelly gases like methane and hydrogen sulfide can result from their action.

When flora ferment undigested carbohydrates, short-chain fatty acids are made. These new nutrients become food for colonocytes. Excess fatty acids can also be absorbed into the bloodstream as a source of fuel for the body and can easily be stored as fat. Some flora produce vitamin K, necessary for blood clotting, which is then absorbed into the bloodstream. This important bacterial mechanism is the main source of vitamin K and assures a ready supply. Bacteria in the colon eventually expire. When they do so, they become part of stool. Dead bacteria make up to a third of the bulk of stool. If the normal bacteria are not thriving, there will be fewer dead ones in turn, so that the amount of stool will be reduced. This is an indication of poor colon health. Stool that has reached the sigmoid colon is moved into the rectum where it is formed for exit through the anus.

Appendices

Appendix I: Unsafe Foods and Ingredients

Appendix II: Gluten-Free Diet Self-Management Three Step Process

Appendix III: Sample of Foods Commonly Allowed and Not Allowed on a GF Diet

APPENDIX I
Unsafe Foods and Ingredients

Persons with celiac disease should discuss gluten-free choices with a health care specialist or dietitian skilled in celiac disease. In all cases where there is an **Ingredient List** on commercially prepared foods, the celiac or responsible person must carefully read the package looking for the word "gluten" or anything derived from wheat, barley, rye, and oats.

Unprocessed	Processed	Fermented/Brewed
Whole grain - Wheat berries, rye, oat groats, rolled oats, barley, pearl barley.	**Thickeners -** Starch from wheat, rye, barley, oat. Modified food starch from wheat. Oat gum. Maltodextrin from wheat/barley.	**Fermented -** Regular soy sauce/tamari from fermented wheat and soy. Barley malt vinegar.
Cracked grain - Wheat, barley, rye, oats.	**Syrups -** Barley malt syrup & oat syrup.	**Brewed -** Beer, ale, porter are made using barley.
Meals/coarsely gound grain - Wheat meal, matzo, oat meal, rye meal, barley meal.	**Protein polymers -** Hydrolized vegetable protein (HVP) and texturized vegetable protein (TVP) from wheat.	
Flours/ finely milled grains - Wheat flour: whole wheat flour, graham flour, all-purpose flour, bread flour, cake flour, pastry flour, semolina flour, durum flour and gluten (high protein or vital wheat gluten) flour. Other strains of wheat: emmer flour, kamut flour, spelt flour (also called dinkel), farro flour, and einkorn flour. Rye flour, Barley flour Oat flour, Triticale flour (wheat /rye hybrid).	**Cooked products -** Seitan (100% gluten) Regular pasta, all types Regular noodles, all types Udon noodles Panko noodles Ramen noodles Couscous Bulgar (parboiled wheat).	
Germ - Wheat germ and wheat germ oil.	**Flavoring -** Barley malt, extract & malt flavoring	
Bran - Wheat bran, oat bran.		

Chart AI-1.1 How unsafe grains may be used as ingredients in making food.

Recognizing Celiac Disease Signs, Symptoms, Associated Disorders & Complications

Appendix II
Gluten-Free Diet Self-Management Three Step Process

Developed by Jean E. Guest, MS, RD, LMNT
Provided by Celiac Sprue Association - USA

Although the gluten-free diet (GFD) is recognized as the only treatment for celiac disease (CD) there is controversy over the exact definition of a GFD. The GFD evolved over many years and is based primarily on anecdotal, observational, and inferential information. There are few clinical studies in the scientific literature regarding the GFD. Due to the variable nature of symptoms and manifestations associated with CD the best management approach is a personalized GFD. Actually the GFD is not just a diet but a lifestyle. With this in mind the Celiac Sprue Association has developed A Three Step Approach to Self-Management in CD.

What is Self-Management?

Self-management is a key concept of the Health Belief Model. The Health Belief Model promotes behaviors associated with understanding and maintaining good health. Self-management is defined as having confidence in one's ability to take action. By establishing and achieving goals, gaining and applying knowledge, providing and receiving support, and reducing anxiety it is more likely that people with CD will be successful in establishing a healthy lifelong gluten-free lifestyle. CSA encourages people with CD to utilize self-management principles.

Why Use A Three Step Approach?

The needs of individuals with CD are unique, dynamic, and change over time. People with newly diagnosed CD have different needs than those diagnosed longer. Initiating a gluten-free lifestyle means adjusting to new ways of shopping, cooking, eating, traveling, socializing and just plain living. Despite advances in research and knowledge some areas of CD remain controversial due to a lack of definitive information. This often leaves people confused and uncertain about applying information to their individual needs. The intent of a Three Step Approach in Self-Management is to provide guidelines for applying research and knowledge to a gluten-free lifestyle plan which adapts to the changing needs of people with CD.

STEP 1 – FOUNDATION

Step 1-Foundation is the basis of a gluten-free lifestyle. Begin Step-1 Foundation by identifying CD resources and educational materials to become knowledgeable about symptoms, diagnosis, and treatment. Establish partnerships with health care professionals experienced in CD who can identify and monitor individual medical and nutritional health needs. People who are newly diagnosed need to consider being evaluated for problems associated with nutrient deficiencies common in CD (i.e., osteoporosis, dental enamel defects, altered mental/emotional status). It is also important to partner with the celiac community by joining local and national support (advocacy) groups. Support groups allow individuals to share their knowledge and experiences as well as to ease the transition into and maintenance of a gluten-free lifestyle.

Initate Step 1 –

Although some sources of gluten are obvious, others are not. Be aware of "hidden" sources of gluten by understanding the definitions of "gluten-free", other words for gluten, and reading labels. Incorporate self-monitoring techniques such as a daily diary, notebook, or calendar to identify gluten exposure by content, contact, and contamination. Examine everything that may come into contact with the gastrointestinal tract. Keep in mind that the gastrointestinal tract begins with the lips so be aware of gluten exposure through hand to mouth contact.

Develop a gluten-free care plan by identifying 30-50 food and beverage items that are known to be gluten-free or are naturally gluten-free. List the gluten-free food and beverage items in a daily diary or notebook, and be certain to include personal preferences. Use the gluten-free care plan as the basis of the GFD. Review the list to assure that all nutrient groups as well as food items appropriate for each meal are included and make adjustments if needed. Due to the lack of information on nutrient enrichment in gluten-free foods people with CD should take a gluten-free vitamin and mineral supplement daily.

Carbohydrate intolerances are linked to CD with lactose intolerance being the most common. Lactose intolerance may be transient (especially in children) or it may be permanent. Nutrients excluded from a gluten-free care plan due to intolerance or allergy should be replaced through identified nutrient supplementation. In the case of lactose intolerance calcium with vitamin D supplementation may be needed to meet individual calcium requirements.

Step 2 –

Foundation should be strictly followed until remission is achieved. A minimum of two to four months following diagnosis is usually necessary. Some individuals may need to maintain Step 1 - Foundation longer. Most people with CD achieve remission within six months to a year although a few people take longer.

Individuals with typical CD symptoms such as diarrhea, constipation, bloating, lethargy, weight loss, or poor linear growth (in children) should record them daily in a diary or notebook. People with atypical symptoms such as anemia, osteoporosis, or thyroid dysfunction (which are not as obvious) may need to monitor individual response to the GFD by following serum markers specific to their particular problem in addition to serum antibody activity. Measurement, frequency, and interpretation of serum antibody and specific serum markers must be done in partnership with a physician.

STEP 2 – EXPANSION

Begin Step 2 – Expansion when symptoms or serum antibody levels indicate that the full benefits of Step 1 – Foundation have been achieved. The purpose of Step 2 – Expansion is to encourage an increase in knowledge of CD and to advance the level of self-management. Networking with the celiac community may help decrease the uncertainty and confusion some individuals experience while adjusting to CD. However, adjustment and integration of the CD lifestyle varies individually. Developing an evaluation and decision-making process for new, questionable, or controversial information/items is recommended.

Initiate Step 2 –

Expansion by adding new items (foods, beverages, personal care items, etc.) to meet individual lifestyle needs. Monitor immune response to new items. Reactions may occur immediately, up to 14 days after exposure, or longer in the case of delayed reactions. It is recommended that one new item be added approximately every two weeks. Individuals choosing to utilize a faster approach may do so. If or when a reaction occurs it is recommended that any items introduced within the past two weeks should be eliminated for about 4-8 weeks. Re-introduction of potential immune response triggers should be done one at a time waiting two weeks between introductions. Utilize self-monitoring tools to record time, date, item, reaction, duration, and comments to assess individual tolerance.

Advance to Step 3 –

Maintenance when clinical symptoms are in remission and satisfactory gluten-free lifestyle choices are achieved. People experiencing symptoms or whose serum antibody activity indicates exposure to immune-response trigger(s) should explore the possibility of unintentional gluten exposure, true food allergies, additional nutrient intolerances, or other autoimmune disorders. Remember to utilize self-management team partners (doctor, dietitian, support group) as needed to assess and evaluate health and well being.

STEP 3 – MAINTENANCE

Step 3 – Maintenance begins when remission is achieved, nutritional status is stable, and lifestyle needs are met. Step 3 – Maintenance includes integration of self-management into daily routines through periodic re-assessment, updating, and application of new knowledge into individual lifestyle plans. Most people achieving Step 3 – Maintenance understand their individual response(s) to situations such as stress, illness, or reactivation of symptoms (i.e., inadvertent gluten exposure). During these times it may be necessary to revisit Steps 1 or 2. People at Step 3 – Maintenance serve as good role models for people with newly diagnosed CD. Continuing to partner with a health care professionals and support groups is essential in reinforcing and sustaining a healthy gluten-free lifestyle.

SUMMARY

A Three Step Approach to Self-Management provides guidelines for people with CD. Self-management in CD is the best way to assure that individual needs are considered and met. If people with CD do not take control of their disease it will take control of them.

References

Arentz-Hansen H, Fleckenstein B, Molberg O, Scott H, Koning F, Jung G, Roepstorff P, Lundin KE, Sollid LM, The molecular basis for oat intolerance in patients with celiac disease, PLoS Med, Oct; 1(1):e1,2004, Epub Oct 19, 2004.

Dicke WK, Van De Kamer JH, Weijers HA, Celiac disease, Adv Pediatr, 57; 9:277-318, 1957.

Janz NK, Champion VL., Strecher VJ, The health belief model, In K Glanz, BK Rimer, FM Lewis (Ed.), Health behavior and health education, 3rd edition (p.p. 45-66), San Francisco, CA: Jossey-Bass.

Kagnoff MF, Two genetic loci control the murine immune response to A-gliadin, a wheat protein that activates coeliac sprue, Nature, Mar 11; 296(5853):158-60, 1982.

Shan L, Molberg O, Parrot I, Hausch F, Filiz F, Gray GM, Sollid LM, Khosla C, Structural basis for gluten intolerance in celiac sprue, Science, Sep 27; 297(5590):2275-9, 2002.

Thompson T, Thiamin, riboflavin, and niacin contents of the gluten-free diet: is there cause for concern?, J Am Diet Assoc, Jul; 99(7):858-62, 1999.

United States Department of Health and Human Services, National Institutes of Health, Consensus Development Conference on Celiac Disease, 2004.

Appendix III:
Sample of Foods Commonly Allowed and Not Allowed on a GF Diet

The following comparison of common foods believed to be those that can be safely eaten and those that must be strictly avoided may serve as a general list. Persons with celiac disease should discuss gluten-free choices with a health care specialist or dietitian skilled in celiac disease.

In all cases, where there is an **Ingredient List** on commercially prepared foods, celiacs must carefully read the package looking for the word "gluten" or anything derived from wheat, barley, rye, and oats. Note: foods that claim "wheat-free" may, in fact, contain one of the other gluten-containing grains.

As of 2006, the "Food Allergen Labeling and Consumer Act of 2003" requires food manufacturers of food sold in the United States to clearly state in "plain English" on the packaging if the product contains wheat. Small amounts such ingredients as colorings, flavorings, and seasonings are included.

Plain means no gluten ingredients are added to the food.
**Commercially prepared means the product is made by a company for the purpose of selling it.*

Food Group	Allowed	Not Allowed
Fruit	All plain* fresh, frozen, or dried fruit; canned fruit in natural juice. Pie fillings thickened with cornstarch, tapioca, or arrowroot.	Commercially prepared** canned or prepared fruits/pie fillings thickened with flour.
Vegetables	All plain*, fresh, frozen, or canned vegetables. GF sauced vegetables; vegetables thickened with cornstarch, tapioca or arrowroot such as sweet & sour red beets.	Commercially prepared **creamed vegetables and vegetables in sauce thickened with flour. Vegetables with regular bread crumbs or battered and fried; salads with croutons or with dressing thickened using flour or oat gum.
Meat, fish, seafood, fowl	Plain* fresh, canned, or frozen beef, pork, ham, lamb, rabbit, or other meat, seafood, fish, poultry, turkey, or other birds. Bacon; hotdogs, cold cuts; scrapple and sausage made with safe fillers and binders. Canned fish, poultry, seafood, meat in brine or plain water. GF breaded, battered or otherwise prepared.	Commercially prepared** meat, fish, seafood, and fowl or other bird, such as are breaded/battered (fried), blended, or injected with solution (as in turkeys/chickens/hams). Any of the following that use gluten-containing fillers: cold cuts, hotdogs, scrapple, meat loaf, sausage, meatballs, meat patties; canned meat, fish, poultry, or seafood using hydrolyzed vegetable protein. Imitation crab, other meat using wheat gluten or seitan.

Food Group	Allowed	Not Allowed
Eggs	Fresh eggs boiled, poached, fried, or plain* scrambled.	Commercially prepared** dried or frozen egg products using flour or wheat starch. Souffle, omelet or scrambled eggs thickened with flour or pancake batter.
Milk and milk products	Plain* fresh or evaporated milk including goat and sheep milk. Plain sour cream, light/heavy cream; plain yogurt.	Malted milk, commercially prepared** chocolate and flavored milk containing gluten. Yogurt thickened with wheat starch, hydrolized protein added, or with granola added.
Cheese	Plain* aged, chunk cheese, such as cheddar, Swiss, edam, parmesan, romano, and manchego; cottage cheese, cream cheese, and specially prepared GF spreads/mixes.	Cheese product thickened or stabilized with oat gum or wheat starch, such as spread/sauce for nachos or macaroni. Some veined cheeses aged with moldy bread, such as bleu cheese, stilton, roquefort, and gorgonzola.
Pasta and noodles	Specially prepared GF pasta and noodles made with rice, corn, potato, or other safe flour. Bean thread, rice, and wheat-free buckwheat noodles.	Regular pasta such as penne, spaghetti, lasagna, and macaroni. Couscous. Regular noodles using wheat flour.
Naturally GF starch dishes	Plain* rice, wild rice, sweet potatoes, potatoes, yams, buckwheat or kasha, millet, and hominy or polenta.	Commercially prepared** flavored or seasoned rice, wild rice, kasha, or other GF food using wheat starch/flour, oat gum, or hydrolized or texturized wheat protein. Frozen French fries and potato products dusted with flour at the plant and/or coated with seasoned flour at the restaurant. Potatoes stuffed with a flour thickened filling.
Breads, yeast raised buns, pizza	Specially prepared GF.	Regular.

Food Group	Allowed	Not Allowed
Flatbreads and tortillas	Specially prepared GF flatbreads. Plain* corn tortillas.	Regular flatbreads/flour tortillas. Corn tortillas with flour or barley added.
Quickbreads	Plain* corn muffins and corn bread. GF muffins, GF English muffins, GF scones, GF biscuits, GF breads like Irish soda bread, banana, apple, & date/nut bread.	Regular quickbreads.
Baked goods	GF cakes, pies, cookies, brownies, pastries, tarts, croisants, and Danish.	Regular baked goods.
Doughnuts and fried dough.	Specially prepared GF doughnuts and fried bread dough.	Regular doughnuts and fried bread dough.
Pancakes, waffles, and crepes	Plain* buckwheat pancakes. GF pancakes, waffles, and crepes.	Regular pancakes, waffles, and crepes. Buckwheat pancakes made with flour.
Cereals	All plain* cereals made from safe foods, such as rice, corn, buckwheat, millet, and amaranth, and are not coated with malt or malt flavoring.	Regular cereal made from wheat, rye, barley, and oats such as wheat flakes, wheat puffs, shredded wheat, wheat germ, cream of wheat, and oatmeal. Any cold cereals coated with malt syrup or malt flavoring to keep them crisp, including safe grains such as crispy rice or corn flakes. Granolas, muesli, and kashi.
Soups	Homemade broth and soup, and stew using safe ingredients and thickened with cornstarch.	Most canned and dry mix soups and stews. Boullion and boullion cubes using hydrolyzed wheat protein.
Legumes	Any, such as plain* beans, peas, lentils, chickpeas, peanuts, and soybeans.	Any made with unsafe ingredients such as baked beans thickened with flour or oat gum, coated or blended with breadcrumbs, or flavored with soy sauce, vinegar, or malt.

Food Group	Allowed	Not Allowed
Snacks	Plain* corn, potato, soy, and vegetable chips. Specially made GF breadsticks, pretzels, and crackers. Trail mix made with GF ingredients. Plain nuts and seeds. Plain fruit bars.	Regular wheat, rye, barley, and oat-based crackers, crisps, and pretzels. Trail mix with wheat nuggets or oat granola. Seasoned roasted nuts. Seeds with unsafe flavoring.
Beverages	Plain*coffee, tea, cocoa, and fruit juices. Wine made in USA, vodka distilled from grapes or potatoes, sake, vermouth, cognac, and tequilla.	Some sodas. Malted milk, commercially made drinks with unsafe grains such as Ovaltine, Postum, and Tang. Herbal teas flavored with barley malt; root beer; some flavored coffees. Some instant decaffeinated coffee. Beer, ale, porter and stout.
Cold Desserts	GF ice cream, frozen yogurt, sherbet, and sorbet. Gelatin, junket, and custard. Puddings, such as rice and tapioca, thickened with cornstarch or arrowroot.	Ice cream and sherbets made with gluten stabilizers, cookie dough, cookies, or other cereal additives. Ice cream cones. Pudding mixes and puddings thickened with flour, wheat starch, or oat gum.
Sweeteners	Crystalline fructose, honey, maltitol, sorbitol, rice & maple syrup, and pure fruit spreads.	Rice syrup with flour and some corn and pancake syrups using wheat, barley malt or oat gum.
Condiments	Apple cider vinegar, rice vinegar, and wine vinegar and products made from them such as mayonnaise, mustard, and catsup. Tamari made from soy only. Soy sauce made from soy only.	Soy sauce made from soy and wheat; hoisin sauce. Barley malt vinegar.
Fats	Butter and any oil other than wheat germ oil.	Wheat germ oil. Non-dairy cream substitutes; some commercial salad dressings using wheat germ oil.

Food Group	Allowed	Not Allowed
Sweets	GF candy and fruit bars.	Commercially prepared** candies dusted with flour to keep from sticking, fillings thickened with flour, wafers and other cereal parts made from unsafe grains, and addition of oats or oat gum or malt flavoring/syrup. Twizzler's red licorice and Goetz's Cow Tales are examples using wheat flour. Licorice, some gum drops, and some chewing gum.
Deli or salad bar foods	Plain* salads/vegetables without croutons or breadcrumbs. **Caution:** may be contaminated by use of utensils used for unsafe foods or by spillage onto them.	Regular tuna, egg, chicken, seafood, fish, and ham salad. Pasta salads. Breaded foods/battered foods. Sauced foods.
Nutritional bars	Specially prepared GF.	Regular bars.
Thickeners	Cornstarch, arrowroot, potato starch, and tapioca starch. Zanthan gum, guar gum, carob bean gum, locust bean gum, gum Arabic, cellulose, and car-rageenan. Agar (gelatin).	Wheat starch/flour, hydrolized wheat protein, oat gum.
Flavorings	Maltodextrin (not made from wheat or barley), most spices and herbs.	Barley malt, malt, malt extract, and malt syrup, oat syrup. Some dry curry powder and some spice blends and extracts.
Miscellaneous	Active dry yeast, bicarbonate of soda, GF baking powder, cream of tartar. Specially prepared communion wafers.	Instant dry yeast. Some baking powders. Standard communion wafers.

Chart AIII-1.1 Sample of Foods Allowed and Not Allowed on a Gluten-Free Diet. Adapted from Safe and Unsafe Foods chart provided in "Celiac Disease." National Digestive Diseases Information Clearinghouse. (NIH Publication No. 98-4269) April 1998.

Glossary

Amino acid – A group of 20 different kinds of small molecules that link together in long chains to form proteins. Often referred to as the "building blocks" of proteins.[47] An amino acid is an organic compound composed of both an amino (NH2) group and a carboxyl (COOH) group. Amino acids are the end products of protein digestion and, as such, are absorbed into the bloodstream for the purpose of building our unique proteins.

Antibody – A protein of the immune system called immunoglobulin. Each antibody consists of 4 polypeptides, comprised of about 100 amino acids, forming a Y shaped molecule. The site on the antibody that binds with an antigen is at the tips of the Y. Each antibody is unique and defends the body against the one specific antigen it recognizes. Types of antibodies involved in celiac disease include:

Immunoglobulin A – This type is the main antibody in intestinal and respiratory mucin and saliva for the purpose of preventing invading organisms from entering the body.

Immunoglobulin G – This type is the main antibody in blood for toxins and organisms.

Antigen, immunogen type – A protein or polysaccharide macromolecule that provokes the immune system to produce antibodies.[47]

Apoptosis – Programmed cell death, the body's normal method of disposing of damaged, unwanted, or unneeded cells.[47]

Biopsy – The obtaining of a tissue sample for microscopic examination, usually to establish a diagnosis.

Carbohydrate – An organic compound composed of carbon, oxygen, and hydrogen. Carbohydrates include glucose, sugars, starches, dextrins, and celluloses from plants and glucose, glycogen, and lactose from animals. The simple sugars, glucose, galactose, and fructose, are the end products of carbohydrate digestion, and as such, are absorbed into the bloodstream and used as a basic source of energy.

Cell – The basic unit of any living organism. It is a small, watery, compartment filled with chemicals and a complete copy of the organism's genome.[47]

Colonocytes – Cells that form the surface lining of the large intestine.

Enterocytes – Cells that form the surface lining of the small intestine.

Erythrocytes – Mature red blood cells that contain hemoglobin for the purpose of carrying oxygen to other cells. Nutrients necessary for the proper formation of erythrocytes are essential amino acids, vitamin B_{12} and folic acid. Nutrients necessary for the production of hemoglobin are iron, cobalt, and copper.

Lymphocyte – A small white blood cell that plays a major role in defending the body against disease. There are two main types of lymphocytes: B cells, which make antibodies that attack bacteria and toxins, and T cells, which attack body cells themselves when they have been taken over by viruses or become cancerous.[47]

B lymphocytes (B cells) – A subpopulation of lymphocytes derived from the bone marrow, make up 10% of all lymphocytes. When B cells come in contact with a foreign antigen, they are stimulated by T cells to mature. Mature B cells differentiate into plasma cells or memory cells that produce antibodies. Plasma cells are the only source of immunoglobulin antibodies. Memory cells enable the body to quickly produce antibodies to previously identified foreign invaders.

T lymphocytes (T cells) – A subpopulation of lymphocytes derived from the thymus gland, make up 75% of all lymphocytes. T cells stimulate B cells to begin antibody production for attaching to antigens, making them easier to digest by white cells.

Chromosomes – One of the threadlike "packages" of genes and other DNA in the nucleus of a cell. Different kinds of organisms have different numbers of chromosomes. Humans have 23 pairs of chromosomes, 46 in all: 44 autosomes and two sex chromosomes. Each parent contributes one chromosome to each pair, so children get half of their chromosomes from their mothers and half from their fathers.[47]

Collagen – A strong, fibrous, insoluble protein in connective tissue, including skin, deep fascia, tendons, ligaments and bone.

Crypt – A small cavity between villi extending into the epithelial surface of the small intestine.

DNA –The chemical inside the nucleus of a cell that carries the genetic instructions for making living organisms. Abbreviation for deoxyribonucleic acid, the molecule that contains the genetic code for all life forms except for a few viruses. It consists of two long, twisted chains made up of nucleotides. Each nucleotide contains one base, one phosphate molecule, and the sugar molecule deoxyribose. The bases in DNA nucleotides are adenine, thymine, guanine, and cytosine.[48]

Endomysium – Loose, irregular connective tissue that lies between muscle cells, covering muscle fibers and holding them together.

Endoscopy – A procedure to inspect the hollow organs of the upper digestive tract by use of an endoscope. An endoscope is a medical device consisting of a long, thin tube and an optical device. Observable organs include the esophagus, stomach, and proximal small intestine.

Enteropathy – Any disease of the intestine, including celiac disease (gluten sensitive enteropathy).

Enzyme – A substance (usually a protein) that speeds up, or catalyzes, a chemical reaction without being permanently altered or consumed. Enzymes carry out the thousands of chemical reactions that go on in a cell. Enzymes help make other molecules, including DNA. Enzymes also break food down and deliver and consume the energy that powers the cell. Other kinds of proteins, called regulatory proteins, preside over the many interactions that determine how and when genes do their work and are copied. Regulatory proteins also supervise enzymes and the give-and-take between cells and their environment.[48]

Epitope –The part of an antigen to which an antibody binds.[47]

Essential fatty acid – A component together with glycerol in a 3 to 1 ratio that makes up fat. Alpha-linolenic acid (ALA), linoleic acid (LA) and arachidonic acid (AA) are not made by the body. These 3 essential fatty acids are necessary for health and must be obtained in the diet. Docosahexaenoic acid (DHA) and eicosapentaenoic acid (EPA) can be made from ALA and arachidonic acid can be made from LA if there is sufficient amounts present. DHA, EPA, and AA should be included in a healthy diet.

Genes –The functional and physical unit of heredity passed from parent to offspring. Genes are pieces of DNA, and most genes contain the information for making a specific protein.[47]

Genetic marker – A segment of DNA with an identifiable physical location on a chromosome and whose inheritance can be followed. A marker can be a gene, or it can be some section of DNA with no known function. Because DNA segments that lie near each other on a chromosome tend to be inherited together, markers are often used as indirect ways of tracking the inheritance pattern of a gene that has not yet been identified, but whose approximate location is known.[47]

Genetic screening – Testing a population group to identify a subset of individuals at high risk for having or transmitting a specific genetic disorder.[47]

Genome – All the DNA contained in an organism or a cell, which includes both the chromosomes within the nucleus and the DNA in mitochondria.[47]

Genotype –The genetic identity of an individual that does not show as outward characteristics.

Glutamine – A non-essential amino acid needed for maintaining health of the intestinal lining.

Gluten sensitive enteropathy – Another name for celiac disease.

Haplotype – A haplotype is the set of SNP (single nucleotide polymorphism) alleles along a region of a chromosome. Theoretically there could be many haplotypes in a chromosome region, but recent studies are typically finding only a few common haplotypes. Some SNP alleles are the actual functional variants that contribute to the risk of getting a disease. Individuals with such a SNP allele have a higher risk for that disease than do individuals without that SNP allele. Most SNPs are not these functional variants, but are useful as markers for finding them. To find the regions with genes that contribute to a disease, the frequencies of many SNP alleles are compared in individuals with and without the disease. When a particular region has SNP alleles that are more frequent in individuals with the disease than in individuals without the disease, those SNPs and their alleles are associated with the disease. These associations between a SNP and a disease indicate that there may be genes in that region that contribute to the disease.[49]

Histology – The study of the microscopic structure of tissue.

Histopathology – The study of diseased microscopic structure.

Human leukocyte antigen (HLA) – A distinguishing series of proteins that exist on the surface of every white blood cell to help the cell discriminate between "friendly" cells and "foreign" matter like bacteria and viruses.

Humoral immunity – A term that refers to antibody production. The aspect of immunity that is mediated by secreted antibodies that are produced by B cells. Secreted antibodies bind to antigens, flagging them for destruction.

Immunoglobulin – See "antibody".

Inherited – Transmitted through genes from parents to offspring.[47]

Lamina propria –The thin layer of areolar connective tissue, blood vessels and nerves that lie just below the epithelium (surface lining of the intestine).

Locus – *(pl. loci)* The place on a chromosome where a specific gene is located.[47]

Lymphocytosis – Abnormal increase in the number of lymphocytes. See "Lymphocyte" under "Cells" p. 54.

Lymphokines – A distinct signaling protein released by lymphocytes.

Pathophysiology –The study of how normal physiological processes are altered by disease.

Peptide – Two or more amino acids joined by a peptide bond.[47]

Phenotype – The observable traits or characteristics of an organism, for example hair color, weight, or the presence or absence of a disease. Phenotypic traits are not necessarily genetic.[47]

Prevalence –The number of cases of a disease present in a specified population at a given time.

Prognosis – The prediction of the course and end of a disease and the estimate of recovery.

Protease – An enzyme that digests proteins.[47]

Protein – A molecule or complex of molecules consisting of subunits called amino acids. Proteins are the cell's main building materials, and they do most of a cell's work. Thanks to proteins, cells and the organisms they form develop, live their lives, and create descendants. Proteins are big, complicated molecules that must be folded into intricate three-dimensional shapes in order to work correctly. To perform its many functions, a cell constantly needs new copies of proteins. Although proteins do lots of jobs well, they cannot make copies of themselves.[48]

Transglutaminase – An enzyme in endomysium tissue that combines with gliadin to form the epitope that is the autoantigen in celiac disease.

Ultrasound procedure –The direction of inaudible sound waves in the frequency range of 10,000 to 10 billion cycles/ sec for the purpose of outlining the shape of various tissues and organs in the body and so permitting "visualization" of them on the monitor screen.

Villus – *(pl. villi)* Minute structures of the intestinal mucosa numbering in the millions that project into the intestinal lumen for the purpose of absorbing passing nutrients into the blood and lymph system. Site of specific enzymes that digest the sugars lactose, sucrose, and maltose and finish digestion of peptides.

Part 2
Health Manifestations of Celiac Disease

Section A
Nutrient Deficiencies in Celiac Disease

HOW TO USE THIS SECTION

Step 1: Review nutrient deficiencies and their symptoms to identify deficits that are present at diagnosis and those that persist or arise after starting a gluten free diet.

Step 2: Search Section B charts (p. 87-259) to identify manifestations caused by nutrient deficiencies.

Step 3: Incorporate dietary sources listed under individual nutrient deficiency into the diet and determine whether nutrient supplementation is necessary.

Section A is comprised of three parts: a diagram, an index, and a chart.

- The diagram shows the relationships of nutritional deficiencies in the chart.
- The index alphabetically lists each nutritional deficiency with its corresponding ID number.
- The chart presents basic information about nutritional deficiencies in celiac disease.

The chart information is organized in seven columns:

1. **Affected System:** lists the primary body system(s) impacted by the deficiency.
2. **Affected Nutrient:** lists the nutrient classification of the deficiency.
3. **ID No:** lists the number assigned to the manifestation for cross-referencing with Alphabetical Index A.
4. **Manifestation:** lists the name of the nutrient deficiency.
5. **Type:** identifies the manifestation's relationship to celiac disease as being a sign, symptom, associated disorder or complication.

   (S)   Classic sign or symptom
   (AT)   Atypical sign or symptom
   (AD)   Associated disorder
   (C)   Complication

6. **Current Medical Information:** organizes current medical information according to prevalence, description, signs or symptoms, CD-related cause and response to gluten-free diet.

   [P]   Prevalence data from research studies and case reports of new associations.
   [D]   Brief description of the characteristics of the manifestation.
   [M]   List of the signs and symptoms of the manifestation as related to CD.
   [C]   CD-related cause(s) of the manifestation.
   [R]   Gives known response of the deficiency to the gluten-free diet and suggests when nutrient supplementation is advised.

7. **Dietary Sources of Nutrient:** lists common foods containing the deficient nutrient.

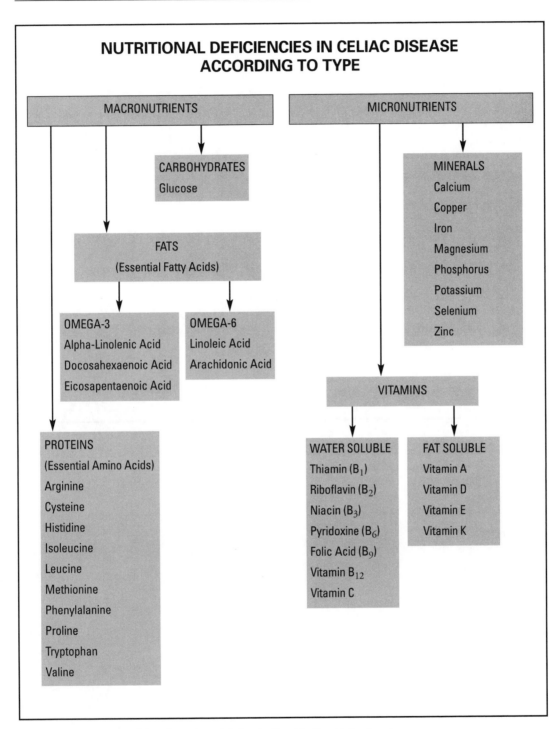

NUTRITIONAL DEFICIENCIES IN CELIAC DISEASE ACCORDING TO TYPE

MACRONUTRIENTS

MICRONUTRIENTS

CARBOHYDRATES

Glucose

MINERALS

Calcium

Copper

Iron

Magnesium

Phosphorus

Potassium

Selenium

Zinc

FATS

(Essential Fatty Acids)

OMEGA-3

Alpha-Linolenic Acid

Docosahexaenoic Acid

Eicosapentaenoic Acid

OMEGA-6

Linoleic Acid

Arachidonic Acid

VITAMINS

PROTEINS

(Essential Amino Acids)

Arginine

Cysteine

Histidine

Isoleucine

Leucine

Methionine

Phenylalanine

Proline

Tryptophan

Valine

WATER SOLUBLE

Thiamin (B_1)

Riboflavin (B_2)

Niacin (B_3)

Pyridoxine (B_6)

Folic Acid (B_9)

Vitamin B_{12}

Vitamin C

FAT SOLUBLE

Vitamin A

Vitamin D

Vitamin E

Vitamin K

Diagram 1.1: Layout of the 26 nutrient deficiencies listed in Part 2, Section A.

Section A: Alphabetical Index
Nutrient Deficiencies in Celiac Disease

ID No.	Manifestation
2	Alpha-Linolenic Acid (ALA) Deficiency
5	Arachidonic Acid (AA) Deficiency
7	Calcium Deficiency
8	Copper Deficiency
3	Docosahexaenoic Acid (DHA) Deficiency
4	Eicosapentaenoic Acid (EPA) Deficiency
15	Essential Amino Acid Deficiency
1	Glucose Deficiency
9	Iron Deficiency
6	Linoleic Acid (LA) Deficiency
10	Magnesium Deficiency
11	Phosphorus Deficiency
12	Potassium Deficiency
13	Selenium Deficiency
16	Vitamin A Deficiency
20	Vitamin B_1 (Thiamin) Deficiency
21	Vitamin B_2 (Riboflavin) Deficiency
22	Vitamin B_3 (Niacin) Deficiency
23	Vitamin B_6 (Pyridoxine) Deficiency
24	Vitamin B_9 (Folic Acid) Deficiency
25	Vitamin B_{12} Deficiency
26	Vitamin C Deficiency
17	Vitamin D Deficiency
18	Vitamin E Deficiency
19	Vitamin K Deficiency
14	Zinc Deficiency

Health Manifestations of Celiac Disease (CD)
Section A: Nutrient Deficiencies

Affected System	Affected Nutrient	ID No.	Manifestation	Type[+]	Current Medical Information [++]	Dietary Sources
Blood Nervous Sensory Skeletal Urinary	Carbohydrate	1	Glucose Deficiency [1,2]	(S)	[P] Common in people with untreated CD.[1] [D] Glucose deficiency is characterized by alterations in nervous system function and tissues that require glucose and cannot metabolize fatty acids, including erythrocytes, leukocytes, bone marrow, eye, renal medulla, and peripheral nerves. In polymer form, glucose is present as starch and cellulose and is found in all edible disaccharides, such as sucrose, lactose, and maltose. Glucose makes up a large part of the total solid content of fruits and vegetables.[2] [M] Marked by neurologic symptoms involving hypoglycemia with irritability, difficulty concentrating, dizziness, restlessness, headache, visual disturbances, faintness, nervousness, hunger, fatigue, and in some people, violent behavior. Metabolic symptoms include weakness and failure to gain weight in a child. [C] Results from limited mucosal surface for absorption of monosaccharides and maldigestion of disaccharides due to disaccharidase deficiency secondary to diffuse villous injury in CD. [R] CD-related glucose deficiency responds quickly to GFD.	Honey, syrups, all edible disaccharides, fruit, vegetables, and starches. Glycogen from meat sources. Lactose from milk sources.

[+] (S) = Classic sign/symptom; (AT) = Atypical sign/symptom; (AD) Associated Disorder; (C) = Complication.

[++] [P] = Prevalance; [D] = Description; [M] = Sign/symptom; [C] = CD related cause; [R] = Response to gluten Free diet (GFD).

Affected System	Affected Nutrient	ID No.	Manifestation	Type[+]	Current Medical Information [++]	Dietary Sources
Blood Cardiovascular Immune Integumentary Nervous Reproductive Sensory	Essential Fatty Acids: omega-3 series of highly unsaturated fatty acids (HUFA)	2	Alpha-Linolenic Acid (ALA) Deficiency [2,3,4,5]	(S)	[P] Serum concentration was reduced in 45% of study subjects with CD. [3] [D] Functional deficiencies or imbalances of alpha-linolenic acid (ALA) contribute to a wide range of developmental and psychiatric conditions, reduced learning and behavioral changes, raised blood pressure, fluid imbalance, changes in vascular membrane lipid composition, neurologic disorders, increased blood clotting and inflammatory responses, and tumor growth. ALA must be obtained in the diet. If sufficient amounts are present in the body, ALA can be used to synthesize eicosapentaenoic acid and docosahexaenoic acid, two other omega-3 fatty acids. [4] ALA enhances the formation of vasodilator prostaglandins (PGs), acting as endogenous (self-made) antihypertensive agents. [5] As a component of lipoproteins and a precursor of leukotrienes and series 3 PGs, ALA reduces the synthesis of aggressive inflammatory response cytokines by interfering with the conversion of arachidonic acid, an opposing omega-6 fatty acid. This process suppresses the activation of cytokines in the cell membrane. ALA appears to inhibit tumor growth by limiting the production of prostaglandin E2, which suppresses immune responses. [2] ALA exerts a specific preventive effect against atherosclerosis, cardiovascular heart disease and stroke. ALA lowers triglycerides by inhibiting the synthesis of VLDL (very low density lipoprotein) and apolipoprotein B-100 and by decreasing postprandial lipemia (abnormal fat in the bloodafter meals). [2] Study evaluating lipid metabolism in patients with CD revealed a drop of serum total lipids, phospholipids, cholesterol, beta-lipoproteins, elevated triglycerides, and free fatty acids. Changes in fatty acid composition of blood serum manifested by derangement of HUFA ratio, omega-3 to omega-6 fatty acids. In all patients, there was low activity of lipolytic blood enzymes lipase and tributyrinase. [3] [M] Marked by hypertension, atherosclerosis, elevated triglycerides, inflammation, short bleeding time, impaired vision, dry eye syndrome, peripheral neuropathy, mental and behavioral disorders, apathy, excessive thirst, split fingernails, and ear problems. [C] Results from malabsorption in CD and lack of necessary vitamin and mineral cofactors (including zinc, magnesium, manganese, and vitamins B_3, B_6, and C). [R] CD-related deficiency responds to GFD containing ALA. Supplementation is suggested. [4]	Richest source of ALA is flaxseed meal or flaxseed oil. Good sources are soybean oil, canola oil, walnuts, butternuts, red and black current seeds, chia seeds, soybeans, and dark green vegetable leaves.

[+] (S) = Classic sign/symptom; (AT) = Atypical sign/symptom; (AD) Associated Disorder; (C) = Complication.

[++] [P] = Prevalence; [D] = Description; [M] = Sign/symptom; [C] = CD related cause; [R] = Response to cause; [R] = Response to gluten Free diet (GFD).

Health Manifestations of Celiac Disease (CD)
Section A: Nutrient Deficiencies

Affected System	Affected Nutrient	ID No.	Manifestation	Type+	Current Medical Information++	Dietary Sources
Blood Cardiovascular Immune Integumentary Nervous Reproductive Sensory	Essential Fatty Acids: omega-3 series of highly unsaturated fatty acids (HUFA)	3	Docosahexaenoic Acid (DHA) Deficiency [2,3,4,5,6]	(S)	[P] Common in study subjects with untreated CD.[3] [D] Functional deficiency or imbalance of docosahexaenoic acid (DHA) is characterized by altered visual and cognitive development during early brain development and brain function through-out life and functional disturbances of blood clotting, inflammatory responses, and vascular health.[4] DHA is crucial in brain structure and is abundant in the brain. DHA is a key component of neuronal membranes together with arachidonic acid (a major omega-6 fatty acid), making up 15- 20% of the brain's dry mass and more than 30% of the retina. DHA is particularly concentrated in highly active membranes such as nerve synapses and photoreceptors of the retina. Sufficient DHA is important for the normal growth and development of the fetal brain.[4] DHA should be obtained in the diet but can usually be synthesized in the body from sufficient alpha-linolenic acid.[2] DHA exerts a specific preventive effect against hypertension by enhancing endothelial nitric oxide synthesis and suppressing the production of transforming growth factor-B. It inhibits the formation of TXA2, a potent vasoconstrictor and platelet aggregator, and enhances that of PGI3, a vasodilator and platelet anti-aggregator.[5] DHA exerts a preventive effect agains atherosclerosis, cardiovascular heart disease and stroke by lowering triglycerides through inhibiting VLDL (very low density lipoprotein) and synthesis of apoprotein B-100 and by decreasing postprandial lipemia (abnormal fat in the blood after meals).[2] Study investigating the effects of DHA as supplements in patients after myocardial infarction (heart attack) demonstrated a clinically important and statistically significant benefit.[6] [M] Marked by slow and/or faulty thinking, inability to concentrate, apathy, brain atrophy, essential hypertension, atherosclerosis, elevated blood triglycerides, hypertension, and bleeding problems. [C] Results from malabsorption in CD and lack of necessary vitamin and mineral cofactors (including zinc, magnesium, manganese, and vitamins B₃, B₆, and C). [R] CD-related deficency responds to nutritious GFD. Supplementation is suggested. For brain function, direct intake of the preformed DHA is likely to be most effective, as alpha-linolenic acid to DHA conversion may be limited.	Highest sources of DHA are salmon oil, cod liver oil, menhaden oil, then herring oil. Good sources are Atlantic mackerel, Muroaji scad, bluefin tuna, king mackerel, lake trout, albacore, tuna, lake whitefish, Atlantic salmon, sprat, anchovy, Atlantic herring, and bluefish. Human milk contains DHA, but cow's milk does not.

+ (S) = Classic sign/symptom; (AT) = Atypical sign/symptom; (AD) Associated Disorder; (C) = Complication.

++ [P] = Prevalance; [D] = Description; [M] = Sign/symptom; [C] = CD related cause; [R] = Response to gluten Free diet (GFD).

Health Manifestations of Celiac Disease (CD)
Section A: Nutrient Deficiencies

Affected System	Affected Nutrient	ID No.	Manifestation	Type[+]	Current Medical Information [++]	Dietary Sources
Blood Cardiovascular Immune Integumentary Nervous Reproductive Sensory	Essential Fatty Acids: omega-3 series of highly unsaturated fatty acids (HUFA)	4	Eicosapentaenoic Acid (EPA) Deficiency [2,3,4,5,6]		[P] Common in study subjects with untreated CD.[3] [D] Deficiency of eicosapentaenoic acid (EPA) is characterized by functional disturbances of attention, cognition, behavior, and mood, alterations in skin integrity, blood clotting, and immune responses, imbalances in eicosanoid production, and difficulties with appetite or digestion, temperature regulation and sleep. EPA should be obtained in the diet, but can be synthesized in the body if sufficient alpha-linolenic acid is present.[4] EPA is crucial for normal brain function. This omega-3 fatty acid is an important substrate for the eicosanoids, a large group of highly bioactive hormone-like substances including prostaglandins, leukotrienes, and thromboxanes in their actions to inhibit clotting, counter vasoconstriction, and interfere with the inflammatory effect of opposing eicosanoids derived from arachidonic acid, an omega-6 fatty acid. EPA opposes arachidonic acid in acting as second messenger in chemical neurotransmitter systems as well as contributing to numerous other aspects of cell signaling.[4] EPA exerts a specific preventive effect against hypertension by enhancing endothelial nitric oxide synthesis in blood vessels and suppressing the production of transforming growth factor-B. Nitric oxide relaxes blood vessel walls. EPA inhibits the formation of TXA_2, a vasoconstrictor and platelet aggregator, and enhances that of PGI_3, a vasodilator and platelet anti-aggregator.[5] EPA exerts a preventive effect against atherosclerosis, cardiovascular heart disease and stroke. EPA lowers triglycerides by inhibiting very low density lipoprotein, and apoprotein B-100 synthesis and by decreasing postprandial lipemia, or abnormal fat in the blood after a meal. Study investigating the effects of EPA as supplements in patients after myocardial infarction (heart attack) demonstrated a clinically important and statistically significant benefit.[6] [M] Marked by hypertension, atherosclerosis, elevated triglycerides, depression, apathy, bipolar disorder, the schizophrenia spectrum disorders, ADHD, dyslexia, dyspraxia, the autistic spectrum disorders, dry eye syndrome, eczema, psoriasis, dry skin, PMS, short bleeding time, excessive thirst, and sleep disorders. [C] Results from malabsorption in CD and lack of necessary vitamin and mineral cofactors (including zinc, magnesium, manganese, and vitamins B_3, B_6, and C). [R] CD-related deficiency responds to nutritious GFD. Direct intake of preformed EPA is likely to be most effective, as alpha linolenic acid to EPA conversion may be limited.[4]	Highest sources of EPA are menhaden fish oil, cod liver oil, salmon oil, and herring oil. Rich sources are fatty marine fish: sardines in oil, Pacific herring, mackerel, Chinook salmon, sablefish, Atlantic herring, Atlantic sturgeon, then halibut, sockeye salmon, anchovy, mullet. Lesser amounts are in high omega-3 eggs, common periwinkle, conch and Pacific oyster.

[+] (S) = Classic sign/symptom; (AT) = Atypical sign/symptom; (AD) Associated Disorder; (C) = Complication.

[++] [P] = Prevalence; [D] = Description; [M] = Sign/symptom; [C] = CD related cause; [R] = Response to gluten Free diet (GFD).

Health Manifestations of Celiac Disease (CD)
Section A: Nutrient Deficiencies

Affected System	ID No.	Manifestation	Affected Nutrient	Type[+]	Current Medical Information [++]	Dietary Sources
Blood Cardiovascular Immune Integumentary Nervous Reproductive Sensory	5	Arachidonic Acid (AA) Deficiency [2,3,4]	Essential Fatty Acids: omega-6 series of highly unsaturated fatty acids (HUFA)	(S)	[P] Serum concentration was reduced in 100% of study subjects with CD.[3] [D] Arachidonic acid (AA) deficiency or imbalance is characterized by alterations in brain development, brain function, and vision, and impaired inflammatory response to injury or invasion, blood clotting response, inflammatory response, blood flow regulation, autoimmune reactivity, and reproduction. Structurally, arachidonic acid is a key component of neuronal membranes together with DHA, a major omega-3 fatty acid, making up 15-20% of the brain's dry mass and more than 30% of the retina. Arachidonic acid is particularly concentrated in highly active membranes such as nerve synapses and photoreceptors in the retina. It is crucial to brain growth, and mild deficiencies are associated with low birth weight and reduced head circumference. It also plays a role in the cellular processes underlying learning and memory. Arachidonic acid is an important substrate for the eicosanoids, a large group of highly bioactive hormone-like substances including prostaglandins, leukotrienes, and thromboxanes. They are primary mediators of late stage inflammation and blood clotting. Arachidonic acid has an opposing action to EPA, an omega-3 fatty acid, in acting as second messenger in chemical neurotransmitter systems as well as contributing to numerous other aspects of cell signaling. Arachidonic acid should be obtained in the diet, but can usually be synthesized in the body from linoleic acid.[4] [M] Marked by faulty memory, thinking, and learning, apathy, low blood pressure, poor inflammatory response, prolonged bleeding, excessive thirst, and low birth weight and reduced head circumference in infants. In children, growth retardation and short stature may develop. [C] Results from malabsorption in CD and lack of necessary vitamin and mineral cofactors (including zinc, magnesium, manganese, and vitamins B₃, B₆, and C). [R] CD-related deficency responds to nutritious GFD. Supplementation is suggested.[4]	Sources of arachidonic acid include meat and dairy proucts. AA is a component of breast milk.
Blood Cardiovascular Digestive Immune Integumentary Nervous Reproductive Sensory	6	Linoleic Acid (LA) Deficiency [2,3,4,5]	Essential Fatty Acids: omega-6 series of highly unsaturated fatty acids (HUFA)	(S)	[P] Common in study subjects with untreated CD.[3] [D] Linoleic acid (LA) deficiency or imbalance is characterized by impaired growth in infants and children, skin integrity, clot formation, blood vessel constriction, reproduction, and inflammatory response. Linoleic acid is a precursor for synthesis of prostaglandins and leukotrienes, substances needed for the inflammatory response to injury or invasion.[4] Linoleic acid is a precursor in the formation of potent vasoconstrictors and platelet aggregators involved in blood clotting.[5] Linoleic acid is an essential fatty acid that must be obtained in the diet. It can be used in the body to synthesize arachidonic acid.[2] [M] Marked by poor inflammatory response to injury, prolonged bleeding time, low blood pressure, skin disorders, fatty liver, excessive thirst, apathy, infertility, in children, growth retardation and short stature. [C] Results from malabsorption in CD and lack of necessary vitamin and mineral cofactors (including zinc, magnesium, manganese, and vitamins B₃, B₆, and C). [R] CD-related deficency responds to nutritious GFD. Linoleic acid supplementation is suggested.[4]	Rich sources of linoleic acid include vegetable oils: safflower, corn, sunflower oil, and ground nut oils. Plant sources include nuts, seeds, soy products, fortified orange juice.

[+] (S) = Classic sign/symptom; (AT) = Atypical sign/symptom; (AD) Associated Disorder; (C) = Complication.

[++] [P] = Prevalance; [D] = Description; [M] = Sign/symptom; [C] = CD related cause; [R] = Response to gluten Free diet (GFD).

Health Manifestations of Celiac Disease (CD)
Section A: Nutrient Deficiencies

Affected System	Affected Nutrient	ID No.	Manifestation	Type+	Current Medical Information ++	Dietary Sources
Blood Cardiovascular Digestive Immune Integumentary Glandular Nervous Reproductive Sensory	Minerals	7	Calcium Deficiency [1,7,8]	(S)	[P] 100% of study subjects with untreated CD.[7] [D] Calcium deficiency is characterized by bone and tooth demineralization and impaired nerve conduction, muscle contraction, blood clotting, blood pressure regulation, glycogen to glucose conversion, many hormone actions, many enzyme activities, and acetylcholine synthesis. Bone density should be measured in adults at diagnosis.[1] Calcium opposes phosphorus as a buffer to maintain acid-alkaline balance of the blood and is required for neuromuscular transmission and activity, to maintain cell permeability for the activation of body enzymes, and for milk production in the nursing of infants. Calcium absorption depends on the ionization of calcium salts in the acidic environment of stomach juice. Ionized calcium is absorbed by active transport in the duodenum where an acid medium prevails and by passive transfer throughout the remainder of the small bowel where the pH is alkaline, providing there is adequate absorptive surface area. Active transport is controlled throughout the action of vitamin D, which increases calcium uptake at the brush border and stimulates production of calcium binding protein.[2] Study investigating calcium at diagnosis and after one year GFD demonstrated significantly abnormal levels of calcium in all women with untreated CD.[7] Study investigating receptors for calcitrol, the active metabolite of vitamin D, demonstrated that calcium malabsorption in CD does not result from the absence of vitamin D receptors, but rather from reduction of vitamin D regulated proteins and functions essential for active calcium absorption that are located in the enterocytes of the villi.[8] [M] Marked by poor development of bones and teeth, rickets in children, osteomalacia in adults, osteoporosis, bone pain, easy fractures; muscle spasms/cramps advancing to tetany, mild encephalopathy; hypertension, anxiety, irritability, insomnia, excessive bleeding, pre-eclampsia in pregnancy, changes in saliva composition. Cataracts in chronic deficiency. Seizures and laryngospasm when severe. [C] Results from malabsorption in CD: ionized calcium being rendered unabsorbable due to binding with unabsorbed fatty acids in the formation of soaps, inadequate absorptive surface area, reduction of vitamin D regulated proteins needed for active transport, and low blood albumin. [R] CD-related deficiency responds to GFD.[7] Patients with decreased axial bone density should obtain 1200 mg calcium and 400 mg of vitamin D daily.[1]	Rich sources of calcium from plant sources include fortified orange juice, bok choy, rice, English walnuts, and green leafy vegetables such as collards, turnip greens, beet greens, and dandelion. Animal sources such as milk and dairy products, canned salmon, sardines, and crab.

+ (S) = Classic sign/symptom; (AT) = Atypical sign/symptom; (AD) Associated Disorder; (C) = Complication.

++ [P] = Prevalence; [D] = Description; [M] = Sign/symptom; [C] = CD related cause; [R] = Response to gluten Free diet (GFD).

Health Manifestations of Celiac Disease (CD)
Section A: Nutrient Deficiencies

Affected System	Affected Nutrient	ID No.	Manifestation	Type[+]	Current Medical Information [++]	Dietary Sources
Blood Cardiovascular Glandular Muscular Nervous Skeletal	Minerals	8	Copper Deficiency [2,9,10]	(S)	[P] Increased frequency in people with untreated CD.[9] In genetically normal people, acquired, environmental, or dietary abnormalities rarely cause clinically significant copper deficiency.[10] [D] Copper deficiency is characterized by altered blood cell formation, elastin formation (component of arteries), bone mineralization, and pigmentation of hair and skin. Progressive brain degeneration and failure to make normal blood cells can result in death. Almost all the copper in the body is present as a component of copper proteins.[9] It is required for hemoglobin, iron absorption and transport, ceruloplasmin production, bone maintenance, adrenal hormone production, maintenance of myelin sheath, inactivation of histamine, and pigmentation of hair and skin. Copper absorption occurs in the small intestine. Entry at the mucosal surface is by facilitated diffusion. Exit at the basolateral membrane is primarily by active transport.[2] Study investigating copper uptake from an oral test dose of copper sulphate solution close to the recommended daily dietary intake demonstrated significantly reduced uptake in patients with CD. Copper deficiency and proximal intestinal disease should be suspected in patients with otherwise unexplained anemia, especially neutropenia.[9] [M] Marked by anemia, leukopenia, neutropenia, and bone abnormalities especially demineralization, and apathy. Later symptoms are subperiosteal bleeding, loss of pigmentation of hair and skin, hair curliness, and loose skin. [C] Results from malabsorption in CD and possible increased biliary loss. [R] CD-related deficiency responds to nutritious GFD. Treatment must be directed at the cause of the deficiency, usually with the addition of 2 to 5mg of cupric ion daily.[9]	Rich sources of copper from animal sources include meat, organs, and shellfish. Plant sources include chocolate, nuts, brown rice, legumes, and dried fruits.

[+] (S) = Classic sign/symptom; (AT) = Atypical sign/symptom; (AD) Associated Disorder; (C) = Complication.

[++] [P] = Prevalance; [D] = Description; [M] = Sign/symptom; [C] = CD related cause; [R] = Response to gluten Free diet (GFD).

Health Manifestations of Celiac Disease (CD)
Section A: Nutrient Deficiencies

Affected System	Affected Nutrient	ID No.	Manifestation	Type+	Current Medical Information ++	Dietary Sources
Blood Cardiovascular Digestive Glandular Immune Integumentary Muscular Nervous Reproductive Sensory Skeletal	Minerals	9	Iron Deficiency [1,2,10, 11,12,13]	(S)	[P] Common in people with untreated CD.[1] Of the general population, it is the most common nutritional deficiency in the world,[10] but does not respond to treatment in persons with untreated CD. [D] Iron deficiency is characterized by impaired red blood cell formation, free-radical disposal, oxygenation of cells, immune response to infection, enzyme activity, cognitive performance, digestion, nail structure, and fetal health.[2] CD induces malabsorption and deficiency of iron essential for fetal organogenesis (organ formation).[11] Iron deficiency has been implicated in elevated prolactin hormone characterized by altered estrogen production in women and androgen production in men.[12] Iron is involved in hemoglobin synthesis, myoglobin activity, and numerous heme and nonheme enzymes. Its redox properties function in the respiratory transport of O_2 and CO_2 and it is an active component of cytochromes involved in cellular respiration. Humoral (antibody production) and cellular immunity requires iron for adequate concentrations of circulating T lymphocytes, mitogenic response, natural killer cell activity, and production of interleukin 1 and 2. Two iron-binding proteins - plasma transferrin and lactoferrin in breast milk - appear to protect against infection by withholding iron from microorganisms that need it for proliferation. Iron is involved in the function and synthesis of neurotransmitters and, possibly, myelin. Heme iron, obtained from animal food, is absorbed across the brush border then by active transport into the blood. Nonheme iron binds with apoprotein after entering the enterocyte to be ferried to the basolateral membrane and exited by active transport. Vitamin C is needed for absorption.[2] Study measuring IgG and IgA isotypes and IgG subclasses demonstrated significantly decreased transferrin saturation, mean corpuscular volume, and mean corpuscular hemoglobin in patients with positive IgA gliadin antibodies.[13] [M] Marked by pallor, fatigue, susceptibility to bacterial infection, reduced learning, inattention, apathy, sensorimotor incompetence, visual impairment, reduced memory, anxiety, anorexia, dysphagia, a pale, smooth and sore tongue, koilonychia, loss of vitality, infertility, and defects in fetal development. [C] Results from malabsorption of iron in CD. Deficiency of vitamin C impairs absorption. [D] CD related deficiency responds to GFD; iron supplementation is required.[10]	Rich animal sources of heme iron include liver, oyster, seafoods, organ meats, meat, fish, poultry, and egg yolks. Iron is not well absorbed from plants, but good sources of nonheme iron include brown rice, legumes, fortified cereal, and wines.

+ (S) = Classic sign/symptom; (AT) = Atypical sign/symptom; (AD) Associated Disorder; (C) = Complication.

++ [P] = Prevalance; [D] = Description; [M] = Sign/symptom; [C] = CD related cause; [R] = Response to gluten Free diet (GFD).

Recognizing Celiac Disease Signs, Symptoms, Associated Disorders & Complications

Health Manifestations of Celiac Disease (CD)
Section A: Nutrient Deficiencies

Affected System	Affected Nutrient	ID No.	Manifestation	Type[+]	Current Medical Information [++]	Dietary Sources [++]
Cardiovascular Digestive Glandular Muscular Nervous Skeletal	Minerals	10	Magnesium Deficiency [2,14,15]	(S)	[P] Common in study subjects with untreated CD.[14] [D] Magnesium deficiency is characterized by decreased parathyroid hormone (PTH) secretion and action and impaired nerve conduction, muscle contraction, bone density, and metabolism. The major function of magnesium may be to stabilize the structure of adenosine triphosphate (ATP) in ATP-dependent enzyme reactions. Magnesium is a cofactor for more than 300 enzymes involved in the metabolism of food components and synthesis of many products. It is required for neuro-muscular transmission and activity, working in concert and against the effects of calcium. In normal muscle contraction, calcium acts as a stimulator and magnesium acts as a relaxer. Magnesium may be absorbed along the entire length of the small intestine, but most absorption occurs in the jejunum. A carrier facilitated mechanism operates when ingested amounts are low. Simple diffusion operates throughout the length of the small intestine when ingested amounts are high.[2] Study investigating the magnesium status in patients at diagnosis demonstrated that magnesium deficiency was present in all patients with classical CD, but only in 1/5 of patients with CD on a GFD and 1/5 of patients with silent CD.[14] Study investigating magnesium status and bone mass in clinically asymptomatic CD patients on GFD and their response to magnesium therapy demonstrated that CD patients have reduction in intracellular free Mg^{2+}, despite being clinically asymptomatic. Bone mass also appears to be reduced. Magnesium therapy resulted in a rise in parathyroid hormone, suggesting that the intracellular magnesium deficit was impairing parathyroid hormone secretion. Bone mineral density increased in response to magnesium therapy.[15] [M] Marked by anorexia, nausea, vomiting, hypertension, muscle pain/spasm, chronic fatigue, weakness, premenstrual syndrome, constipation, bone pain, headache, depression, irritability, personality change, confusion, anxiety, insomnia, and decreased parathyroid hormone. Contributes to osteoporosis. Serious neuromuscular disturbances may develop including tetany, cardiac dysrhythmias, myocardial ischemia, and seizures. [C] Results from malabsorption in CD, being rendered unabsorbable due to binding with unabsorbed fatty acids in the formation of soaps, and shift in electrolyte balance from loss of potassium in diarrhea. [R] CD-related deficiency responds to nutritious GFD in most patients.[14,15] Supplementation may be needed.	Rich plant sources of magnesium include, soybeans, buckwheat, black-eyed peas, almonds, cashews, kidney beans, lima beans, Brazil nuts, pecans, whole grains, peanuts, walnuts, and bananas. Rich animal sources are halibut, then haddock, with lesser amounts in other fish, shellfish and chicken.

[+] (S) = Classic sign/symptom; (AT) = Atypical sign/symptom; (AD) Associated Disorder; (C) = Complication.

[++] [P] = Prevalance; [D] = Description; [M] = Sign/symptom; [C] = CD related cause; [R] = Response to gluten Free diet (GFD).

Health Manifestations of Celiac Disease (CD)
Section A: Nutrient Deficiencies

Affected System	Affected Nutrient	ID No.	Manifestation	Type[+]	Current Medical Information [++]	Dietary Sources
Body - Composition Cardiovascular Digestive Glandular Muscular Nervous Reproductive Skeletal	Minerals	11	Phosphorus Deficiency [2,7]	(S)	[P] Found in 100% of study subjects with untreated CD.[7] [D] Phosphorus deficiency is characterized by alterations in blood acid-alkaline balance and serious neuromuscular, hematologic, renal, skeletal, and dental abnormalities. Symptoms result primarily from decreased synthesis of adenosine triphosphate (ATP), the main energy source in cells, and phosphocreatine, a secondary energy source for muscle contraction. Severe deficiency has widespread and ultimately fatal consequences due to its widespread role in body functions. Most phosphates are absorbed in the inorganic state. Most absorption occurs within one hour in the proximal portion of the duodenum where the milieu is acidic. Organically bound phosphates are hydrolyzed and released as inorganic phosphates through action of the enzyme, alkaline phosphatase.[2] Study investigating the effect of GFD on mineral and bone metabolism in women with CD at diagnosis and after one year of GFD demonstrated, by use of strontium testing, significantly abnormal levels of phosphorus in all women.[7] [M] Marked by loss of appetite, muscle weakness, weight loss, low milk production in lactating women. Dysrathria (clumsy speech), paresthesia, confusion advances to stupor, seizures and coma. Contributes to osteoporosis. In children, imperfect bone and teeth development, rickets, and retarded growth occur. Osteomalacia developes in adults. [C] Results from phosphate malabsorption in CD, deficiency of 1,25 (OH)2 D3 (vitamin D) which increases absorption of phosphorus, depletion in vomiting and diarrhea, and increased parathyroid hormone which increases renal excretion. [R] CD-related deficiency responds to nutritious GFD.	Good animal sources of phosphorus include dairy products and liver with lesser amounts in crabmeat, beef, chicken, clams, and fish. Very rich plant sources include peanuts, almonds, cashews, walnuts, filbert nuts, macadamia nuts, and pecans. Good amounts are in chickpeas, lentils, lima beans, cocoa, and chocolate.

Recognizing Celiac Disease Signs, Symptoms, Associated Disorders & Complications

[+] (S) = Classic sign/symptom; (AT) = Atypical sign/symptom; (AD) Associated Disorder; (C) = Complication.

[++] [P] = Prevalance; [D] = Description; [M] = Sign/symptom; [C] = CD related cause; [R] = Response to gluten Free diet (GFD).

Health Manifestations of Celiac Disease (CD)
Section A: Nutrient Deficiencies

Affected System	Affected Nutrient	ID No.	Manifestation	Type[+]	Current Medical Information [++]	Dietary Sources
Blood Body - Composition Cardiovascular Digestive Muscular Nervous Pulmonary Skeletal	Minerals	12	Potassium Deficiency [2,4,7]	(S)	[P] Found in 100% of study subjects with untreated CD.[7] [D] Potassium deficiency is characterized by dehydration that may result in vascular collapse, muscular malfunction that may result in paralytic ileus, paralysis, respiratory hypoventilation or failure, metabolic acidosis resulting from diarrhea, and altered nerve conduction.[2] Potassium is the most important positively charged ion (electrolyte) within cells. It is required for electrolyte balance, acid-alkali balance, fluid balance, nerve and muscle function, enzyme activities, red cell transport of carbon dioxide, protein synthesis, bone structure, and stability of cell structure. Potassium is readily absorbed by the small intestine.[4] [M] Marked by fatigue, low blood pressure, dizziness, loss of appetite, thirst, vomiting, tremor, muscle aches/spasm, weakness of the lower extremities, drowsiness, confusion, anxiety, personality changes, mental depression, and bone pain. Contributes to osteoporosis. Severe symptoms include premature ventricular and atrial contractions of the heart, tetany, myoclonic jerks, and convulsions. [C] Results from depletion in diarrhea and vomiting. [R] CD-related deficiency resolves on nutritious GFD.	Good animal sources of potassium are milk and dairy, beef, poultry, and fish. Plant sources are much higher. Good sources are bananas, beans, pumpkin, chick peas and endive.
Cardiovascular Glandular Immune Muscular Skeletal	Minerals	13	Selenium Deficiency [2,10,16,17]	(S)	[P] Increased frequency in study subjects with untreated CD. [16,17] In the general population, selenium deficiency is rare.[10] [D] Selenium deficiency is characterized by alterations in any of its functions, including anti-oxidant, DNA repair, protective role against cancer, immune system enhancement, thyroid hormone activation, production of prostaglandins, and glutathione perioxidase enzyme.[2] Selenium is absorbed in the upper segment of the small intestine.[16] Study investigating selenium in whole blood, plasma, and leukocytes in patients with biopsyconfirmed CD on GFD demonstrated significantly lower concentrations of selenium than controls.[16] Study investigating serum levels of free carnitine and selenium in children with CD having type 3 duodenal lesions demonstrated that selenium and carnitine levels are decreased in children with CD, with and without diarrhea.[17] [M] Marked by muscle weakness, loss of vitality, hypertension, cardiomyopathy, thyroid disorders, testosterone deficiency, lowered resistance to infection, and predisposition to cancer. Contributes to osteoporosis.[2] [C] Results from malabsorption in CD.[17] [R] CD-related deficiency responds to selenium-containing GFD and may require supplementation.	Richest source of selenium is Brazil nuts. The richest animal source is kidney, then tuna, oyster, liver, clams, turkey dark meat, fish and shrimp. A rich plant source is sunflower seeds.

[+] (S) = Classic sign/symptom; (AT) = Atypical sign/symptom; (AD) Associated Disorder; (C) = Complication.

[++] [P] = Prevalance; [D] = Description; [M] = Sign/symptom; [C] = CD related cause; [R] = Response to gluten Free diet (GFD).

Health Manifestations of Celiac Disease (CD)
Section A: Nutrient Deficiencies

Affected System	Affected Nutrient	ID No.	Manifestation	Type[+]	Current Medical Information [++]	Dietary Sources
Blood Body - Composition Cardiovascular Digestive Glandular Immune Integumentary Muscular Nervous Reproductive Sensory Skeletal	Minerals	14	Zinc Deficiency [2,12, 18,19,20,21]	(S)	[P] Common in people with untreated CD.[18] [D] Zinc deficiency is characterized by alterations in any of its functions, including energy metabolism, immune function, growth, hemoglobin, carbon dioxide transport, hormone activity, insulin storage, many enzyme activities, prostaglandin function, synthesis of collagen, male fertility, protein synthesis, and vitamin A metabolism.[2] Disturbed zinc metabolism results in vitamin A deficiency.[18] Zinc deficiency has been implicated in elevated prolactin hormone, characterized by altered estrogen production in women and androgen production in men.[12] Zinc is absorbed throughout the small intestine, including the ileum.[19] A carrier absorption mechanism operates at low zinc intraluminal concentrations and a passive mechanism involving paracellular movement at high intake. Exit step is by active transport. Protein increases zinc absorption while copper, iron, calcium, and folic acid decrease zinc absorption.[2] Study investigating zinc nutritional status in adults with biopsy-proved CD demonstrated depression of plasma zinc and lowered taste discrimination among the untreated patients. Some patients who were in clinical remission on the GFD also had impaired zinc nutrition.[2] [M] Marked by low energy, fatigue, slow wound healing, frequent infections, nervousness, depression, anorexia, impaired taste and smell, skin rashes and disorders including eczema, acne, psoriasis, photophobia, male infertility, and white spots in fingernails. In children and youths, anemia, hypogonadism, and short stature develop. Zinc-deficiency syndrome in pregnancy includes increased maternal morbidity, abnormal taste sensations, abnormally short or prolonged gestations, inefficient labor, atonic bleeding, and increased risks to fetus such as malformations, growth retardation, prematurity, and perinatal death.[21] Severe deficiency results in immunologic disorders including thymic atrophy, deficient thymic hormone, lymphopenia, and worsening of diarrhea.[2] [C] Results from malabsorption in CD. [R] CD-related deficiency responds to zinc-containing GFD. Supplementation in some patients on GFD may be required.[20]	Highest animal source of zinc is the oyster. Rich meat sources include canned salmon, beef, liver, turkey neck, shellfish, poultry, and fish. Good plant choices include soybeans, pumpkin seeds, dry peas, dry beans, brown rice, and sunflower seeds.

[+] (S) = Classic sign/symptom; (AT) = Atypical sign/symptom; (AD) Associated Disorder; (C) = Complication.

[++] [P] = Prevalance; [D] = Description; [M] = Sign/symptom; [C] = CD related cause; [R] = Response to gluten Free diet (GFD).

Health Manifestations of Celiac Disease (CD)
Section A: Nutrient Deficiencies

Affected System	Affected Nutrient	ID No.	Manifestation	Type[+]	Current Medical Information [++]	Dietary Sources

All Systems	Proteins	15	Essential Amino Acid Deficiency [1,2]	(S)	[P] Common in patients with untreated CD.[1]
					[D] Deficiency of essential amino acids is characterized by impairment in growth and repair of body tissues, maintenance of osmotic pressure in blood vessels, performance as a carrier for many substances in the blood, and neurotransmitter production and function.[2] Deficiency of any essential amino acid results in inefficient utilization.
					    Of 20 amino acids making up human proteins that are part of all cell membranes, 10 are essential amino acids used as substrates for protein synthesis, and must be derived from the diet. These include arginine, methionine, cysteine, histidine, isoleucine, leucine, phenylalanine, proline, tryptophan, and valine.
					    Methionine is required to make homocysteine and also for conversion to S-adenosylmethionine (SAM). Glutathione is made from cysteine (a source of sulfur in metabolism). Histidine is required for the binding of zinc in signaling proteins. Muscle metabolism requires isoleucine. Leucine is required for protein synthesis, normal growth and metabolism. Phenylalanine is converted to tyrosine for synthesis of norepinephrine, epinephrine, and dopamine. Proline is required for triple helix, and is a significant constituent of collagens. Tryptophan is required for normal growth and development, and for conversion to the neurotransmitters, serotonin/melatonin, and to niacin. Valine is required for muscle metabolism, and in infants, normal growth.[2]
					[M] Marked by fluid retention and malnutrition including muscle wasting, weakness, poor muscle tone, fatigue, loss of vitality, anxiety, insomnia, dermatitis, hunger, weight loss, wasting of subcutaneous fat and muscle, flaky skin, thinning hair, discoloration of hair (black or brown turns reddish), apathy, diminished intellect, susceptibility to infection, infertility, and impaired growth in children.[2]
					[C] Results from protein maldigestion and malabsorption in CD, including B complex vitamins.
					[R] CD-related deficiency quickly responds to a strict GFD.
						Rich animal sources of essential amino acids include meat, poultry, seafood, fish, eggs, and dairy.
						
						Rich plant sources of protein include tree nuts, soybeans, peanuts, legumes, and seeds.[4]

[+] (S) = Classic sign/symptom; (AT) = Atypical sign/symptom; (AD) Associated Disorder; (C) = Complication.

[++] [P] = Prevalance; [D] = Description; [M] = Sign/symptom; [C] = CD related cause; [R] = Response to gluten Free diet (GFD).

Health Manifestations of Celiac Disease (CD)
Section A: Nutrient Deficiencies

Affected System	Affected Nutrient	ID No.	Manifestation	Type[+]	Current Medical Information [++]	Dietary Sources
Blood Digestive Immune Integumentary Pulmonary Reproductive Sensory Skeletal Urinary	Vitamins - fat soluble	16	Vitamin A Deficiency [1,2,18,22]	(S)	[P] Common in people with untreated CD.[1] [D] Vitamin A deficiency is characterized by alterations in the regulation and maintainance of a wide range of essential metabolic processes. Altered functions include 1) immune response with resulting impairment of numbers and responsiveness of T lymphocytes and susceptibility to bacterial, viral, and parasitic infections; 2) eye tissues with resulting changes to conjunctiva, cornea, and retina; 3) vision with resulting decreased production of visual pigments for cells of the retina; 4) development and maintenance of epithelial cells with resulting keratinization (thickening) and loss of skin and mucous membrane integrity with increased susceptibility to microbe invasion; 5) gene regulation with resulting adverse growth and development of tissues in general; 6) reproduction for conceiving and producing children with resulting loss of fertility; 7) and cell regulation of bone growth with resulting diminished stature. The absorption of vitamin A compounds requires their initial digestion. Preformed vitamin A and carotenoids (precursors of vitamin A) from food are released from protein in the stomach as retinol esters. The retinol esters are hydrolized in the small intestine to retinol. In the blood plasma retinol levels depend on the adequate presence of amino acids and zinc.[2] Study investigating vitamin A status in children with CD demonstrated a significant reduction of mean retinol acytransferase activity in older children with CD.[22] [M] Marked by repeat infections and poor recovery. Visual problems include nightblindness, impaired dark visual adaptation, dryness of the bulbar conjunctiva, chronic conjunctivitis, dryness of the cornea with haziness, cataracts, dysfunction of the retina, Bitot's spots, xerophthalmia and blindness. Dermatologic problems include dry, scaly, rough skin and plugged hair follicles - "goose flesh." Mucous problems include dry mouth, poor digestion, and diminished mucous production in the digestive tract, lungs, and urinary tract. Impairment of sperm formation in males and spontaneous abortion in females occur. In children, growth retardation is the most common sign and xerophthalmia is the major cause of blindness. Child mortality can be 50% or more. [C] Results from malabsorption in CD and as a consequence of disturbed zinc metabolism.[18] [R] CD-related deficiency responds to nutritious GFD.	Rich sources of vitamin A are found in preformed animal foods only. Liver is by far the highest source, then oysters, cod and halibut. Good sources are milk, cheese, butter, eggs, and fish. Plants are sources of carotenoids. Exceptionally rich sources include pumpkin, carrots, and sweet potatoes. Excellent vegetable are dark green leafy plants such as beet greens,

[+] (S) = Classic sign/symptom; (AT) = Atypical sign/symptom; (AD) Associated Disorder; (C) = Complication.

[++] [P] = Prevalance; [D] = Description; [M] = Sign/symptom; [C] = CD related cause; [R] = Response to gluten Free diet (GFD).

Health Manifestations of Celiac Disease (CD)
Section A: Nutrient Deficiencies

Affected System	Affected Nutrient	ID No.	Manifestation	Type[+]	Current Medical Information[++]	Dietary Sources
Digestive Glandular Immune Integumentary Muscular Nervous Skeletal	Vitamins - fat soluble	17	Vitamin D Deficiency [1,2]	(S)	[P] Common in people with untreated CD.[1] [D] Vitamin D deficiency is characterized by impaired bone mineralization, proximal muscle weakness and alterations in the maintenance of calcium and phosphorus homeostasis, metabolic functions, and male reproduction. Vitamin D deficiency is implicated in psoriasis. In the small intestine, vitamin D enhances the active transport of calcium across the small intestinal lining, which involves stimulation of the synthesis of calcium-binding protein (calbindin) in the mucosal brush border. This also involves the stimulation of intestinal phosphate transport, perhaps involving acid phosphatase, which is also induced. Vitamin D increases magnesium, zinc and other mineral absorption from the intestine. Vitamin D functions in conjunction with parathyroid hormone and estrogen to regulate the mobilization and deposition of calcium and phosphorus in bones, increases kidney tubular reabsorption of both calcium and phosphate for the purpose of maintaining plasma calcium within a narrow range of concentration, is essential for the functional maintenance of membranes, and is involved in the functions of several organs including skin, muscles, the pancreas, nerves, the parathyroid gland, and the immune system. Absorption of vitamin D from the small intestine along with lipids is by micelle-dependent diffusion.[2] [M] Marked by bone pain, easy fractures, osteopenia/osteoporosis (bone thinning), osteomalacia (bone softening) in adults, affecting the spine with vertical shortening of the vertebrae, the pelvis with flattening and narrowing of the pelvic outlet and the lower extremities with bowing of the long bones; muscle weakness, defective coordination for walking, osteomalacic myopathy, and spasm; psoriasis; decreased male fertility. In young children, development of rickets with bone bending of the weak shaft and delayed walking in 1 to 4 year olds. In older children, walking is painful with development of bowlegs and knock-knees.[2] [C] Results from malabsorption in CD. [R] CD-related deficiency responds to GFD. Supplementation produces rapid resolution of symptoms.[2]	Rich sources of vitamin D from animal sources include fish liver oil and egg yolk. Very good sources include herring, salmon, mackerel, sardines, tuna, fortified milk and butter.

[+] (S) = Classic sign/symptom; (AT) = Atypical sign/symptom; (AD) Associated Disorder; (C) = Complication.

[++] [P] = Prevalance; [D] = Description; [M] = Sign/symptom; [C] = CD related cause; [R] = Response to gluten Free diet (GFD).

Health Manifestations of Celiac Disease (CD)
Section A: Nutrient Deficiencies

Affected System	Affected Nutrient	ID No.	Manifestation	Type[+]	Current Medical Information [++]	Dietary Sources
Cardiovascular Muscular Nervous Reproductive Sensory	Vitamins - fat soluble	18	Vitamin E Deficiency [1,2,11,16,23, 24,25,26]	(S)	[P] Common in people with untreated CD. [1] [D] Vitamin E deficiency is characterized by impaired reproduction, altered neurologic function seen as ataxias and peripheral neuropathies, abnormal platelet aggregation (blood clumping), dry, rough skin, and impaired antioxidant protection resulting in more rapid injury and death in cells exposed to oxidant stress. [34] In males, vitamin E supports the correct differentiation and function of epidydimal epithelium, spermatid maturation and secretion of proteins by the prostate. [11] It is essential for normal cerebellar function and integrity of peripheral nerves. Vitamin E plays a role in maintaining healthy skin, wound healing, defense against infections, and protects red blood cells from hemolysis. Vitamin E is absorbed in the upper small intestine by highly variable micelle-dependent diffusion. [2] Study investigating the role of oxidative stress in CD demonstrated that the level of markers of oxidative stress derived for both protein (carbonyl groups) and lipids (thiobarbituric acid-reactive substances) were significantly higher in asymptomatic CD patients, whereas lipoproteins and alphatocopherol (vitamin E) were significantly lower. These data indicate that in CD even when asymptomatic, a redox imbalance persists, probably due to malabsorption. [23] Study investigating vitamin E status in patients with active CD and patients on a GFD demonstrated that plasma concentrations of vitamin E were significantly lower in untreated CD patients. Vitamin E correction may offer benefit to newly diagnosed and those who fail to adhere to a strict GF diet. [24] Study investigating vitamin E in the treatment of dysmenorrhea demonstrated that vitamin E relieves the pain of primary dysmenorrhea and reduces blood loss. [25] Case report of CD in 2 patients with common variable immunodeficiency disease (CVID) having free radical mediated neuronal damage induced by vitamin E deficiency recommends all CVID patients with evidence of enteropathy should be screened for vitamin E deficiency, as early detection and consequent treatment may prevent, halt or reverse the neurological sequelae. [26] [M] Marked by loss of deep tendon reflexes, impaired vibratory and sensory sensations, changes in balance and coordination, weakness, retinopathy, abnormal clots, increased risk of cancer and atherosclerosis. Infertility occurs in males. Dysmenorrhea and reproductive disorders occur in females. [C] Results from malabsorption in CD and pancreatic insufficiency. [R] CD-related deficiency responds to GFD. Supplementation is suggested. [24]	Animal sources are low in vitamin E with small amounts in salmon, butter, and chicken. Rich plant sources include sunflower oil, almonds, corn oil, avocado, olive oil, beans, apricots, plant leaves and brown rice.

[+] (S) = Classic sign/symptom; (AT) = Atypical sign/symptom; (AD) Associated Disorder; (C) = Complication.

[++] [P] = Prevalance; [D] = Description; [M] = Sign/symptom; [C] = CD related cause; [R] = Response to gluten Free diet (GFD).

Health Manifestations of Celiac Disease (CD)
Section A: Nutrient Deficiencies

Affected System	Affected Nutrient	ID No.	Manifestation	Type+	Current Medical Information ++	Dietary Sources
Blood Reproductive Skeletal	Vitamins - fat soluble	19	Vitamin K Deficiency 1,2,11, 27	(S)	[P] Common in patients with untreated CD.[1] [D] Vitamin K deficiency is characterized by impaired clotting function and bone mineralization.[2] CD induces malabsorption and deficiency of factors essential for fetal organogenesis (organ formation), including vitamin K.[11] Most of the vitamers K are absorbed across the small intestine by micelle-dependent diffusion which requires a minimum of dietary fat as well as adequate biliary and pancreatic function.[2] Study investigating the behavior of K-dependent factors after vitamin K administration in untreated children with CD demonstrated that all parameters return to normal in 15 days on a GFD when intestinal absorption is regained. However, Vitamin K administration determined a rapid increase in clotting activity of all K-dependent factors after 24 hours for severely compromised, newly diagnosed patients on a GFD.[27] [M] Marked by abnormal bleeding, including easy bruising, nosebleeds, bleeding gums, gastrointestinal bleeding, excessive menstrual bleeding, and blood in the urine. Contributes to osteoporosis. [C] Results from malabsorption in CD, diarrhea. [R] CD-related deficiency responds quickly to GFD.	Animal sources of vitamin K are low, of which beef and pork are best. Rich plant sources include green leafy vegetables such as broccoli, cabbage, turnip greens, spinach, seaweed, and dark lettuce.

+ (S) = Classic sign/symptom; (AT) = Atypical sign/symptom; (AD) Associated Disorder; (C) = Complication.

++ [P] = Prevalance; [D] = Description; [M] = Sign/symptom; [C] = CD related cause; [R] = Response to gluten Free diet (GFD).

Health Manifestations of Celiac Disease (CD)
Section A: Nutrient Deficiencies

Affected System	Affected Nutrient	ID No.	Manifestation	Type[+]	Current Medical Information [++]	Dietary Sources
Body-Composition Cardiovascular Digestive Muscular Nervous Reproductive Sensory	Vitamins - water soluble	20	Vitamin B$_1$ (Thiamin) Deficiency [1,2]	(S)	[P] Common in patients with untreated CD.[1] [D] Thiamin deficiency is characterized by impairment in carbohydrate metabolism, cardiac and neural function. Cocarboxylase, the functional form of thiamin, serves as coenzyme in energy metabolism, being involved in the metabolism of pyruvate and other a-keto acids which enter the Krebs cycle to generate energy. It is similarly required for the conversion of a-ketoglutarate and the 2- keto-carboxylates derived metabolically from the amino acids methionine, leucine, isoleucine, and valine. Thiamin pyrophosphate also serves as the coenzyme for transketolase, which catalyzes 2-carbon fragment exchange reactions in the oxidation of glucose by the hexose monophosphate shunt. Thiamin is absorbed from the proximal small intestine both by active transport at low doses and passive transport at doses greater than 5mg per day. Absorption is inhibited by folate deficiency. It must be supplied in the diet daily.[2] [M] Marked by anorexia, weight loss, poor concentration/memory, difficulty recalling information, low morale, irritability, anxiety, sleep disturbances, apathy, mental confusion, weakness, fatigue, indigestion, abdominal discomfort, constipation, pain over heart, ophthalmoplegia, and decreased urine output. Late syndromes include: Beriberi "dry" causes changes in both legs: loss of feeling in toes, burning of the feet, muscle cramps in the calves and tenderness, and pain in the legs. Later, loss of knee jerk reflex, tense calf muscles, and atrophy of calf and thigh muscles occur. Beriberi "wet" causes heart muscle disease: vasodilatation and warm extremities, tachycardia, and sweating. Cardiomegaly leads to heart failure with edema of face, legs, trunk and serous cavities with lung congestion, high blood pressure, distended neck veins, fatigue and inactivity. Cerebral beriberi (Wernicke Kosakoff syndrome) results from acute deficiency on top of chronic deficiency: confusion, dementia, loss of speech sounds from the larynx, and confabulation, then loss of immediate memory, disorientation, nystagmus, staggering walk, coma and death. [C] Results from malabsorption in CD. [R] CD-related thiamin deficiency responds quickly to nutritious GFD.	Rich animal sources of thiamin include pork, whole milk or 2%, salmon, halibut, chicken, beef, and egg. Plant sources include pecans, sunflower seeds, filberts, walnuts, watermelon, chestnuts, beans, peanuts, avocado, peas, and whole grain rice.

[+] (S) = Classic sign/symptom; (AT) = Atypical sign/symptom; (AD) Associated Disorder; (C) = Complication.

[++] [P] = Prevalance; [D] = Description; [M] = Sign/symptom; [C] = CD related cause; [R] = Response to gluten Free diet (GFD).

Health Manifestations of Celiac Disease (CD)
Section A: Nutrient Deficiencies

Affected System	Affected Nutrient	ID No.	Manifestation	Type[+]	Current Medical Information [++]	Dietary Sources
Blood Digestive Integumentary Muscular Sensory	Vitamins - water soluble	21	Vitamin B$_2$ (Riboflavin) Deficiency [1,2]	(S)	[P] Common in people with untreated CD.[1] [D] Riboflavin deficiency is characterized by impaired metabolism of carbohydrates, amino acids, and lipids and antioxidant protection. Deficiency first manifests in tissues with rapid cellular turnover, such as skin and epithelia and results in shortened life span of red blood cells. The flavin coenzymes, flavin adenine nucleotide and flavin adenine mononucleotide, are versatile redox factors, catalyze oxidation-reduction reactions, serve as hydrogen carriers in the mitochondrial electron transport system, and are coenzymes of dehydrogenases that catalyze the initial oxidations of fatty acids and of several intermediates in glucose metabolism. They are required for the conversion of pyridoxine to its functional form and the biosynthesis of niacin from the amino acid tryptophan. Riboflavin appears to combat oxidative damage to the cell. Riboflavin is absorbed in free form by a carrier-mediated process in the proximal small intestine. It is not stored in any appreciable degree and must be supplied in the diet daily.[2] [M] Marked by loss of visual acuity, tearing, burning and itching of eyes, photophobia, inflammation of conjunctiva, oral soreness and burning of lips, mouth and tongue, cheilosis, purplish swollen tongue, hypertrophy or atrophy of tongue papillae, normocytic and normochromic anemia, and seborrhea dermatitis.[2] Predisposes to cataracts. [C] Results from malabsorption in CD. [R] CD-related deficiency resolves quickly on nutritious GFD.	Sources of riboflavin include liver, milk, yogurt, clams, egg, pork, cheese, beef, chicken, trout, brewer's yeast, spinach, brown rice, orange, and apple.

[+] (S) = Classic sign/symptom; (AT) = Atypical sign/symptom; (AD) Associated Disorder; (C) = Complication.

[++] [P] = Prevalance; [D] = Description; [M] = Sign/symptom; [C] = CD related cause; [R] = Response to gluten Free diet (GFD).

Health Manifestations of Celiac Disease (CD)
Section A: Nutrient Deficiencies

Affected System	Affected Nutrient	ID No.	Manifestation	Type+	Current Medical Information ++	Dietary Sources ++

Body - Composition Cardiovascular Digestive Immune Integumentary Muscular Nervous Reproductive Sensory Urinary	Vitamins - water soluble	22	Vitamin B$_3$ (Niacin) Deficiency [1,2,28]	(S)	[P] Common in people with untreated CD.[1]
					[D] Niacin deficiency is characterized by impaired carbohydrate, fatty acid and amino acid metabolism, and oral and esophageal mucous membrane integrity. Advances to pellegra.
					    Niacin is a component of the pyridine nucleotide coenzymes nicotinamide adenine dinucleotide (NAD) and nicotinamide adenine dinucleotide phosphate (NADP) which are present in all cells. NADH and NADPH are co-substrates of more than 200 enzymes involved in metabolism. The NADH dependent reactions are involved in intracellular respiration, whereas most reactions dependent on NADPH serve biosynthetic functions, e.g. fatty acids, sterols. Niacin can be synthesized from the amino acid tryptophan.
					    Dietary niacin must be digested to release the absorbable forms, nicotinimide and nicotinic acid, which are absorbed from the small intestine by carrier-mediated facilitated diffusion.[2]
					    Case report describes presentation of CD in a 70 year old man with no prior GI symptomatology or positive family history. Triggering of all symptoms followed a recent myocardial infarction and infective endocarditis. Presentation was marked by more than 20% weight loss and pellagra-like lesions despite nearly normal examination and laboratory tests.[28]
					[M] Marked by muscle weakness, anorexia, distorted taste, indigestion, scarlet swollen tongue with burning of the mouth, throat, and esophagus, abdominal discomfort and distention, followed by nausea, vomiting and diarrhea - serious and may be bloody from ulceration. Nervous symptoms include dizziness, poor memory, anxiety, apathy, depression, disorientation, confabulation, neuritis, tremors, and hyperactivity in children. Skin can be cracked, itchy, pigmented red rash advancing to crusting skin eruptions sensitive to sunshine, itchy red wet areas from chafing, and inflammation of mucous membranes of vagina and urethra.
					[C] Results from malabsorption in CD.
					[R] CD-related deficiency responds quickly to nutritious GFD.
						Richest animal source of niacin is liver. Good sources include oyster, milk, yogurt, clams, pork, cheese, beef, chicken, egg, human milk, and trout. The richest plant source is almonds. Good sources include brewer's yeast, black eyed peas, spinach, peanuts, chestnuts, avocado, asparagus, broccoli, soybeans, beans, brown rice, and orange juice.

+ (S) = Classic sign/symptom; (AT) = Atypical sign/symptom; (AD) Associated Disorder; (C) = Complication.

++ [P] = Prevalance; [D] = Description; [M] = Sign/symptom; [C] = CD related cause; [R] = Response to gluten Free diet (GFD).

Health Manifestations of Celiac Disease (CD)
Section A: Nutrient Deficiencies

Affected System	Affected Nutrient	ID No.	Manifestation	Type[+]	Current Medical Information [++]	Dietary Sources
Blood Cardiovascular Digestive Immune Integumentary Muscular Nervous Reproductive	Vitamins - water soluble	23	Vitamin B$_6$ (Pyridoxine) Deficiency [2]	(S)	[P] Common in people with untreated CD. [D] Pyridoxine deficiency is characterized by impairment in any of its functions including metabolism of amino acids and for the biosynthesis of the neurotransmitters serotonin, epinephrine, norepinephrine, and y-aminobutyric acid, the vasodilator and gastric secretagogue histamine, and the porphyrin precursor of heme. Pyridoxine is required for the conversion of tryptophan to niacin, the release of glucose from glycogen, the biosynthesis of sphingolipids in the myelin sheaths of nerve cells, and in the modulation of steroid hormone receptors. The various forms of pyridoxine appear to be absorbed by passive diffusion primarily in the jejunum and ileum.[2] [M] Marked by anemia, increased homocysteine leading to atherosclerosis, lymphopenia, seborrhea dermatosis, glossitis, stomatitis, cheilosis, peripheral neuropathies, weakness, sleeplessness, irritability, depression, apathy and impaired cell mediated immunity. Convulsions in infancy. [C] Results from malabsorption in CD. [R] CD-related deficiency responds to GFD.	Animal sources of pyridoxine are more available for absorption than plant sources and include beef liver, chicken, halibut, pork, whole milk or 2%, and egg. Good plant sources include banana, potato, avocado, sunflower seeds, brown rice, prunes, white rice, peanut butter, Brussels sprouts, orange, cauliflower, tomato and apple.

[+] (S) = Classic sign/symptom; (AT) = Atypical sign/symptom; (AD) Associated Disorder; (C) = Complication.

[++] [P] = Prevalance; [D] = Description; [M] = Sign/symptom; [C] = CD related cause; [R] = Response to gluten Free diet (GFD).

Health Manifestations of Celiac Disease (CD)
Section A: Nutrient Deficiencies

Affected System	Affected Nutrient	ID No.	Manifestation	Type[+]	Current Medical Information [++]	Dietary Sources
Blood Body - Composition Cardiovascular Digestive Glandular Immune Integumentary Muscular Nervous Reproductive Sensory	Vitamins - water soluble	24	Vitamin B$_9$ (Folic acid) Deficiency [1,2,11,12] [29,30,31]	(S)	[P] Common in patients with untreated CD.[1] [D] Folic acid deficiency is characterized by impairment in any of its functions including many varied metabolic reactions involving amino acids, biosynthesis of DNA and RNA which reduce the division of red and white blood cells and the cells lining the stomach, intestine, vagina, and uterus.[4] CD induces malabsorption and deficiency of factors essential for organogenesis including folic acid.[11] Folate deficiency has been implicated in elevated prolactin hormone characterized by altered estrogen production in women and androgen production in men.[12] There is a subgroup of patients with epilepsy who developed the syndrome of CD, epilepsy, and cerebral calcifications which may be related to underlying folate deficiency.[30] Study investigating folate compounds and their breakdown compounds demonstrated that 5-methyltetrahydrofolate is poorly absorbed by patients with CD and the availability for biological utilization of the major dietary folate compounds will depend on the amount of gastric acidity and of the ascorbate in the intestinal chyme. Many folate compounds may be unavailable for metabolic utilization in the body.[29] Case report describes pathological changes in the syndrome of CD: folate deficiency, bilateral occipital calcifications, and intractable epilepsy. A child with this disorder had a field defect correlating with active lateralized epileptic discharges and asymmetrical lesions. A cortical vascular abnormality with patchy pial angiomatosis, fibrosed veins, and large jagged microcalcifications was found on resection of the right occipital lobe.[31] [M] Marked by megaloblastic anemia, thrombocytopenia leading to risk of bleeding, neutropenia leading to risk of infection, hyperhomocysteinemia leading to atherosclerosis, glossitis, stomatitis, diarrhea, malabsorption, weakness, depression, apathy, psychiatric disorders, polyneuropathy, and neurological abnormalities including seizures, migraine, and intracranial hypertension. In men, impotence, hypogonadism, and reduced semen quality may develop. In women, infertility, toxemia of pregnancy, miscarriage, abruptio placenta, restless leg syndrome, and congenital malformations can result. [C] Results from malabsorption in CD. [R] CD-related deficiency responds to GFD.	The richest animal source of folic acid is by far liver, followed by lamb and veal. Good sources are beef, egg yolk, shrimp, oysters, clams, and cheese. Plant sources are rich in folates especially lentils, beans, chickpeas, spinach, turnip greens, black eyed peas, active dry yeast, broccoli, asparagus, collard greens, avocado, oranges, and green leafy vegetables.

[+] (S) = Classic sign/symptom; (AT) = Atypical sign/symptom; (AD) Associated Disorder; (C) = Complication.

[++] [P] = Prevalance; [D] = Description; [M] = Sign/symptom; [C] = CD related cause; [R] = Response to gluten Free diet (GFD).

Health Manifestations of Celiac Disease (CD)
Section A: Nutrient Deficiencies

Affected System	Affected Nutrient	ID No.	Manifestation	Type+	Current Medical Information++	Dietary Sources
Blood Body - Composition Cardiovascular Digestive Integumentary Muscular Nervous Sensory	Vitamins - water soluble	25	Vitamin B$_{12}$ Deficiency [2,32,33]	(S)	[P] Vitamin B$_{12}$ deficiency is common in untreated celiac disease.[32,33] Low B$_{12}$ is common in CD without concurrent pernicious anemia, and may be a presenting manifestation.[33] [D] Vitamin B$_{12}$ deficiency is characterized by impaired metabolism of all cells. Vitamin B$_{12}$ functions in two coenzyme forms: adenosylcobalamin (for methyl-CoA mutase and leucine mutase) and methylcobalamin (for methionine synthetase). These forms of the vitamin play important roles in the metabolism of proprionate, amino acids, and single carbons. These steps are essential for normal function in the metabolism of all cells, especially for those of the GI tract, bone marrow, and nervous tissue. Concentrations should be measured routinely before supplementation.[32] B$_{12}$ status should be known before folic acid replacement is started.[33] Vitamin B$_{12}$ is absorbed in the ileum by active transport and, at low efficiency (about 1%), by simple diffusion. The active process is mediated by intrinsic factor which is present in gastric secretions.[2] Study investigating the prevalence of vitamin B$_{12}$ deficiency in patients with CD demonstrated that vitamin B$_{12}$ deficiency is common in untreated CD and concentration should be measured routinely before hematinic replacement.[32] [M] Marked by increase in plasma and urinary levels of homocysteine (leading to atherosclerosis), methylmalonicacid, and aminoisocaproate, megaloblastic anemia giving a lemon yellow tint to skin, pallor, thrombocytopenia in half of severe cases leading to risk of bleeding, neutropenia leading to risk of infection, apathy, anorexia, distorted taste, beefy red, smooth tongue with burning, intermittent diarrhea and constipation, poorly localized abdominal pain, considerable weight loss, muscle stiffness and generalized weakness in legs, numbness with tingling and burning in feet. Spasticity and ataxia, depression, and impaired thinking occur later. Late signs include paranoia, hallucinations, confusion, and delirium. [C] Results from malabsorption in CD and is not due to autoimmune gastritis.[33] [R] CD-related deficiency normalizes on GFD. Supplementation may be required by symptomatic patients.[32]	Rich animal sources of vitamin B$_{12}$ include clams, beef liver, oysters, crab, tuna, beef, halibut, milk 2%, pork, egg, cheese, chicken, and yogurt. Plant sources include some sea vegetables.

+ (S) = Classic sign/symptom; (AT) = Atypical sign/symptom; (AD) Associated Disorder; (C) = Complication.

++ [P] = Prevalance; [D] = Description; [M] = Sign/symptom; [C] = CD related cause; [R] = Response to gluten Free diet (GFD).

Health Manifestations of Celiac Disease (CD)
Section A: Nutrient Deficiencies

Affected System	Affected Nutrient	ID No.	Manifestation	Type+	Current Medical Information ++	Dietary Sources

Blood
Body - Composition
Cardiovascular
Digestive
Glandular
Immune
Integumentary
Muscular
Nervous
Pulmonary
Reproductive
Sensory
Skeletal
	Vitamins - water soluble	26	Vitamin C Deficiency [1,2]	(S)	[P] Common in people with untreated CD.[1]
					[D] Vitamin C deficiency is characterized by impairment in its metabolic functions as an enzyme cofactor, an antioxidant protector against free radicals, and a reactant with metal. Each of these functions involves the reduction/oxidation properties of the vitamin. Gingival (gum) inflammation is due to defects in epithelial basement membrane and peridontal collagen fiber synthesis. Scurvy may develop in 45 to 80 days.
					    Vitamin C is a co-substrate for at least 8 enzymes, of which it is best characterized in the role of the hydroxilation of proline to form hydroxyproline in the synthesis of collagen. It is needed for absorption of non-heme iron and is involved in the transfer of iron from plasma transferrin to liver ferritin. It is needed for the making of neurotransmitters (serotonin and nor-epinephrine), and for adrenal gland activity under stress. Vitamin C promotes resistance to infection through the immunologic activity of leukocytes, the production of interferon, the process of inflammatory reaction, or the integrity of mucous membranes. It is important for lung function.
					    Vitamin C is absorbed by active transport as well as passive diffusion.[2]
					[M] Marked by swollen ulcerated and bleeding gums and eventual tooth loss from infection, impaired wound healing, bleeding including bruising, petechiae, nosebleeds, conjunctival hemorrhage, and splinter hemorrhages in nails, loss of muscle, weakness, fatigue, anemia, rheumatic pains in legs, arthritis resembling rheumatoid arthritis, lethargy, irritability, depression, hysteria, hypochondria and coiling of hair in skin with hyperkeratosis of folicles (bumps). Edema of lower extremities appears late.
					    In infants, weakness of bone, teeth, cartilage, and connective tissue, edema, and hemorrhages occur (due to gluten in formula).
					[C] Results from malabsorption in CD.
					[R] CD-related deficiency responds quickly to GFD.
						Rich sources of vitamin C include orange juice, fresh broccoli, citrus fruits, papaya, strawberries, yellow peppers, kiwi, cantaloupe, honeydew, and cranberry juice.

+ (S) = Classic sign/symptom; (AT) = Atypical sign/symptom; (AD) Associated Disorder; (C) = Complication.

++ [P] = Prevalance; [D] = Description; [M] = Sign/symptom; [C] = CD related cause; [R] = Response to gluten Free diet (GFD).

Recognizing Celiac Disease Signs, Symptoms, Associated Disorders & Complications

Part 2
Health Manifestations of Celiac Disease

Section B
Signs, Symptoms, Associated Disorders
& Complications of Celiac Disease

HOW TO USE THIS SECTION

Step 1: Review list of manifestations to identify health problems. Review identified manifestations to determine relationship to celiac disease and whether nutritional deficiencies could be the cause.

Step 2: If a deficient nutrient is listed as cause, refer to Section A charts (p. 57-86) for dietary sources to incorporate into diet and determine whether nutrient supplementation is necessary.

Step 3: For manifestations not caused by nutrient deficiencies, which do not resolve by the elimination of gluten, implement appropriate medical treatment.

Section B is comprised of two parts: an index and a chart.

- The index alphabetically lists each manifestation with its corresponding ID number.
- The chart presents basic information about 309 manifestations of celiac disease.

The chart information is organized in seven columns:

1. **Affected System:** lists the primary body system(s) impacted by the manifestation.
2. **Affected Organ:** lists the organ affected by the manifestation.
3. **ID No:** lists the number assigned to the manifestation for cross-referencing with Alphabetical Index B.
4. **Manifestation:** lists the name of the manifestation.
5. **Type:** identifies the manifestation's relationship to celiac disease as being a sign, symptom, associated disorder or complication.

   (S)   Classic sign or symptom
   (AT)   Atypical sign or symptom
   (AD)   Associated disorder
   (C)   Complication

6. **Current Medical Information:** organizes current medical information according to prevalence, description, signs or symptoms, CD-related cause and response to gluten-free diet.

   [P]   Prevalence data from research studies and case reports of new associations.
   [D]   Brief description of the characteristics of the manifestation.
   [M]   List of the signs and symptoms of the manifestation as related to CD.
   [C]   CD-related cause(s) of the manifestation.
   [R]   Gives known response of the deficiency to the gluten-free diet and suggest when nutrient supplementation is advised.

7. **Deficient Nutrient:** lists deficient nutrient(s) leading to the manifestation. Please refer to Chart A to learn more about nutritional deficiencies involved in individual manifestations.

Section B: Alphabetical Index
Signs, Symptoms, Associated Disorders & Complications of Celiac Disease

ID No.	Manifestation
103	Abdominal Distention, Chronic
104	Abdominal Pain, Chronic
278	Abortions, Spontaneous
132	Addison's Disease
295	ADHD (Attention Deficit Hyperactive Disorder) and Learning Disabilities
147	Allergic Rhinitis
159	Alopecia Areata
160	Alopecia, Diffuse
264	Amenorrhea, Secondary
49	Anemia, Folic Acid Deficiency
50	Anemia, Iron Deficiency
289	Anemia, Latent in Intestinal Enzymopathies of Small Intestine
290	Anemia, Refractory Iron Deficiency in Childhood
276	Anemia, Severe Iron Deficiency in Pregnancy
51	Anemia, Vitamin B_{12} Deficiency
62	Angina Pectoris
71	Anorexia
27	Anti-Endomysium Antibodies (EMA) Present
28	Anti-Gliadin Antibodies (AGA) Present
148	Antiphospholipid Syndrome
29	Anti-tissue Transglutaminase Antibodies (tTG) Present
222	Anxiety, Chronic Maladaptive
57	Aortic Vasculitis causing Midaortic Syndrome
223	Apathy
73	Aphthous Ulcers and Non-Aphthous Ulcers - Canker Sores
257	Arthritis, Enteropathic
299	Arthritis, Juvenile Idiopathic
258	Arthritis, Psoriatic
259	Arthritis, Recurrent Monoarthritis
149	Asthma
204	Ataxia, Gait Disturbance
205	Ataxia, Gluten
206	Ataxia, Progressive Myoclonic
58	Atherosclerosis
294	Autism and Learning Disabilities
30	Autoimmune - Associated Autoimmune Antibodies Present
99	Autoimmune Cholangitis (Antimitochondrial Antibody-Negative Primary Biliary Cirrhosis)
150	Autoimmune Disorders in CD
151	Autoimmune Disorders in Dermatitis Herpetiformis
133	Autoimmune Hepatitis
152	Autoimmune Polyglandular Syndromes
145	Autoimmune Thyroiditis (Hypothyroidism)
238	Bitot's Spots
239	Blepharitis, Unexplained

ID No.	Manifestation
240	Bloodshot Eyes, Chronic
241	Blurred Vision, Unexplained
31	Bone Alkaline Phospahatase (BALP), Elevated
251	Bone Fractures
252	Bone Pain
209	Brain Atrophy
230	Bronchiectasis
231	Bronchoalveolitis
68	Cachexia
105	Cancer, Adenocarcinoma of Small Intestine
87	Cancer, Esophageal Small Cell Carcinoma
179	Cancer, Melanoma
84	Cancer, Post-Cricoid Carcinoma
85	Cancer of the Esophagus
82	Cancer of the Pharynx
300	Cancer Predisposition in Children
107	Candida Albicans Mucosal Infection
106	Carbohydrate Malabsorption
63	Cardiomegaly
64	Cardiomyopathy, Idiopathic Dilated
242	Cataracts
210	Cerebral Perfusion Abnormalities
74	Cheilosis
280	Childbirth - Puerperium Complicated by CD
277	Childbirth - Short Duration of Breast Feeding
32	Cholesterol, Low
207	Chorea
304	Chronic Bullous Dermatosis of Childhood
33	Coagulation Factors, Low
123	Colitis, Collagenous
124	Colitis, Lymphocytic
125	Colitis, Ulcerative
122	Colonic Volvulus and Ulcerative Jejunoileitis
153	Common Variable Immunodeficiency
283	Congenital Anomalies
127	Constipation Alternating with Diarrhea
126	Constipation, Chronic
65	Coronary Artery Disease
211	Cortical Calcifying Angiomatosis
128	Crohn's Disease
188	Cryptic Intestinal T-cell Lymphoma (Refractory Sprue)
168	Cutaneous Vasculitis
169	Cutis Laxa, Generalized Acquired
285	Cystic Fibrosis
92	Delayed Gastric Emptying
308	Delayed Puberty in Boys
302	Delayed Puberty in Girls
212	Dementia

ID No.	Manifestation
75	Dental Enamel Defects
224	Depression
170	Dermatitis Herpetiformis
305	Dermatitis Herpetiformis in Childhood
171	Dermatomyositis
296	Developmental Delay
138	Diabetes, Gastrointestinal Complications in Type I Diabetes Mellitus
303	Diabetes Mellitus, Juvenile Type 1
136	Diabetes Mellitus, Type 1
137	Diabetic Instability
108	Diarrhea, Acute
109	Diarrhea, Chronic
281	Down Syndrome
110	Duodenal Erosions in the Second Part of the Duodenum
250	Dysgeusia - Abnormal Taste
269	Dysmenorrhea
270	Dyspareunia
86	Dysphagia - Difficulty Swallowing
59	Ecchymosis - Easy Bruising
173	Eczema
172	Edema
111	Edema, Intestinal
213	Emicrania - Headache
189	Enteropathy-Associated T cell Lymphoma (EATL)
214	Epilepsy
219	Epilepsy, Occipital Lobe Epilepsy with Cerebral Calcifications
60	Epistaxis, Unexplained
174	Erythema Elevatum Diutinum (EED)
175	Erythema Nodosum
88	Esophageal Motor Abnormalities
287	Failure to Thrive and Growth Retardation
215	Fatigue, Chronic / Lassitude
216	Fatigue, Chronic Syndrome
306	Fecal Occult Blood in Stool (Children)
176	Follicular Hyperkeratosis
112	Food Allergy, IgE and Non IgE
129	Gas, Excessive
93	Gastric Ulcer
94	Gastric Ulcerations, Multiple
95	Gastritis, Collagenous
96	Gastritis, Lymphocytic
89	Gastroesophageal Reflux Disease (GERD)
130	Gastrointestinal Bleeding, Occult
113	Gluten Sensitive Enteritis
298	Glycogenic Acanthosis
146	Grave's Disease (Hyperthyroidism)
76	Gums, Bleeding and/or Swollen
161	Hair Diameter Lower and Cuticolar Erosion Scores Higher

ID No.	Manifestation
177	Hangnail
90	Heartburn
97	Helicobacter Pylori Infection
288	Hematologic, Abnormal Values in Childhood
52	Hemochromatosis
135	Hepatic Granulomatous Disease
158	Hives - Urticaria, Chronic
34	Homocysteine, Elevated
141	Hyperparathyroidism, Primary
142	Hyperparathyroidism, Secondary
35	Hyperprolactinemia
61	Hypertension, Reversible - reversible high blood pressure
36	Hypertransaminasemia
37	Hypocalcemia - low blood calcium
260	Hypocalciuria - low calcium in urine
38	Hypocupremia - low blood copper
39	Hypoglycemia - low blood sugar
272	Hypogonadism, Unexplained in Adults
40	Hypokalemia - low blood potassium
195	Hypokalemic Rhabdomyolysis in Celiac Disease and Dermatitis Herpetiformis
41	Hypomagnesemia - low blood magnesium
143	Hypoparathyroidism, Idiopathic
42	Hypophosphatemia - low blood phosphorus
53	Hypoprothrombinemia
194	Hyposplenism - low spleen function
301	Hypotonia
178	Ichthyosis, Acquired
54	Idiopathic Thrombocytopenic Purpura
154	IgA Deficiency
261	IgA Nephropathy
100	Impaired Gall Bladder Motility
273	Impotence
225	Inability to Concentrate
72	Increased Appetite
114	Increased Intestinal Permeability
265	Infertility, Female
274	Infertility, Male
226	Insomnia
284	Intrauterine Growth Retardation
227	Irritability
131	Irritable Bowel Syndrome (IBS)
115	Jejunitis, Chronic Ulcerative
309	Juvenile Autoimmune Thyroid Disease
243	Keratoconjunctivitis Sicca
244	Keratomalacia
164	Koilonychia
116	Lactose Intolerance
83	Laryngospasm

ID No.	Manifestation
295	Learning Disabilities and ADHD (Attention Deficit Hyperactive Disorder)
249	Loss of Smell
69	Loss of Vitality
232	Lungs Cavities or Abcess
192	Lymphadenopathy
187	Lymphoma, B cell non-Hodgkin Lymphoma (NHL)
190	Lymphomas, Extraintestinal Lymphomas
191	Lymphocytosis, Intraepithelial in Small Bowel Samples
43	Macroamylasemia
44	Macrocytosis
45	Macrolipasemia
117	Maltose Intolerance
266	Menarche, Late
267	Menopause, Early
193	Mesenteric Lymph Node Cavitation and Hyposplenism
217	Migraine Headaches
118	Milk Intolerance (Bovine Beta Casein Enteropathy)
218	Multiple Sclerosis
196	Muscle Pain and Tenderness
197	Muscle Spasm and Muscle Cramps
198	Muscle Wasting
199	Muscle Weakness
246	Myopathy, Ocular
200	Myopathy, Osteomalacic
162	Nails, Dry and Brittle that Chip, Peel, Crack or Break Easily
163	Nails, Horizontal & Vertical Ridges; Fragile Nails
166	Nails, Rounded with Curved Ends, Dark and Excessively Dry
165	Nails, Subungual Splinter Hemorrhages
167	Nails, White Spots and White Bands in Nails
203	Nervous System Disorders
55	Neutropenia, Granulocytic Hypersegmentation
245	Night Blindness (Nyctalopia)
134	Non-Alcoholic Fatty Liver Disease
66	Obesity
279	Obstetrical Complications
77	Oral Mucosal Lesions, Chronic
253	Osteitis Fibrosa Cystica
254	Osteomalacia
255	Osteonecrosis
291	Osteopenia in Childhood
256	Osteoporosis
139	Pancreatic Insufficiency
144	Parathyroid Carcinoma
307	Penicillin V Impaired Absorption in Children
229	Peripheral Neuropathy
180	Pityriasis Rubra Pilaris
46	Plasma Proteins, Low
91	Plummer-Vinson Syndrome affecting Esophagus

ID No.	Manifestation
233	Pneumococal Septicemia
201	Polymyositis
119	Postbulbar Duodenal Ulceration and Stenosis
268	Premenstrual Syndrome, (PMS)
101	Primary Biliary Cirrhosis
102	Primary Sclerosing Cholangitis
220	Progressive Multifocal Leukoencephalopathy
47	Prolonged Prothrombin Time
181	Prurigo Nodularis (Hyde's Prurigo)
182	Pruritic Skin Rash
183	Psoriasis
234	Pulmonary Hemosiderosis, Idiopathic
235	Pulmonary Permeability, Increased
262	Renal Calculus
292	Rickets
155	Sarcoidosis
228	Schizophrenic Spectrum Disorders
184	Scleroderma
185	Seborrhea
293	Short Stature
156	Sjögren's Syndrome
120	Small Bowel Intussusception
275	Sperm abnormalities
286	Spina Bifida
140	Steatorrhea
297	Stroke in Childhood
121	Sucrose Intolerance and Sucrosemia
157	Systemic Lupus Erythematosus
202	Tetany
78	Tongue, Beefy Red, Smooth, Burning
79	Tongue, Fiery Red, Smooth, Swollen, Sore
80	Tongue, Magenta, Swollen
81	Tongue, Pale, Smooth, Burning
56	Transient Erythroblastopenia
208	Tremors
236	Tuberculosis, Increased Susceptibility
237	Tuberculosis, Non-Response to Treatment
282	Turner's Syndrome
263	Urinary Tract Infection (UTI)
247	Uveitis, Bilateral
271	Vaginitis
221	Vasculitis of the Central Nervous System
186	Vitiligo
98	Vomiting
67	Weight Gain, Unexplained
70	Weight Loss, Unexpected
248	Xerophthalmia
48	Zincemia

Health Manifestations of Celiac Disease (CD)
Section B: Signs, Symptoms, Associated Disorders and Complications

Affected System	Affected Organ	ID No.	Manifestation	Type+	Current Medical Information++	Deficient Nutrient
Blood System	Blood component	27	Anti-Endomysium Antibodies (EMA) Present [1,2,3,4]	(S)	[P] CD occurs in 1% of the general population.[2] A healthy population usually tests negative for EMA.[3] 100% of study patients with abdominal symptoms had positive EMA antibodies present.[4] [D] Anti-endomysium antibodies are connective tissue autoantibodies that are highly sensitive and specific to CD, making their abnormal presence in the blood useful for identifying CD. A negative test result does not rule out the possibility of CD. Patients with IgA deficiency will test negative for IgA-EMA antibodies.[3] EMA-IgA assay may be especially predictive in populations who have a high prevalence of other causes of flat mucosa. In this instance, a biopsy indicating villous atrophy with a positive EMA test would differentiate CD from conditions such as cow's milk enteropathy and other enteropathies.[3] Study investigating the usefulness of IgG- and IgA-antigliadin antibodies, IgA-endomysial antibodies, and intestinal permeability tests in diagnosing CD in 102 adult patients with nonspecific abdominal symptoms demonstrated the advantage of IgA-EMA for screening CD. 100% of patients, in whom CD was later confirmed by biopsy, had IgA-EMA present, except in the case of patients with IgA deficiency or dermatitis herpetiformis. In these patients, the permeability test could improve noninvasive differential diagnosis.[4] [M] Marked by positivity to IgA-EMA antibody assay, with or without abdominal symptoms. [C] Results from exposure to gluten in susceptible individuals. [R] A strict GFD results in disappearance of these antibodies, usually diminishing within weeks.[3]	Not applicable.
Blood System	Blood component	28	Anti-Gliadin Antibodies (AGA) Present [1,2,3,5]	(S)	[P] CD occurs in 1% of the general population.[2] Sensitivity of IgA anti-gliadin antibody test is 31-100% and specificity is 85-100%.[3] [D] Anti-gliadin antibodies (AGA) are produced against grain peptides, making their abnormal presence in the blood useful for identifying CD in combination with EMA. There is significant variability in the accuracy of antibodies to gliadin, whether IgA or IgG, and these tests are less specific in young children.[3] Antibodies to gliadin have been shown to have a greater sensitivity in some studies.[3] Importantly, their presence is valuable for detecting gluten sensitivity reactions resulting from gliadin leaking into the blood secondary to increased intestinal permeability, whether caused by, or separate from, CD. Study measuring antigliadin antibodies of the IgG and IgA isotypes and IgG subclasses revealed that a significantly higher proportion of the AGA-positive individuals had diarrhea and chronic fatigue and showed significantly decreased transferrin saturation, mean corpuscular volume, mean corpuscular hemoglobin, and folic acid concentrations compared with AGA-negative controls. Persistent or recurrent headaches were more common in AGA-positive patients. These findings raise the possibility that a subclinical form of gluten intolerance may be relatively common.[5] [M] Marked by positivity to anti-gliadin antibody assay. [C] Results from exposure to gluten in susceptible patients. [R] A strict GFD results in disappearance of these antibodies.	Not applicable.

+ (S) = Classic sign/symptom; (AT) = Atypical sign/symptom; (AD) Associated Disorder; (C) = Complication.

++ [P] = Prevalance; [D] = Description; [M] = Sign/symptom; [C] = CD related cause; [R] = Response to gluten Free diet (GFD).

Health Manifestations of Celiac Disease (CD)
Section B: Signs, Symptoms, Associated Disorders and Complications

Affected System	Affected Organ	ID No.	Manifestation	Type[+]	Current Medical Information [++]	Deficient Nutrient
Blood System	Blood component	29	Anti-tissue Transglutaminase Antibodies (tTG) Present [1,2,3,6]	(S)	[P] CD occurs in 1% of the general population.[2] Anti-tissue transglutaminase antibodies are highly sensitive and specific to CD.[2] [D] Anti-tissue transglutaminase antibodies (anti-tTG) are connective tissue autoantibodies. Tissue transglutaminase is the autoantigen in endomysium. Their abnormal presence in the blood is useful for identifying CD. A negative test result does not rule out the possibility of CD. Patients with IgA deficiency will test negative for IgA-tTG.[3] Study investigating the diagnostic performance of serologic tests for the diagnosis and screening of CD demonstrated the pooled specificity of transglutaminase antibody (tTG)-guinea pig (GP) and tTG-human recombinant (HR) were between 95% and 99%. The pooled sensitivity of tTG-GP in adults and children was 90% and 93%, respectively. The sensitivity of tTG-HR was 98% and 96%, respectively. The sensitivity of these tests appears to be lower than reported when milder histologic grades are used to define CD (below 90%). The positive predictive value of these tests is likely lower than reported when the tests are applied to low prevalence populations.[6] [M] Marked by positivity to tTG antibody assay, with or without abdominal symptoms. [C] Results from exposure to gluten in susceptible patients. [R] A strict GFD results in disappearance of these antibodies, usually diminishing within weeks.[3]	Not applicable.
Blood System	Blood component	30	Associated Autoimmune Antibodies Present [7]	(AD)	[P] Prevalence of associated autoimmune antibodies in CD is 14% vs. 2.8% in healthy controls. The rate for those diagnosed with CD at less than two years is 5.1%, 17% at 2 to 10 years, and 23.6% for those over 10 years of age.[7] [D] Associated autoimmune antibodies indicate the presence of autoimmune diseases that occur more often in people with CD than expected in the general population. Study investigating the relationship between the prevalence of autoimmune disorders in 909 patients with CD and the duration of exposure to gluten demonstrated that the prevalence of autoimmune disorders in CD is related to the duration of exposure to gluten. Prevalence of autoimmune disorders in CD increased with increasing age at diagnosis.[7] [M] Marked by positive serology for autoantibodies. [C] Results from an autoimmune mechanism. [R] Response to GFD varies by individual autoimmune disorder.	Not applicable.

+ (S) = Classic sign/symptom; (AT) = Atypical sign/symptom; (AD) = Associated Disorder; (C) = Complication.

++ [P] = Prevalance; [D] = Description; [M] = Sign/symptom; [C] = CD related cause; [R] = Response to gluten Free diet (GFD).

Health Manifestations of Celiac Disease (CD)
Section B: Signs, Symptoms, Associated Disorders and Complications

Affected System	Affected Organ	ID No.	Manifestation	Type+	Current Medical Information ++	Deficient Nutrient
Blood System	Blood component	31	Bone Alkaline Phosphatase (BALP), Elevated [1,8,9]	(S)	[P] Common serology result in patients with untreated CD.[8] [D] Elevated bone alkaline phosphatase (BALP) an enzyme present in bone, is one of the most frequently used biochemical markers of bone activity. BALP is released from bone tissue that is being broken down. Determination of BALP activity can predict bone loss in secondary osteoporosis associated with CD, and is helpful in diagnosing CD and monitoring antiresorptive therapy.[8] Study investigating calcium absorption and bone mineral density (BMD) in treated adult celiac patients after a prolonged, over 4 years, treatment with a GFD demonstrated significant inverse correlations between 1) serum parathyroid hormone (PTH) and femoral neck or total body BMD, 2) PTH and duration of GFD, and 3) fractional calcium absorption and alkaline phosphatase. Increased calcium intake could potentially compensate for the reduced fractional calcium intake but may not normalize the BMD. Serum calcium and serum 25(OH)D (vitamin D) concentrations did not differ from controls. In addition, the inverse correlation between PTH and time following treatment is suggestive of a long-term benefit of gluten withdrawal on bone metabolism in CD patients.[9] [M] Marked by osteopenia/osteoporosis. [C] Results from calcium malabsorption in CD.[9] [R] CD-related elevated BALP normalizes on GFD.[9] Calcium supplementation may be required.	Calcium.

+ (S) = Classic sign/symptom; (AT) = Atypical sign/symptom; (AD) Associated Disorder; (C) = Complication.

++ [P] = Prevalance; [D] = Description; [M] = Sign/symptom; [C] = CD related cause; [R] = Response to gluten Free diet (GFD).

Section B   *Signs, Symptoms, Associated Disorders & Complications*   97

Health Manifestations of Celiac Disease (CD)
Section B: Signs, Symptoms, Associated Disorders and Complications

Affected System	Affected Organ	ID No.	Manifestation	Type[+]	Current Medical Information [++]	Deficient Nutrient
Blood System	Blood component	32	Cholesterol, Low 1,10,11,12	(S)	[P] Common serology result in 17.9% of untreated CD patients.[10] [D] Low cholesterol is characterized by altered production of bile and steroid hormones including estrogen, testosterone and adrenalin, and has been linked to depression and increased incidence of cancer. Cholesterol is essential to structure and function of cell membranes. Level between 185-200 mg is desirable. Study investigating the association of cholesterol malabsorption with cholesterol and lipoprotein metabolism by determining low-density lipoprotein (LDL) apolipoprotein (apo) B kinetics simultaneously with measurements of cholesterol absorption and synthesis before and during the GFD, demonstrated that cholesterol absorption, cholesterol synthesis, hepatic B/E receptor activity, and LDL apo B transport rate are closely associated with each other and that their levels can change markedly with no detectable change in serum levels of LDL cholesterol or apo B. The basal condition was characterized by low cholesterol absorption, enhanced cholesterol synthesis, and high removal and transport rate of LDL apo B. The GFD markedly improved cholesterol absorption and decreased intestinal influx of cholesterol, fecal neutral steroids, and cholesterol synthesis. Only plasma high-density lipoprotein (HDL) was enhanced by the GFD proportionately to cholesterol absorption. The plasma LDL apo B level remained unchanged because of simultaneous decreases in the fractional catabolic rate (FCR) and transport of LDL apo B. As cholesterol absorption was improved by GFD, the FCR and transport rate for LDL apo B was decreased, and reductions were closely related to the decrease in synthesis.[11] Study defining the correlates of CD in 100 anemic adults without overt malabsorption demonstrated that among patients with hypochromic anemia, plasma cholesterol in the high-to-normal range could be used to exclude the presence of CD. Within the entire cohort of anemic patients (100%) plasma cholesterol inversely related to prevalence of CD. All anemic CD patients had plasma cholesterol less than 156mg/100ml. Compared to anemic patients without CD, anemic patients with CD had significant or borderline significant differences for plasma cholesterol, albumin, and body mass index but not for blood hemoglobin, mean corpuscular volume, plasma iron, and ferritin.[10] Study investigating prolonged prothrombin time (PT) in celiac adults with untreated CD-demonstrated that patients with prolonged PT had significant lower values of cholesterol.[12] [M] Marked by effects on hormone production and symptoms related to low bile salt production - steatorrhea and crampy pain after fatty meals. [C] Results from low cholesterol absorption, enhanced cholesterol synthesis, and high removal and transport rate of LDL apo B.[11] [R] GFD enhances HDL cholesterol levels without change in LDL levels.[11]	Cholesterol.

[+] (S) = Classic sign/symptom; (AT) = Atypical sign/symptom; (AD) Associated Disorder; (C) = Complication.

[++] [P] = Prevalance; [D] = Description; [M] = Sign/symptom; [C] = CD related cause; [R] = Response to gluten Free diet (GFD).

Health Manifestations of Celiac Disease (CD)
Section B: Signs, Symptoms, Associated Disorders and Complications

Affected System	Affected Organ	ID No.	Manifestation	Type[+]	Current Medical Information [++]	Deficient Nutrient
Blood System	Blood component	33	Coagulation Factors, Low[1,13]	(S)	[P] Common serology result in untreated CD patients with malabsorption.[13] [D] Low coagulation factors are characterized by altered secondary coagulation resulting in impaired clot formation. These vitamin K-dependent factors are PT, PTT and Factors II, IX, X. Study investigating the behavior of vitamin K-dependent factors after vitamin K administration in 37 untreated celiac children randomized on the initial day of a GFD into a group who received a single 10 mg, intramuscular dose of Phytonadione, a vitamin K medication, and a group who did not receive vitamin K administration, demonstrated that after 15 days on GFD when intestinal absorption is regained, all parameters returned to normal. Vitamin K administration determined a rapid increase in clotting activity of all K-dependent factors after 24 hours for severely compromised newly diagnosed CD patients on a GFD. On the contrary, the children not treated had levels similar to those of acute stage on day 7, reaching normal limits on day 15. Vitamin K deficiency not only seems constant in children with CD, but also seems responsible for the hemocoagulative deficit of the K-dependent factors. Vitamin K-dependent factors can be used as short term indexes of improved intestinal absorption and celiac children with severely compromised nutritional status can be treated with vitamin K (10 mg dose).[13] [M] Marked by deep ecchymosis, hematoma, and easy bleeding after trauma. [C] Results from vitamin K deficiency state in CD.[13] [R] CD-related low coagulation factors normalize on a GFD.[13]	Vitamin K.

+ (S) = Classic sign/symptom; (AT) = Atypical sign/symptom; (AD) Associated Disorder; (C) = Complication.

++ [P] = Prevalance; [D] = Description; [M] = Sign/symptom; [C] = CD related cause; [R] = Response to gluten Free diet (GFD).

Health Manifestations of Celiac Disease (CD)
Section B: Signs, Symptoms, Associated Disorders and Complications

Affected System	Affected Organ	ID No.	Manifestation	Type+	Current Medical Information ++	Deficient Nutrient
Blood System	Blood component	34	Homocysteine, Elevated [14,15,16]	(S)	[P] Celiac patients show a higher total plasma status than the general population.[14] [D] Elevated homocysteine, or hyperhomocysteinemia, is characterized by altered endothelial function of blood vessels. Homocysteine, an amino acid, briefly formed in the breakdown of methionine, is normally converted to cystathione and then to cysteine by means of a vitamin B_6 dependent enzyme. In the reverse, conversion of homocysteine to the amino acid methionine requires an enzyme dependent on adequate folic acid and vitamin B_{12} levels. Insufficient methionine levels and/or inefficiency in this process results in elevated homocysteine plasma levels that are toxic to blood vessels. Folic acid, vitamin B_{12} and vitamin B_6 are involved in the metabolic removal of homocysteine, but folic acid deficit occurs the most often.[15] Study investigating the vitamin nutrition status of patients 45 to 64 years old with diagnosed CD in biopsy proven remission who were on a GFD for 10 years, demonstrated half of the patients showed a poor vitamin status. Plasma levels of folate were low in 37% and pyridoxal 5'-phosphate levels were low in 20% and accounted for 33% of the variation of the total plasma homocysteine level. The mean daily intakes of folate and vitamin B_{12}, but not of pyridoxine (vitamin B_6), were significantly lower in CD patients than in controls. This may have clinical implications considering the linkage between vitamin deficiency, elevated total plasma homocysteine levels and cardiovascular disease. Follow-up should include review of vitamin status.[14] Case report of a 49 year old woman with uncomplicated sustained hypertension describes investigation of raised homocysteine levels with low vitamin B_{12} level and endothelial dysfunction and subsequent diagnosis of CD. Treatment of CD normalized her blood pressure (BP) with parallel normalization of homocysteine levels and endothelial function. These observations suggest that subclinical CD related hyperhomocysteinemia might cause endothelial dysfunction, potentially giving rise to a reversible form of hypertension. In addition, this case study supports the notion that irrespective of etiology, endothelial dysfunction may be the precursor of hypertension. This highlights the need to resolve co-existing vascular risk factors in patients with hypertension.[16] [M] Marked by arteriosclerosis, coronary heart disease, cerebral vascular disease and reversible hypertension.[15,16] [C] Results from vitamin cofactor malabsorption in CD (folic acid, vitamin B_{12}, and vitamin B_6). [R] CD-related hyperhomocysteinemia resolves on a strict GFD with supplementation.	Folic acid, Vitamin B_6, Vitamin B_{12}.

+ (S) = Classic sign/symptom; (AT) = Atypical sign/symptom; (AD) Associated Disorder; (C) = Complication.

++ [P] = Prevalance; [D] = Description; [M] = Sign/symptom; [C] = CD related cause; [R] = Response to gluten Free diet (GFD).

Health Manifestations of Celiac Disease (CD)
Section B: Signs, Symptoms, Associated Disorders and Complications

Affected System	Affected Organ	ID No.	Manifestation	Type[+]	Current Medical Information[++]	Deficient Nutrient
Blood System	Blood component	35	Hyperprolactinemia [1,17,18]	(S)	[P] 100% prevalence in untreated celiac patients.[17] [D] Hyperprolactinemia, or elevated prolactin hormone produced by the anterior pituitary gland, is characterized by altered estrogen production in women and androgen production in men. The real mechanism by which CD produces these changes is unclear, but factors such as malnutrition, iron, folate and zinc deficiencies have all been implicated.[18] In addition, in men gonadal dysfunction is believed to be due to reduced conversion of testosterone to dihydrotestosterone caused by low levels of 5 alphareductase in CD. This leads to derangement of the hypothalmic-pituitary axis.[18] Study investigating serum prolactin levels of CD patients on unrestricted gluten containing diet (group 1) and CD patients on GFD (group 2) vs. controls, demonstrated hyperprolactinemia in all patients of group 1 and one patient in group 2 who had severe villous atrophy, showing a positive correlation between serum prolactin levels (SPL) and duration of symptoms. A positive correlation also existed in group 2 between SPL and degree of villous atrophy. Serum prolactin estimation may provide an additional marker of disease activity and may be a more viable option economically.[17] Correction of deficient dietary elements can lead to return of fertility in both sexes.[18] [M] Marked in women by delayed menarche, amenorrhea, early menopause, recurrent abortions, and a reduced pregnancy rate. In men it can cause hypogonadism, immature secondary sex characteristics, and reduced semen quality.[18] Contributes to osteoporosis. [C] Results from unclear mechanism; malnutrition and micronutrient deficiencies in CD are implicated.[18] [R] CD-related hyperprolactinemia responds to GFD.[17]	Folic acid, Iron, Zinc.

+ (S) = Classic sign/symptom; (AT) = Atypical sign/symptom; (AD) Associated Disorder; (C) = Complication.

++ [P] = Prevalance; [D] = Description; [M] = Sign/symptom; [C] = CD related cause; [R] = Response to gluten Free diet (GFD).

Health Manifestations of Celiac Disease (CD)
Section B: Signs, Symptoms, Associated Disorders and Complications

Affected System	Affected Organ	ID No.	Manifestation	Type+	Current Medical Information ++	Deficient Nutrient
Blood System	Blood component	36	Hypertransaminasemia 1,3,19	(AT)	[P] Frequent in untreated celiac patients.[19] [D] Hypertransaminasemia, or elevated liver enzymes, is characterized by hepatocellular (liver cell) injury and correlates with increased intestinal permeability (gut leakiness) in CD.[3] Study investigating the prevalence and potential pathogenetic (disease-causing) factors of hypertransaminasemia in 178 patients with CD prior to the initiation of a GFD and assessment of the course of transaminases on a GFD, demonstrated that hypertransaminasemia before GFD is frequent in celiac patients, correlates with intestinal permeability and normalizes on a GFD in most patients. Aspartate aminotransferase (AST) and/or alanine aminotransferase (ALT) were found increased in the blood of 40% of patients prior to initiation of GFD. Of 5 selected study patients who underwent liver biopsy, mild to moderate hepatitis with septal fibrosis was found in 2 and minimal lymphocytic infiltrates of the portal tracts without inflammation of the bile ducts was found in 3 patients. Underlying CD should be considered in cases of persistently elevated liver function tests of unknown origin.[19] [M] Marked by mild liver disease. [C] Results from gluten exposure in CD. [R] CD-related ALT and AST normalize in most CD patients within one year on a GFD.[19]	Not applicable.

+ (S) = Classic sign/symptom; (AT) = Atypical sign/symptom; (AD) Associated Disorder; (C) = Complication.

++ [P] = Prevalance; [D] = Description; [M] = Sign/symptom; [C] = CD related cause; [R] = Response to gluten Free diet (GFD).

Affected System	Affected Organ	ID No.	Manifestation	Type+	Current Medical Information++	Deficient Nutrient
Blood System	Blood component	37	Hypocalcemia [1,20,21,22,23]	(S)	[P] Significantly abnormal serology result in all study patients at diagnosis of CD.[20] [D] Hypocalcemia, or low plasma calcium, is characterized by altered muscle contraction, nerve conduction, hormone release, blood coagulation, and bone health. Study investigating the effect of GFD on mineral and bone metabolism in CD women on GFD and, using the strontium test to assess intestinal calcium absorption, demonstrated mean strontium absorption was markedly decreased and 61% of CD patients had low values. After GFD, all biochemical variables and strontium absorption normalized whereas BMD did not. At diagnosis, the patients frequently had intestinal calcium malabsorption with an early renal compensatory mechanism. After GFD, the normalization of calcium absorption and the decrease of mid-molecule parathyroid hormone suggested a normalization of mineral metabolism.[20] Case report of a 40 year old woman with hypocalcemia and generalized tonic-clonic seizures describes subsequent diagnosis of CD. Hypocalcemia was corrected and convulsions disappeared, but the EEG showed persistent occipital epileptiform activity. Patients with CD and low calcium are particularly at risk for convulsions, therefore even a mild degree of hypocalcemia in these patients should be corrected as soon as possible.[21] Case report of a 36 year old woman with isolated hypocalcemia despite a normal vitamin D status and absence of steatorrhea describes subsequent diagnosis of asymptomatic CD. Patient had hypocalciuria, secondary hyperparathyroidism, and osteopenia that were refractory to pharmacologic calcium and cholecalciferol supplementation. The GFD resulted in correction of all biochemical abnormalities and a substantial increase in BMD. Primary intestinal malabsorption of calcium without concomitant vitamin D deficiency is possible in CD because of the preferential involvement of the proximal small intestine early in the disease process. Discussion: the diagnosis of calcium malabsorption was considered despite the absence of GI symptoms because the serum 25-hydroxyvitamin D level seemed inappropriate for the degree of hypocalcemia, and the PTH and 1 alpha-hydroxylase responses to hypocalcemia appeared intact. Correction was demonstrated after dietary gluten withdrawal.[22] Case report of an elderly woman describes investigation of presenting laryngospasm secondary to severe hypocalcemia and hypomagnesemia in CD. The malabsorption syndrome was responsible for low levels of vitamin D causing the electrolyte imbalance.[23] [M] Marked by muscle spasms, lethargy, insomnia, confusion, hypertension, excessive bleeding, bone pain; mild encephalopathy, paresthesia, tetany (muscle cramps including carpalpedal spasm, irritability, apprehension, nervousness), pre-eclampsia in pregnancy and cataracts (prolonged). If severe, laryngospasm or generalized seizures. May be asymptomatic. [C] Results from calcium malabsorption in CD, with or without vitamin D deficiency, low albumin, hypomagnesemia and idiopathic hypoparathyroidism. [R] CD-related hypocalcemia normalizes on a GFD.[20,22]	Calcium, Protein, Vitamin D.

+ (S) = Classic sign/symptom; (AT) = Atypical sign/symptom; (AD) Associated Disorder; (C) = Complication.

++ [P] = Prevalance; [D] = Description; [M] = Sign/symptom; [C] = CD related cause; [R] = Response to gluten Free diet (GFD).

Affected System	Affected Organ	ID No.	Manifestation	Type+	Current Medical Information ++	Deficient Nutrient
Blood System	Blood component	38	Hypocupremia 24,25	(S)	[P] Increased frequency in untreated CD patients.24 [D] Hypocupremia, or low plasma copper, is characterized by altered blood cell formation, elastin formation, bone formation, and pigmentation of hair and skin. Brain degeneration and failure to make normal blood cells can result in death. Study investigating copper uptake during three hours from an oral test dose of copper sulphate solution giving 3 mg Cu++, close to the recommended daily dietary intake, demonstrated that absorption was significantly reduced in patients with proximal intestinal disease compared to normal subjects. Three out of 10 patients had abnormal, and otherwise unexplained, blood counts compatible with the known hematological effects of copper deficiency and were restored to normal levels on GFD. Copper deficiency and CD should be suspected in patients with otherwise unexplained anemia, especially neutropenia.24 Case report of two unrelated infants aged 7 and 7.5 months presenting with severe malnutrition describes copper deficiency in CD suggested by hypocupremia and persistent neutropenia. Rapid and complete correction of these anomalies could only be obtained after addition of oral copper sulfate to the GFD. Mechanisms possibly involved in the development of copper deficiency in young infants with CD are high copper needs in rapidly growing infants and possibly increased biliary and digestive losses. Young infants with severe CD should be monitored for their copper status.25 [M] Marked by anemia, leukopenia, neutropenia, and bone abnormalities especially demineralization; later, subperiosteal bleeding and loss of pigmentation of hair and skin can occur. Apathy. [C] Results from copper malabsorption in CD and possibly increased biliary losses. [R] CD-related hypocupremia and anemia resolve on a GFD in adults. In infants, rapid and complete correction may require addition of oral copper sulfate to the GFD.25	Copper.
Blood System	Blood component	39	Hypoglycemia 1,2	(S)	[P] Common serology result in untreated CD patients. [D] Unexplained hypoglycemia, or low blood glucose, is characterized by altered nervous system function and tissues that require glucose and cannot metabolize fatty acids including erythrocytes, leukocytes, bone marrow, eye, renal medulla, and peripheral nerves. [M] Marked by any or all of these neurologic symptoms: **Sympathetic nervous system** stimulation including faintness, weakness, tremulousness, palpitation, sweating, hunger, difficult concentration, restlessness, fatigue and nervousness; or **Central nervous system** dysfunction including headache, confusion, visual disturbances, weakness, palsy, ataxia, and marked personality changes such as irritability and violent behavior. [C] Results from limited mucosal surface area for absorption of monosaccharides and maldigestion of disaccharides in CD. [R] CD-related hypoglycemia normalizes on GFD.	Glucose.

+ (S) = Classic sign/symptom; (AT) = Atypical sign/symptom; (AD) Associated Disorder; (C) = Complication.

++ [P] = Prevalance; [D] = Description; [M] = Sign/symptom; [C] = CD related cause; [R] = Response to gluten Free diet (GFD).

Health Manifestations of Celiac Disease (CD)
Section B: Signs, Symptoms, Associated Disorders and Complications

Affected System	Affected Organ	ID No.	Manifestation	Type+	Current Medical Information ++	Deficient Nutrient
Blood System	Blood component	40	Hypokalemia [1,20,26]	(C)	[P] Significantly abnormal serology result in all study patients at diagnosis of CD.[20] [D] Hypokalemia, or low plasma potassium level less than 3.5 mEq/L, is characterized by metabolic acidosis and altered nerve conduction and muscle contraction. Rapid potassium loss can result in hypokalemic rhabdomyolysis.[26] Study investigating the effect of GFD on mineral and bone metabolism in women with CD showed significantly abnormal serology result for potassium in all study patients at diagnosis of CD that normalized on GFD.[20] Case report of a 60 year old man presenting with weakness describes hypokalemic rhabdomyolysis caused by CD. The patient's myopathy responded to potassium supplements and his diarrhea and histological changes resolved while on GFD.[26] [M] Marked by fatigue, excessive thirst, muscle weakness/spasm that may progress to paralysis and respiratory failure, hypotension, anxiety, personality changes, bone pain, dizziness, drowsiness, confusion, depression, anorexia, and if severe, cardiac disturbance (premature ventricular and atrial contractions), myoclonic jerks and seizures. Contributes to osteoporosis. Symptoms vary greatly depending on level of potassium. [C] Results from potassium depletion associated with loss from vomiting, diarrhea and steatorrhea in CD.[26] [R] CD-related hypokalemia normalizes on GFD with resolution of diarrhea. Rhabdomyolysis requires potassium therapy.[26]	Potassium.

+ (S) = Classic sign/symptom; (AT) = Atypical sign/symptom; (AD) Associated Disorder; (C) = Complication.

++ [P] = Prevalance; [D] = Description; [M] = Sign/symptom; [C] = CD related cause; [R] = Response to gluten Free diet (GFD).

Health Manifestations of Celiac Disease (CD)
Section B: Signs, Symptoms, Associated Disorders and Complications

Affected System	Affected Organ	ID No.	Manifestation	Type+	Current Medical Information ++	Deficient Nutrient
Blood System	Blood component	41	Hypomagnesemia 20,23,27,28	(S)	[P] Significantly abnormal serology result in all study patients at diagnosis of CD.[20] Low plasma magnesium often occurs in CD, affecting 100% of patients with classical CD, one-fifth of patients with silent CD, and one-fifth of CD patients on a GFD.[27] [D] Hypomagnesemia, or low plasma magnesium, reflecting severe magnesium depletion of stores, is characterized by impaired parathyroid hormone secretion and action, and altered nerve conduction, muscle contraction, and bone density.[28] Laryngospasm correlates with concomitant hypomagnesemia and severe hypocalcemia.[23] Magnesium deficiency often causes hypokalemia and hypocalcemia. Study investigating the effect of GFD on mineral and bone metabolism in women with CD showed significantly abnormal serology result for magnesium in all study patients at diagnosis of CD that normalized on GFD in 12 months.[20] Study evaluating the magnesium status in CD patients, demonstrated deficiency in all patients with classical CD, 1/5th of patients with silent CD, and 1/5th of those on a GFD.[27] Study investigating magnesium status, bone mass and response to magnesium (Mg) therapy in 23 CD patients who were clinically asymptomatic and on a stable GFD, demonstrated that CD patients have reduction in intracellular free Mg2+, despite being clinically asymptomatic on GFD. Bone mass also appears to be reduced. Mg therapy resulted in a rise in parathyroid hormone (PTH) secretion in these patients. Rise in PTH and significant increase in bone density of the femur and femoral neck in response to magnesium therapy over 2 years suggests that Mg depletion may be one factor contributing to osteoporosis in CD.[28] [M] Marked by anorexia, constipation, nausea, vomiting, fatigue, anxiety, insomnia, irritability, weakness, personality change, confusion, hypertension, and serious neuromuscular disturbances including tetany, ataxia, seizures, myocardial ischemia and cardiac dysrhythmia. Contributes to osteoporosis. [C] Results from magnesium depletion in diarrhea/steatorrhea, if present, and magnesium malabsorption in CD.[28] [R] CD-related hypomagnesemia responds to GFD with supplementation.[28]	Magnesium.

+ (S) = Classic sign/symptom; (AT) = Atypical sign/symptom; (AD) Associated Disorder; (C) = Complication.

++ [P] = Prevalance; [D] = Description; [M] = Sign/symptom; [C] = CD related cause; [R] = Response to gluten Free diet (GFD).

Health Manifestations of Celiac Disease (CD)
Section B: Signs, Symptoms, Associated Disorders and Complications

Affected System	Affected Organ	ID No.	Manifestation	Type+	Current Medical Information ++	Deficient Nutrient
Blood System	Blood component	42	Hypophosphatemia [1,20,29]	(S)	[P] Significantly abnormal result in all study patients at diagnosis of CD.[20] [D] Hypophosphatemia, or low plasma phosphate level, is characterized by altered nerve conduction, muscle contraction, and bone structure. Study investigating the effect of GFD on mineral and bone metabolism in women with CD showed significantly abnormal serology result for phosphorus in all study patients at diagnosis of CD that normalized on GFD after 12 months.[20] Case report of a 45 year old woman with painful proximal muscle weakness and hyperreflexia, describes recognition of an increased serum alkaline phosphatase and hypophosphatemia leading to diagnosis of osteomalacia. Identification of iron deficiency anemia and hypocholesteremia implicated previously unrecognized CD with associated vitamin D malabsorption as the cause of the osteomalacia.[29] [M] Marked by anorexia, weight loss, thigh weakness and pain; osteomalacia and serious neuromuscular disturbances may develop, including dysarthria, paresthesia and confusion advances to stupor, seizure and coma. Low milk production in lactating women. [C] Results from phosphorus malabsorption in CD and depletion in vomiting and diarrhea. [R] CD-related hypophosphatemia responds to GFD. Pain resolved and strength improved in reported patient within three months.[29]	Phosphorus.
Blood System	Blood component	43	Macroamylasemia [1,30,31]	(S)	[P] Occurs in approximately 0.4% of general population and 16.9% in CD patients.[30] [D] Macroamylasemia is characterized by altered amylase bound with serum proteins, commonly IgG and/or IgA. Resulting molecule is too large to be filtered by the kidneys and excreted in the urine, causing sustained elevation of amylase levels in the plasma. May present simultaneously with elevated lipase.[30] Reported with recurrent miscarriages and multiple immune disorders,[30] also in Down syndrome with multiple autoimmune abnormalities.[31] Case report of a 34 year old woman describes unrecognized CD and multiple extraintestinal manifestations including recurrent miscarriage, hyperamylasemia and hyperlipasemia of unknown origin, IgA nephropathy, and thyroiditis that disappeared or improved when a correct diagnosis was made and the patient was given a GFD.[30] Case report of a 40 year old patient with Down syndrome with multiple autoimmune abnormalities for 15 years describes macroamylasemia, IgA hypergammaglobulinemia and subsequent diagnosis of CD. Follow-up on GFD showed a transitory decrease in seric immunoglobulin A and macroamylase with persistent autoantibodies and AST elevation.[31] [M] Marked by accumulation of macroamylase complex in the plasma.[30] [C] Results from elevated IgG and/or IgA antibody levels.[30] [R] Macroamylase response varies on GFD.[30]	Not applicable.

+ (S) = Classic sign/symptom; (AT) = Atypical sign/symptom; (AD) Associated Disorder; (C) = Complication.

++ [P] = Prevalance; [D] = Description; [M] = Sign/symptom; [C] = CD related cause; [R] = Response to gluten Free diet (GFD).

Health Manifestations of Celiac Disease (CD)
Section B: Signs, Symptoms, Associated Disorders and Complications

Affected System	Affected Organ	ID No.	Manifestation	Type[+]	Current Medical Information [++]	Deficient Nutrient
Blood System	Blood component	44	Macrocytosis [1,32]	(S)	[P] Common serology result in untreated CD patients. [D] Macrocytosis is characterized by altered blood cell formation resulting in abnormally large erythrocytes (red blood cells). Initial evaluation should include a carefully taken history and physical examination along with a complete hematologic profile, reticulocyte count, and peripheral blood smear. Serum B_{12} and red cell folate determinations and other studies may then be undertaken as appropriate.[32] [M] Marked by anemia. [C] Results from folic acid and/or vitamin B_{12} deficiencies induced by CD. [R] Macrocytosis responds to GFD.	Folic acid, Vitamin B_{12}.
Blood System	Blood component	45	Macrolipasemia [1,30,33]	(S)	[P] 5.9% of patients with macroamylasemia have macrolipasemia. CD found in more than 50% of patients with both macroamylase and macrolipase present.[30] [D] Macrolipasemia is characterized by altered plasma lipase. Lipase bound with polyclonal IgA, forming a molecule too large to be filtered by the kidneys, causes sustained elevation of lipase levels and occurs with or without macroamylasemia.[30] Case report of a patient showing persistently elevated levels of greater than normal molecular weight serum amylase and lipase enzymes. The assay showed amylase was bound to polyclonal IgG and IgA, whereas lipase was bound to polyclonal IgA. If macroamylasemia and macrolipasemia are present, the possibility of CD should be considered.[33] [M] Marked by accumulation of macrolipase complex in the plasma.[30] [C] Results from elevated IgA antibody levels in CD.[30] [R] Macrolipasemia may not resolve on GFD.[30]	Not applicable.

[+] (S) = Classic sign/symptom; (AT) = Atypical sign/symptom; (AD) Associated Disorder; (C) = Complication.

[++] [P] = Prevalance; [D] = Description; [M] = Sign/symptom; [C] = CD related cause; [R] = Response to gluten Free diet (GFD).

Health Manifestations of Celiac Disease (CD)
Section B: Signs, Symptoms, Associated Disorders and Complications

Affected System	Affected Organ	ID No.	Manifestation	Type+	Current Medical Information ++	Deficient Nutrient
Blood System	Blood component	46	Plasma Proteins, Low [1,2,10,34,35,36]	(S)	[P] Common serology result in patients with untreated CD.[2] [D] Low plasma protein levels are symptomatic of malabsorption characterized by altered albumin, transferrin, transthyretin, and retinol-binding protein levels. Low albumin levels (>35g/dl) with half-life of 3 weeks affect maintenance of osmotic pressure in blood vessels and performance as a carrier for many substances in the blood.[34] Low albumin has a high predictive value for the identification of patients with intestinal damage and low predictive value as a marker of absent intestinal damage.[35] Study defining the correlates of CD in 100 anemic adults without overt malabsorption demonstrated that patients with hypochromic anemia had significant albumin difference (-9.4%) compared to CD patients without anemia.[10] Anthropometric, biochemical, and bone densitometric assessment performed in 23 celiac children aged 1 to 12 years at diagnosis and one year after GFD demonstrated that a year of GFD allows virtually complete return in body mass composition. At diagnosis, the patients had height, arm muscle triceps, skin folds, subscapular skin folds, fat area index, and bone mineral content significantly lower than controls. Serum proteins and albumin values rose significantly during the year of GFD.[36] [M] Marked by anxiety, apathy, hunger, increased infection, loss of vitality, fluid retention and malnutrition including muscle/ subcutaneous fat wasting, weight loss, weakness, poor muscle tone, fatigue, infertility and dermatitis.[34] [C] Results from protein maldigestion and malabsorption in CD. [R] CD-related low plasma protein levels quickly respond to a strict GFD. Their levels depend on continued dietary compliance.[35]	Protein.

+ (S) = Classic sign/symptom; (AT) = Atypical sign/symptom; (AD) Associated Disorder; (C) = Complication.
++ [P] = Prevalance; [D] = Description; [M] = Sign/symptom; [C] = CD related cause; [R] = Response to gluten Free diet (GFD).

Health Manifestations of Celiac Disease (CD)
Section B: Signs, Symptoms, Associated Disorders and Complications

Affected System	Affected Organ	ID No.	Manifestation	Type+	Current Medical Information ++	Deficient Nutrient
Blood System	Blood component	47	Prolonged Prothrombin Time [12]	(AT)	[P] 20% prevalence in untreated CD.[12] [D] Prolonged prothrombin time (PT) out of proportion to the partial thromboplastin time (PTT) is significantly related to all the markers of severe malabsorption, including low bone mineral density.[12] Study evaluating the prevalence and associations of prolonged PT in celiac adults demonstrated that vitamin K proteins may play a role in determining or worsening calcium homeostasis disorders in CD. Patients with prolonged PT had lower values of hemoglobin, iron, proteins, cholesterol, and serum aspartate transaminase and significantly higher proportion of diarrhea, weight loss, abdominal pain, and low bone mineral density than controls.[12] [M] Marked by excessive bleeding. [C] Results from vitamin K depletion induced by CD. [R] CD-related prolonged PT resolves on GFD. Some patients require parenteral vitamin K therapy.[12]	Omega-3 fatty acids, Vitamin K.
Blood System	Blood component	48	Zincemia [1,34,36,37,38]	(S)	[P] Common serology result in patients with untreated CD. Present in more than 50% of untreated children with CD.[36] [D] Low plasma zinc is a symptom of malabsorption characterized by altered immunity and defense against infection, reproduction, normal growth, and fetal organogenesis. Severe deficiency causes immunologic disorders.[34] Zinc deficiency might play an important role in the pathogenesis of CD in that it might aggravate the induced disease by allowing calcium to activate intestinal transglutaminase.[37] This opens up a possibility for treating and even preventing CD.[37] Anthropometric, biochemical, and bone densitometric assessment performed in 23 celiac children aged 1 to 12 years at diagnosis and one year after GFD demonstrated that a year of GFD allows virtually complete return in body mass composition. At diagnosis, the patients had height, arm muscle triceps, skin folds, subscapular skin folds, fat area index, and bone mineral content significantly lower than controls. Serum zinc values rose significantly during the year of GFD.[36] [M] Marked by delayed wound healing, increased susceptibility to infections, increased recuperation time, diarrhea, distorted taste and smell, low energy, nervousness, photophobia, anorexia, fatigue, male infertility. Zinc deficiency syndrome in pregnancy includes increased maternal disorders, abortions, abnormal taste sensations, abnormally short or prolonged gestations, inefficient labor, atonic bleeding and increased risk to fetus such as malformations, growth retardation, prematurity and perinatal death.[21 Section A] In children/youth, anemia, hypogonadism, and short stature may develop.[38] [C] Results from zinc depletion and zinc malabsorption in CD. [R] CD-related zincemia usually resolves on GFD, rising significantly in one year to within the normal range for children.[36]	Zinc.

+ (S) = Classic sign/symptom; (AT) = Atypical sign/symptom; (AD) Associated Disorder; (C) = Complication.

++ [P] = Prevalance; [D] = Description; [M] = Sign/symptom; [C] = CD related cause; [R] = Response to gluten Free diet (GFD).

Health Manifestations of Celiac Disease (CD)
Section B: Signs, Symptoms, Associated Disorders and Complications

Affected System	Affected Organ	ID No.	Manifestation	Type[+]	Current Medical Information [++]	Deficient Nutrient
Blood System	Blood plasma and cells	49	Anemia, Folic Acid Deficiency [1,3,5,39]	(S)	[P] Common and a classic presentation of CD.[3] [D] Folic acid deficiency anemia, a megaloblastic anemia, is characterized by defective DNA synthesis of red blood cells. Red blood cell (RBC) folate and/or serum folate levels are decreased and normal plasma methylmalonic acid level with elevated homocysteine level distinguish folic acid deficiency anemia from vitamin B_{12} deficiency anemia.[39] CD should be considered in folate deficiency.[3] Study measuring IgG and IgA isotypes and IgG subclasses demonstrated significantly lower serum folic acid concentrations in patients with positive IgA gliadin antibodies than healthy controls.[5] [M] Marked by weakness, diarrhea, thrombocytopenia, intracranial hypertension and tissue hypoxia including fatigue, headache, lightheadedness, angina, dyspnea, pallor, and tachycardia. Depression and polyneuropathy appear later. Leads to atherosclerosis and infertility in both sexes. [C] Results from folic acid malabsorption in CD.[3] [R] Folic acid deficiency anemia responds to GFD and folic acid supplementation.	Folic Acid.

[+] (S) = Classic sign/symptom; (AT) = Atypical sign/symptom; (AD) Associated Disorder; (C) = Complication.

[++] [P] = Prevalance; [D] = Description; [M] = Sign/symptom; [C] = CD related cause; [R] = Response to gluten Free diet (GFD).

Health Manifestations of Celiac Disease (CD)
Section B: Signs, Symptoms, Associated Disorders and Complications

Affected System	Affected Organ	ID No.	Manifestation	Type[+]	Current Medical Information [++]	Deficient Nutrient
Blood System	Blood plasma and cells	50	Anemia, Iron Deficiency [1,2,3,5,40,41]	(S)	[P] Common and classic presentation of CD.[3] Prevalence of CD in patients with iron deficiency anemia is 2.8%.[40] [D] Iron deficiency anemia (IDA), a microcytic anemia, is characterized by abnormal formation of small, pale red blood cells and iron depletion refractory to oral iron supplementation. Screening for CD recommended in patients with unexplained iron-deficiency anemia.[40] Study investigating the prevalence of CD in patients with IDA supports a referral for endoscopy to exclude CD.[40] Study measuring anti-gliadin antibody IgG and IgA isotypes and IgG subclasses demonstrated significantly decreased transferrin saturation, mean corpuscular volume, and mean corpuscular hemoglobin in patients with positive IgA gliadin antibodies vs. controls.[5] Study evaluating the effect of iron supplementation, in addition to the GFD, on hematological profile of children with CD demonstrated that IDA is commonly associated with CD and the iron deficiency state continues a long time even with iron supplementation.[41] Study defining the correlates of CD in 100 anemic adults without overt malabsorption demonstrated that among patients with hypochromic anemia, plasma cholesterol in the high-to-normal range could be used to exclude the presence of CD. Compared to anemic patients without CD, anemic patients with CD had significant or borderline significant differences for plasma cholesterol, albumin, and body mass index but not for blood hemoglobin, mean corpuscular volume, plasma iron, and ferritin. All anemic CD patients had plasma cholesterol less than 156mg/100ml.[10] [M] Marked by tissue hypoxia including fatigue, headache, lightheadedness, angina, and dyspnea, pallor, tachycardia, and visual impairment, susceptibility to infection, anorexia, anxiety, apathy, loss of vitality, inability to pay attention, reduced memory/learning, sensory motor incompetence, alopecia, infertility, possible difficulty swallowing and koilonychia. [C] Results from iron malabsorption in CD. [R] CD-related iron deficiency anemia responds to GFD rich in iron.[41]	Iron.

[+] (S) = Classic sign/symptom; (AT) = Atypical sign/symptom; (AD) Associated Disorder; (C) = Complication.

[++] [P] = Prevalance; [D] = Description; [M] = Sign/symptom; [C] = CD related cause; [R] = Response to gluten Free diet (GFD).

Health Manifestations of Celiac Disease (CD)
Section B: Signs, Symptoms, Associated Disorders and Complications

Affected System	Affected Organ	ID No.	Manifestation	Type[+]	Current Medical Information [++]	Deficient Nutrient
Blood System	Blood plasma and cells	51	Anemia, Vitamin B_{12} Deficiency [1,2,3,39]	(S)	[P] Common and a classic presentation in patients with untreated CD.[3] [D] Vitamin B_{12} deficiency anemia, a megaloblastic anemia, is characterized by defective DNA synthesis of red blood cells. Decreased serum vitamin B_{12} level and elevated plasma methyl-malonic acid level with elevated homocysteine level distinguish vitamin B^{12} deficiency anemia from folic acid deficiency anemia.[39] CD should be considered in vitamin B_{12} deficiency.[3] [M] Marked by weakness, sore tongue, dysgeusia, paresthesias (numbness/burning feeling of limbs), intermittent diarrhea and constipation, nausea, and hypoxia (including fatigue, headache, light-headedness, dyspnea, pallor, tachycardia, and lemon yellow tint to skin), confusion, impaired thinking, considerable weight loss. Leads to atherosclerosis. Late symptoms include spasticity, ataxia and psychiatric symptoms such as hallucinations. [C] Results from vitamin B_{12} deficiency state induced by CD. [R] CD-related vitamin B_{12} deficiency anemia responds to GFD.	Vitamin B_{12}.
Blood System	Blood plasma and cells	52	Hemochromatosis [1,42]	(AD)	[P] Rare association with CD.[42] [D] Hemochromatosis, a common autosomal recessive disease in the Caucasian population, is characterized by increased iron deposition within the tissues associated with injury. CD and hereditary hemochromatosis are genetic disorders paradoxically associated with altered intestinal absorption of iron. Clinical presentation is modified by co-existence of hemochromatosis and CD.[42] [M] Marked by gray or bronzed skin, weakness, fatigue, cirrhosis, thyroid disorder, cardiovascular complications, arthritis, and hypogonadism. [C] Results from potential genetic linkage.[42] [R] Studies are insufficient to determine effect of GFD.	Not applicable.

[+] (S) = Classic sign/symptom; (AT) = Atypical sign/symptom; (AD) Associated Disorder; (C) = Complication.

[++] [P] = Prevalance; [D] = Description; [M] = Sign/symptom; [C] = CD related cause; [R] = Response to gluten Free diet (GFD).

Affected System	Affected Organ	ID No.	Manifestation	Type[+]	Current Medical Information [++]	Deficient Nutrient
Blood System	Blood plasma and cells	53	Hypo-prothrombinemia [1,43]	(AT)	[P] New association with CD.[43] [D] Hypoprothrombinemia, or low prothrombin level, is an immunologically mediated disorder characterized by altered hemostasis, or ability to stop bleeding. Circulating anticoagulant antibodies interfere with the function of procoagulant phospholipid and non-neutralizing antibodies bind prothrombin. The prothrombin anti-prothrombin complex is rapidly cleared from the blood, preventing formation of thrombin that is essential to clotting. Case report describes a patient with lupus anticoagulant hypoprothrombinemia syndrome and CD. Presence of a neutralizing antiprothrombin antibody was demonstrated by coagulation tests, immunoadsorption, and Western blot analysis. The probable cause for the severe hypoprothrombinemia was clearance of prothrombin-antibody complexes from the circulation. Studies showed the antiprothrombin antibody binding to human prothrombin was phospholipid- and Ca(++)-independent; the antibody did not bind to human thrombin. The proposed mechanism for the neutralizing action of the antibody is impairment of prothrombin activation by the prothrombinase complex, either by steric hindrance of the hydrolysis of prothrombin by factor Xa or by interference of the interaction of prothrombin with factor Va; both reactions are required for efficient conversion of prothrombin to thrombin.[43] [M] Marked by petecchiae, ecchymosis, and risk for hemorrhage and purpura. [C] Results from unclear etiology involving autoimmune mechanism. [R] CD-related hypoprothrombinemia responds to GFD.	Not applicable.

Blood System	Blood plasma and cells	54	Idiopathic Thrombocytopenic Purpura [1,44,45]	(AD)	[P] Uncommon immunological association with CD.
					[D] Idiopathic thrombocytopenia purpura is an immunologically mediated hemorrhagic disorder characterized by destruction of circulating platelets by autoantibodies. Antibodies bind to platelet surface antigens, resulting in their clearance by the reticuloendothelial system.
					    Case report of a patient with inclusion body myositis associated with CD and idiopathic thrombocytopenic purpura purports presence of all three disorders may share an interrelated immune mechanism with CD.[44]
					    Case report of a patient with CD in whom idiopathic thrombocytopenic purpura and associated granulomatous disease developed. The three processes appear linked through autoimmune mechanisms.[45]
					[M] Marked by bleeding from the nose, gums, or digestive tract, petechiae and purpura.[45] See above.
					[C] Results from autoimmune mechanism.[45]
					[R] Spontaneous remission occurs in many patients with or without GFD.
						Not applicable.

[+] (S) = Classic sign/symptom; (AT) = Atypical sign/symptom; (AD) Associated Disorder; (C) = Complication.

[++] [P] = Prevalance; [D] = Description; [M] = Sign/symptom; [C] = CD related cause; [R] = Response to gluten Free diet (GFD).

Health Manifestations of Celiac Disease (CD)
Section B: Signs, Symptoms, Associated Disorders and Complications

Affected System	Affected Organ	ID No.	Manifestation	Type[+]	Current Medical Information [++]	Deficient Nutrient
Blood System	Blood plasma and cells	55	Neutropenia, Granulocytic Hypersegmentation [24,46]	(AD)	[P] Increased frequency in untreated CD. [D] Neutropenia, granulocytic hypersegmentation is a blood disorder characterized by presence of an abnormally low number of neutrophils. Copper deficiency and proximal intestinal disease should be suspected in patients with otherwise unexplained anemias, especially neutropenia.[24] Case report describes hematological abnormalities in a 7 year old child with 2 month history of profound weakness which resolved in 3 weeks on GFD with intravenous supplementation of folic acid. Anemia, marked neutropenia, and hypersegmentation of the granulocytes were due to significant folate deficiency caused by active CD.[46] [M] Marked by profound weakness and predisposition to infection. [C] Results from significant copper and folate deficiencies due to malabsorption in CD. [R] Resolves on GFD with supplementation of folic acid.[46]	Copper. Folic acid.
Blood System	Blood plasma and cells	56	Transient Erythroblastopenia [1,47]	(AD)	[P] Immunological association may be less rare than commonly thought.[47] [D] Transient erythroblastopenia is a disorder of red blood cell formation characterized by brief, reversible disappearance of red blood cell precursors in the bone marrow. [M] Marked by waxy pallor of skin and mucous membranes advancing to severe thrombocytopenia with bleeding into the skin, mucous membranes and white of eye, and life-threatening infections. [C] Results from autoimmune mechanism.[47] [R] Transient erythroblastopenia resolves on GFD.	Not applicable.
Cardiovascular System	Blood vessels	57	Aortic Vasculitis causing Midaortic Syndrome [48]	(C)	[P] New association in untreated CD.[48] [D] Midaortic syndrome is a variety of aortic coarctation, located in the distal thoracic aorta, the abdominal aorta or both, involving the intestinal and renal vessels, usually presenting with renovascular arterial hypertension.[48] Deposition of antigen-antibody immune complexes is involved in CD. Case report describes the case of a young woman who presented with claudication of the lower limbs, therapy-refractory arterial hypertension, and untreated CD. Midaortic syndrome was characterized by severe stenosis of the infrarenal aorta, of both renal arteries and of the inferior mesenteric artery. The underlying condition was assumed to be local vasculitis due to the chronic inflammation of untreated CD. Percutaneous transluminal angioplasty together with implantation of two stents into the infrarenal aorta and the right renal artery was performed and dietary intervention with GFD was started.[48] [M] Marked by arterial hypertension and cramping or pain in leg muscles on walking and relieved by rest. [C] Results from immune mediated vascular inflammation with scarring. [R] GFD resulted in control of vasculitis.[48]	Not applicable.

[+] (S) = Classic sign/symptom; (AT) = Atypical sign/symptom; (AD) Associated Disorder; (C) = Complication.

[++] [P] = Prevalance; [D] = Description; [M] = Sign/symptom; [C] = CD related cause; [R] = Response to gluten Free diet (GFD).

Health Manifestations of Celiac Disease (CD)
Section B: Signs, Symptoms, Associated Disorders and Complications

Affected System	Affected Organ	ID No.	Manifestation	Type[+]	Current Medical Information [++]	Deficient Nutrient
Cardiovascular System	Blood vessels	58	Atherosclerosis [15,34, 39,49]	(C)	[P] Increased prevalence in CD. [D] Atherosclerosis is a disease of medium and large arteries characterized by patchy subintimal thickening, hardening, and loss of elasticity of blood vessels which can reduce or obstruct blood flow. Hypotheses postulate 1) epithelial dysfunction, and 2) lipid accumulation in smooth muscle cells and in foam cells, causing buildup of fatty deposits on the inside walls progressing to fibrous plaque formation - intimal smooth muscle cells surrounded by connective tissue and intracellular and extracellular lipids.[39] 1. Epithelial dysfunction results from elevated homocysteine levels. Homocysteine, an amino acid, briefly formed in the breakdown of the amino acid methionine, is normally converted to cystathione and then to cysteine by means of a vitamin B_6 dependent enzyme. In the reverse, conversion of homocysteine to methionine requires an enzyme dependent on adequate folic acid and vitamin B_{12} levels. Insufficient methionine levels and/or inefficiency in this process results in elevated homocysteine plasma levels that are toxic to blood vessels. Folic acid, pyridoxine, and vitamin B_{12} are involved in the metabolic removal of homocysteine, but folic acid deficit occurs the most often.[15] 2. Lipid accumulation in smooth muscle cells results from elevated plasma triglyceride levels and elevated plasma LDL, the latter being rendered more atherogenic by oxidation. Insufficient antioxident molecules are involved. Omega-3 fatty acids, a component of lipoproteins and a precursor of leukotrienes and series 3 prostaglandins, exert a specific preventive effect against atherosclerosis. Their action lowers tiglycerides by inhibiting VLDL (the main source of LDL), and apolipoprotein B-100 synthesis and by decreasing post prandial lipemia (fat level in blood after eating).[34] Study investigating the role of oxidative stress in CD demonstrated that the level of markers of oxidative stress derived for both protein (carbonyl groups) and lipids (thiobarbituric acid-reactive substances) were significantly higher in asymptomatic CD patients, whereas lipoproteins and alphatocopherol (vitamin E) were significantly lower. These data indicate that in CD even when asymptomatic, a redox imbalance persists; this is probably caused by an absorption deficiency, even if slight. Dietary supplementation with antioxident molecules may offer some benefit and deserves further investigation.[49] [M] Marked by gradual development including hypertension, claudication, and angina on exertion. Acute occlusion of major vessel may be dramatic.[39] [C] Results from hyperhomocysteinemia (deficiencies of co-factors folic acid, vitamin B_{12} and pyridoxine); oxidized LDL cholesterol (deficiency of antioxidants); and elevated triglyceride levels (deficiency of omega-3 fatty acids in CD). [R] Insufficient studies. GFD containing deficient nutrients may resolve nutritional causes of atherosclerosis with normalization of homocysteine, LDL and triglyceride levels.	Folic acid, Omega-3 fatty acids, Selenium, Vitamin B_6, Vitamin B_{12}, Vitamin E.[49]

+ (S) = Classic sign/symptom; (AT) = Atypical sign/symptom; (AD) Associated Disorder; (C) = Complication.

++ [P] = Prevalance; [D] = Description; [M] = Sign/symptom; [C] = CD related cause; [R] = Response to gluten Free diet (GFD).

Health Manifestations of Celiac Disease (CD)
Section B: Signs, Symptoms, Associated Disorders and Complications

Affected System	Affected Organ	ID No.	Manifestation	Type[+]	Current Medical Information [++]	Deficient Nutrient
Cardiovascular System	Blood vessels	59	Ecchymosis/Easy Bruising [2,50]	(S)	[P] Common in people with untreated CD. [2,50] [D] Ecchymosis, or easy bruising, is a feature of secondary hemostasis characterized by superficial subcutaneous bleeding in response to light trauma. Case report of 47 year old man without previously known illness having acute hematomas and swellings on both legs reveals that CD can take a clinically unremarkable course for a long time and may finally become manifest through an isolated abnormality, such as bleeding. Hemoglobin was 5.6g/dl while iron was normal and ferritin reduced. Quick value was below 5% and activated partial thromboplastin time prolonged to 180s. Vitamin A and E concentrations were not demonstrated in the blood of this patient. Four units of erythrocyte concentrate were immediately administered, together with 2000 IU factors II, VII, X, and antihemophilic factor B, and 10mg vitamin K intravenously. [50] [M] Marked by unsightly dark bluish swellings, affecting subcutaneous tissue and occasionally mucosal tissue. [C] Results from vitamin K deficiency induced by CD. [R] CD-related ecchymosis quickly resolves on GFD. [50]	Vitamin K.
Cardiovascular System	Blood vessels	60	Epistaxis, Unexplained [12,34]	(AT)	[P] Common in people with untreated CD. [12] [D] Unexplained epistaxis, or nosebleed, is a feature of secondary hemostasis characterized by fragility of a plexus of vessels in the anteroinferior septum and/or abnormal blood coagulation. [M] Marked by bright red nasal bleeding. [C] Results from nutritional deficiencies induced by CD. [R] Occurrence of CD-related epistaxis resolves on GFD.	Iron, Vitamin C, Vitamin K. [34]

[+] (S) = Classic sign/symptom; (AT) = Atypical sign/symptom; (AD) Associated Disorder; (C) = Complication.

[++] [P] = Prevalance; [D] = Description; [M] = Sign/symptom; [C] = CD related cause; [R] = Response to gluten Free diet (GFD).

Health Manifestations of Celiac Disease (CD)
Section B: Signs, Symptoms, Associated Disorders and Complications

Affected System	Affected Organ	ID No.	Manifestation	Type+	Current Medical Information ++	Deficient Nutrient
Cardiovascular System	Blood vessels	61	Reversible Hypertension [16]	(AD)	[P] New association with CD.[16] [D] Reversible hypertension is an arterial pressure disorder characterized by endothelial dysfunction of vessel walls due to hyperhomocysteinemia causing increased systemic vascular resistance. The vascular endothelium normally maintains a relatively vasodilated state via release of nitric oxide, a process that could be disrupted by hyperhomocysteinemia. Irrespective of etiology, endothelial dysfunction may be the precursor of hypertension. Case report of a patient with unresponsive hypertension describes diagnosis of subclinical CD. Subsequently, homocysteine level normalized with restoration of endothelial function after 15 months of GFD with vitamin B_{12} injection, folic acid and oral iron supplements. Conclusion is that co-existing vascular risk factors should be resolved in patients with hypertension.[16] [M] Marked by sustained, elevated blood pressure. [C] Results from impaired absorption of essential cofactors for normal homocysteine metabolism in CD.[16] [R] CD-related hypertension is reversible on GFD.[16]	Folic acid, Omega-3 fatty acids, Vitamin B_6, Vitamin B_{12}.
Cardiovascular System	Heart	62	Angina Pectoris [1,51,52]	(AD)	[P] New association with CD.[51] [D] Angina pectoris is a coronary syndrome characterized by an oppressive substernal pain or pressure precipitated by exertion and relieved by rest. Oxidized low-density lipoprotein (oxLDL) and oxysterols play an important role in atherogenesis leading to narrowing of arteries that results in angina. Study investigating the relevance of oxysterols and autoantibodies against oxLDL to coronary artery disease in 183 patients undergoing coronary angiography demonstrated oxLDL is immunogenic, and autoantibodies against oxLDL are detectable in serum. Antibodies, but not oxysterol concentrations, were significantly greater in subjects with unstable angina than with stable angina (P<0.01). Concluded that antioxLDL antibody and oxysterol concentrations are associated with coronary artery stenosis, and oxidative stress may be greatly increased in unstable angina.[52] [M] Marked by pain or pressure in the chest which may radiate down the arm or into the jaw, shoulders or neck and may be accompanied by shortness of breath, nausea or vomiting, sweating, anxiety or fear. [C] Results from inadequate blood flow and oxygenation due to atherosclerosis caused by nutritional deficiencies in CD. [R] Occurrence of CD-related angina pectoris responds to GFD.[51]	Folic acid, Omega-3 fatty acids, Selenium, Vitamin B_{12}, Vitamin B_6, Vitamin E.

+ (S) = Classic sign/symptom; (AT) = Atypical sign/symptom; (AD) Associated Disorder; (C) = Complication.

++ [P] = Prevalance; [D] = Description; [M] = Sign/symptom; [C] = CD related cause; [R] = Response to gluten Free diet (GFD).

Health Manifestations of Celiac Disease (CD)
Section B: Signs, Symptoms, Associated Disorders and Complications

Affected System	Affected Organ	ID No.	Manifestation	Type+	Current Medical Information ++	Deficient Nutrient
Cardiovascular System	Heart	63	Cardiomegaly [34]	(AD)	[P] Increased frequency in people with untreated CD. [D] Cardiomegaly is a noninflammatory disorder of the myocardium seen in cardiovascular (wet) beriberi characterized by secondary fatty changes, degeneration, and swelling of the muscle fibers. [M] Marked by vasodilation and warm extremities, tachycardia, and lactic acidosis. Orthopnea, and pulmonary and peripheral edema develop with heart failure. [C] Results from thiamin (vitamin B_1) deficiency.[34] [R] CD-related cardiomegaly responds to GFD.	Vitamin B_1.
Cardiovascular System	Heart	64	Cardiomyopathy, Idiopathic Dilated [1,53,54]	(AD)	[P] CD found in 5.7% patients with idiopathic dilated cardiomyopathy (ICDM).[53] ICDM affects untreated CD patients and those who do not strictly follow GFD.[54] [D] Idiopathic dilated cardiomyopathy is a disorder of myocardial function characterized by dilation of the cardiac chambers and reduction in ventricular contractile function often resulting in symptomatic heart failure. Case report describes 3 patients with ICDM and CD who underwent clinical and laboratory evaluation to establish the effect of a GFD on cardiac performance. Preliminary data suggests that the GFD may have a beneficial effect on cardiac performance in patients with ICDM. Two patients who observed the GFD regimen very strictly, after a 28 month follow-up period, showed an improvement in echocardiographic parameters as well as of cardiological features and quality of life. The third patient did not observe the GFD and presented a worsening in the echocardiographic parameters and cardiological symptoms which required supplementary drug therapy.[54] [M] Marked by weakness, dyspnea, tachycardia, and edema. [C] Results from unclear etiology involving gluten exposure in CD. [R] CD-related ICDM responds to a strict GFD.[54]	Not known.

+ (S) = Classic sign/symptom; (AT) = Atypical sign/symptom; (AD) Associated Disorder; (C) = Complication.

++ [P] = Prevalance; [D] = Description; [M] = Sign/symptom; [C] = CD related cause; [R] = Response to gluten Free diet (GFD).

Health Manifestations of Celiac Disease (CD)
Section B: Signs, Symptoms, Associated Disorders and Complications

Affected System	Affected Organ	ID No.	Manifestation	Type[+]	Current Medical Information [++]	Deficient Nutrient
Cardiovascular System	Heart	65	Coronary Artery Disease [14,49,52]	(AD)	[P] Increased frequency of coronary artery disease (CAD) in people with CD. [D] Coronary artery disease is a disease of medium and large arteries involving 1) epithelial dysfunction and 2) lipid accumulation in smooth muscle cells and in foam cells causing buildup of fatty deposits on the inside walls progressing to fibrous plaque formation. Oxidized low-density lipoprotein (oxLDL) and oxysterols play important roles in atherogenesis. OxLDL is immunogenic, and autoantibodies against oxLDL are detectable in serum. Anti-oxLDL antibody and oxysterol concentrations are associated with coronary artery stenosis, and oxidative stress may be greatly increased in unstable angina.[52] Study investigating the role of oxidative stress in CD demonstrated the level of markers of oxidative stress derived for both protein (carbonyl groups) and lipids(thiobarbituric acid-reactive substances) were significantly higher in CD patients, whereas lipoproteins and alpha-tocopherol (vitamin E) were significantly lower. These data indicate that in CD even when asymptomatic, a redox imbalance persists; this is probably caused by an absorption deficiency.[49] Study assessing the vitamin nutrition status of a series of celiac patients living on a gluten-free diet for 10 years demonstrated that they had a higher total plasma homocysteine level than the general population, indicative of a poor vitamin status. Results suggest that, when following up adults with CD, the vitamin status should be reviewed.[14] [M] Marked by insidious interference with blood flow resulting in angina and thrombosis. [C] Results from atherosclerosis due to nutritional deficiencies including folic acid, vitamin B[12], pyridoxine, selenium, vitamin E and omega-3 fatty acids in CD. [R] GFD resolves the causes of atherosclerosis as risk factor for CD-related CAD.[49]	Folic acid, Omega-3 fatty acids, Selenium, Vitamin B[6], Vitamin B[12], Vitamin E.

+ (S) = Classic sign/symptom; (AT) = Atypical sign/symptom; (AD) Associated Disorder; (C) = Complication.

++ [P] = Prevalance; [D] = Description; [M] = Sign/symptom; [C] = CD related cause; [R] = Response to gluten Free diet (GFD).

Health Manifestations of Celiac Disease (CD)
Section B: Signs, Symptoms, Associated Disorders and Complications

Affected System	Affected Organ	ID No.	Manifestation	Type+	Current Medical Information ++	Deficient Nutrient
Body Composition	Adipose	66	Obesity [2,3,34]	(AT) (C)	[P] Newly recognized presentation of CD.[2] [D] Obesity, a metabolic disorder complicating CD,[3] is characterized by body mass index greater than 30%. Faulty regulation of body weight and concomitant abnormal appetite are recognized features possibly involving nutritional deficiencies in CD. Unsatisfied need for nutrients results in unsatisfied hunger which stimulates appetite. An unexpected source of energy may result from excessive short-chain fatty acid manufacture in the bowel from maldigested macronutrients and their absorption. Restricted energy expenditure is a part of obesity that can be further induced by many of the effects of nutritional deficiencies including low energy, apathy, depression, weakness, pain, impaired metablism and endocrine factors. The GFD commonly results in weight loss of 5 to 8 pounds in the obese patient within the first week. Further weight loss varies and involves weight management strategies involving diet and exercise education. [M] Marked by abnormally large accumulations of body fat. Hunger. [C] Results from unclear etiology in CD possibly involving nutrient deficiencies. [R] CD-related obesity responds to nutritious, balanced GFD.	Calcium, Omega-3 fatty acids, Omega-6 fatty acids, Protein, Vitamin C.[34]
Body Composition	Adipose	67	Weight Gain, Unexplained [2,34]	(AT)	[P] Newly recognized presentation of CD.[2] [D] Unexplained weight gain is a sign of malabsorption characterized by increasing body mass. Unsatisfied need for nutrients results in unsatisfied hunger which stimulates appetite. The GFD commonly results in weight loss of about 5 pounds in the overweight patient within the first week. Further weight loss varies and involves weight management strategies involving diet and exercise education. [M] Marked by increasing fat accumulation. Hunger. [C] Results from unclear etiology in CD, possibly involving nutritional deficiencies. [R] CD-related weight gain responds to a nutritious, balanced GFD.	Calcium, Omega-3 fatty acids, Omega-6 fatty acids, Protein, Minerals, Vitamin C.[34]

+ (S) = Classic sign/symptom; (AT) = Atypical sign/symptom; (AD) Associated Disorder; (C) = Complication.

++ [P] = Prevalance; [D] = Description; [M] = Sign/symptom; [C] = CD related cause; [R] = Response to gluten Free diet (GFD).

Health Manifestations of Celiac Disease (CD)
Section B: Signs, Symptoms, Associated Disorders and Complications

Affected System	Affected Organ	ID No.	Manifestation	Type[+]	Current Medical Information [++]	Deficient Nutrient
Body Composition	All	68	Cachexia [1,10,34,36,55]	(S)	[P] Common in patients at diagnosis of CD.[55] [D] Cachexia is a state of ill health characterized by general malnutrition and loss of lean tissue. Anthropometric, biochemical, and bone densitometric assessment performed in 23 celiac children aged 1 to 12 years at diagnosis and one year after GFD demonstrated that a year of GFD allows virtually complete return in body mass composition. At diagnosis, the patients had height, arm muscle triceps, skin folds, subscapular skin folds, fat area index, and bone mineral content significantly lower than controls. After one year on GFD, no significant difference was found between patients and controls in all parameters studied except in height and arm muscle area, which were very near to the normal expected. Serum hemoglobin, iron, and zinc values were below the normal range in more than half of patients at diagnosis and within the normal range in almost all of them after 1 year of GFD. Serum hemoglobin, iron, zinc, triglycerides, proteins, albumin, and calcium values rose significantly during the year of GFD.[36] Study of 458 patients diagnosed with CD aimed to describe the clinical manifestations of celiac sprue related to malabsorption and to analyze the associations between CD and other diagnoses, found cachexia to be a common nutritional manifestation.[55] Study defining the correlates of CD in 100 anemic adults without overt malabsorption demonstrated that compared to anemic patients without CD, anemic patients with CD had significant or borderline significant differences for plasma cholesterol, albumin, and body mass index but not for blood hemoglobin, mean corpuscular volume, plasma iron, and ferritin.[10] [M] Marked by anorexia, weakness, lethargy, and loss of muscle and weight. [C] Results from protein malabsorption in gluten sensitive enteropathy, with or without diarrhea.[34] [R] CD-related cachexia improves quickly on GFD.	Carbohydrate, Omega-3 fatty acids, Omega-6 fatty acids, Protein, Minerals, Vitamins.[34]
Body Composition	All	69	Loss of Vitality [3,34]	(AD)	[P] Common in people with untreated CD.[3] [D] Loss of vitality is a state of diminished power to live or go on living, interfering with normal functioning and survival. [M] Marked by loss of activity, strength, and reaction. [C] Results from multiple nutritional deficiencies induced by gluten sensitive enteropathy; diarrhea, pain, and indigestion if present. [R] CD-related loss of vitality returns on GFD.	Iron, Omega-3 fatty acids, Omega-6 fatty acids, Protein, Selenium.

[+] (S) = Classic sign/symptom; (AT) = Atypical sign/symptom; (AD) Associated Disorder; (C) = Complication.

[++] [P] = Prevalance; [D] = Description; [M] = Sign/symptom; [C] = CD related cause; [R] = Response to gluten Free diet (GFD).

Health Manifestations of Celiac Disease (CD)
Section B: Signs, Symptoms, Associated Disorders and Complications

Affected System	Affected Organ	ID No.	Manifestation	Type[+]	Current Medical Information[++]	Deficient Nutrient

Body Composition	All	70	Weight Loss, Unexpected [1,3,10,34,36,55]	(S)	[P] Common in people with untreated CD.[55]
					[D] Unexpected weight loss, a classic presentation of CD,[3] is a symptom of malabsorption characterized by abnormal maintenance or loss of fat, muscle and other tissue. Vitamin B_{12} deficiency can cause considerable weight loss.[34]
					  Anthropometric, biochemical, and bone densitometric assessment performed in 23 celiac children aged 1 to 12 years at diagnosis and one year after GFD demonstrated that a year of GFD allows virtually complete return in body mass composition. At diagnosis, the patients had height, arm muscle triceps, skin folds, subscapular skin folds, fat area index, and bone mineral content significantly lower than controls. After one year on GFD, no significant difference was found between patients and controls in all parameters studied except in height and arm muscle area, which were very near to the normal expected. Serum hemoglobin, iron, and zinc values were below the normal range in more than half of patients at diagnosis and within the normal range in almost all of them after 1 year of GFD. Serum hemoglobin, iron, zinc, triglycerides, proteins, albumin, and calcium values rose significantly during the year of GFD.[36]
					  Study defining the correlates of CD in 100 anemic adults without overt malabsorption demonstrated that compared to anemic patients without CD, anemic patients with CD had significant or borderline significant differences for plasma cholesterol, albumin, and body mass index but not for blood hemoglobin, mean corpuscular volume, plasma iron, and ferritin.[10]
					[M] Marked by decreased body mass, decreased serum proteins, and increased stool fat.[34]
					[C] Results from nutritional deficiencies in gluten sensitive enteropathy, and may include diarrhea, vomiting, or nausea.
					[R] CD-related weight loss rapidly improves on GFD.
						Carbohydrate, B-complex Vitamins: (Vitamin B_1, Vitamin B_2, Vitamin B_3, Pantothenic acid, Vitamin B_6, Vitamin B_{12}) Iron, Manganese, Omega-3 fatty acids, Omega-6 fatty acids, Phosphorus, Protein, Vitamin K, Zinc.

Body Composition	Brain: cerebrum	71	Anorexia [1,2,3,34]	(S)	[P] Common in people with untreated CD.[3] [D] Anorexia is a symptom of malabsorption characterized by loss of appetite.[34] [M] Marked by no desire to seek or enjoy food. [C] Results from nutritional deficiencies including zinc, phosphorus, potassium, magnesium, iron, thiamin (vitamin B_1), and niacin (vitamin B_3) induced by CD. Other causes include nausea, vomiting, chronic gastroenteritis, constipation, abdominal bloating, and pain associated with CD. [R] CD-related anorexia improves quickly on GFD. Resolution may take 3-6 months.[3]	Iron, Magnesium, Phosphorus, Potassium, Vitamin B_1, Vitamin B_3, Zinc.

[+] (S) = Classic sign/symptom; (AT) = Atypical sign/symptom; (AD) Associated Disorder; (C) = Complication.

[++] [P] = Prevalance; [D] = Description; [M] = Sign/symptom; [C] = CD related cause; [R] = Response to gluten Free diet (GFD).

Health Manifestations of Celiac Disease (CD)
Section B: Signs, Symptoms, Associated Disorders and Complications

Affected System	Affected Organ	ID No.	Manifestation	Type+	Current Medical Information ++	Deficient Nutrient
Body Composition	Brain: cerebrum	72	Increased Appetite [39]	(AT)	[P] Newly recognized presentation of CD. [39] [D] Increased appetite is a symptom of malnutrition characterized by abnormal desire for food. [39] [M] Marked by unsatisfied hunger and eating larger than usual quantities of food and/or at more frequent intervals. [C] Results from malabsorption in CD. [R] CD-related appetite increase normalizes on GFD.	Carbohydrate, Omega-3 fatty acids, Omega-6 fatty acids, Protein.
Digestive System	Mouth	73	Aphthous Ulcers and Non-Aphthous Ulcers [1,34,56]	(S) (AD)	[P] CD occurs in 3.1% of people with recurrent aphthous ulcers. Aphthous ulcers occurred in 12.5% of untreated CD patients and 3.1% of previously diagnosed patients with CD. Non-aphthus buccal mucosa ulcers occurred in 29.6% of treated CD patients (of whom only 80.4% reported strict adherence to GFD) and 12.5% of untreated CD patients. [56] [D] Aphthous ulcers and non-aphthous ulcers are chronic recurrent disorders of soft mouth tissue characterized by small, painful purpuric, papular, or erosive sores that are often surrounded by erythematous (red) margins. [56] Study investigating histopathology of oral lesions in 128 patients with CD on GFD and 8 patients with newly diagnosed CD compared to 30 healthy controls demonstrated that aphthous and non-aphthous ulcers are common in patients with CD. Clinically, it is important to study the oral cavity of patients suspected of having CD where the only clue to the disease may reside, since no less than 66% of the patients in this study had oral symptoms. Occasional diet laxity was associated neither with the oral lesions and symptoms nor changes in CD serology. This implies that also non-dietary factors may be involved in the clinical course of CD. In this study, even CD patients on a GFD often had oral manifestations that could not be explained by other causes than CD. Note: since raised antibodies were found in those claiming to follow a strict GFD, many patients probably do not follow GFD strictly. [56] [M] Marked by oral pain and difficulty eating. [C] Results probably from contact with gluten, and even minute amounts of gluten may lead to oral manifestations since ingested food first contacts the oral surfaces. The pathogenesis is unclear. [56] [R] Some patients with ulceration respond to a GFD even in the absence of jejunal villous atrophy. [56]	Folic acid, Iron, Vitamin B_{12}. [34]

+ (S) = Classic sign/symptom; (AT) = Atypical sign/symptom; (AD) Associated Disorder; (C) = Complication.

++ [P] = Prevalance; [D] = Description; [M] = Sign/symptom; [C] = CD related cause; [R] = Response to gluten Free diet (GFD).

Health Manifestations of Celiac Disease (CD)
Section B: Signs, Symptoms, Associated Disorders and Complications

Affected System	Affected Organ	ID No.	Manifestation	Type[+]	Current Medical Information [++]	Deficient Nutrient
Digestive System	Mouth	74	Cheilosis [34,56]	(S)	[P] Common in people with untreated CD. [D] Cheilosis is a feature of B-vitamin complex deficiency, especially riboflavin and/or pyridoxine deficiency, characterized by redness of the lips with cracking and weeping in the corner of the mouth. In addition, the damaging effects of CD on the duodenal mucosa may affect the absorption of vitamin B_{12}, folate and iron. It is well known that redness and soreness of the tongue with atrophied papillae is occasionally accompanied by angular stomatitis and less frequently by cheilosis and this constellation is linked to these deficiency states. [56] [M] Marked by local soreness with pain on opening mouth. [C] Results from B-complex deficiency, especially riboflavin (vitamin B_2) and/or pyridoxine (vitamin B_6) deficiency and less frequently, by vitamin B_{12}, folate and iron deficiencies induced by CD. [R] Occurrence of CD-related cheilosis resolves on a nutrient dense GFD.	B-complex: (especially Vitamin B_2, Vitamin B_6,) Folate, Vitamin B_{12}, Iron. [34]

+ (S) = Classic sign/symptom; (AT) = Atypical sign/symptom; (AD) Associated Disorder; (C) = Complication.

++ [P] = Prevalance; [D] = Description; [M] = Sign/symptom; [C] = CD related cause; [R] = Response to gluten Free diet (GFD).

Health Manifestations of Celiac Disease (CD)
Section B: Signs, Symptoms, Associated Disorders and Complications

Affected System	Affected Organ	ID No.	Manifestation	Type[+]	Current Medical Information [++]	Deficient Nutrient
Digestive System	Mouth	75	Dental Enamel Defects [1,56,57,58]	(S)	[P] Severe grade III or grade IV enamel defects occurred in 10.1% of study patients that included both children and adults with CD.[56] Demarcated opacities or hypoplasia occurred in 28% of children with CD vs. 14.8% of controls.[57] Dental enamel defects occurred in 89% of patients with CD and Sjögrens syndrome (SS) and 88% in CD alone compared with only 25% in SS alone.[58] [D] Dental enamel defects are characterized by alteration in the hard, white, dense, inorganic substance covering the crowns of the teeth in genetically determined CD patients. No relation found for calcium concentrations.[57] Study investigating 128 patients on GFD revealed that changes in the permanent teeth may be the only sign of an otherwise symptomless CD. It is important to study the oral cavity of patients suspected of having CD, since no less than 66% of the patients in this study had oral symptoms. In a study by Aine et al., 3% of adult CD patients had grade III - IV enamel defects. In this study, the figure was 10.3%, but this included pediatric patients. In the study of Aine et al., 30% of their children with CD had grade III - IV enamel defects. The difference between the children and adults might indicate that the adults often develop CD after the critical age of 7 years when the crowns of the permanent teeth have developed.[56] Study investigating 82 children with celiac disease for the presence of dental enamel defects and their relation to hypocalcemia or a particular HLA class demonstrated that the presence of HLA DR3 antigen significantly increased the risk of dental lesions, while genotype DR5,7 seemed to protect against enamel defects. A logistic regression analysis of the variables age, serum calcium concentrations, number of affected teeth, type of enamel defect and DR antigens showed that only DR antigens discriminated celiac disease patients with defects from those without enamel defects.[57] Study investigating oral findings in patients with CD and Sjögrens syndrome compared with patients having CD alone and those with SS alone found celiac-type dental enamel defects in 89% in CD and SS and 88% in CD compared with only 25% in SS. The co-occurrence of CD and SS should be recognized because of its effects on dental and oral mucosal health.[58] [M] Marked by demarcated opacities and hypoplasia and associated with yellowing, horizontal grooves, and/or pits on one or more permanent teeth.[56] [C] Results from CD in patients with HLA DR3 genotype before the critical age of 7 years when the crowns of the permanent teeth have developed.[57] Pathogenesis of these oral lesions is not fully understood.[56] [R] GFD is protective against CD-related dental enamel defects in children while the crowns are developing.[56] In patients with both CD and SS, a GFD may alleviate autoimmune inflammation.[58]	Not known.

+ (S) = Classic sign/symptom; (AT) = Atypical sign/symptom; (AD) Associated Disorder; (C) = Complication.

++ [P] = Prevalance; [D] = Description; [M] = Sign/symptom; [C] = CD related cause; [R] = Response to gluten Free diet (GFD).

Health Manifestations of Celiac Disease (CD)
Section B: Signs, Symptoms, Associated Disorders and Complications

Affected System	Affected Organ	ID No.	Manifestation	Type+	Current Medical Information++	Deficient Nutrient
Digestive System	Mouth	76	Gums, Bleeding and/or Swollen[34]	(S)	[P] Common in untreated people with CD. [D] Bleeding or swollen gums, a feature of vitamin C deficiency, is a symptom of malabsorption characterized by alteration in gum integrity that may result in tooth loss. Sponginess indicates inflammation. [M] Marked by oral pain on chewing. Scurvy in adults is characterized by a purplish line while in children it is marked by a red gum line.[34] [C] Results from vitamin C malabsorption in CD. [R] CD-related gum changes resolve on a nutrient dense GFD.	Vitamin C.
Digestive System	Mouth	77	Oral Mucosal Lesions, Chronic[1,56]	(S) (AD)	[P] Common in people with untreated CD and 55.5% of treated patients not following a strict GFD.[56] [D] Chronic oral mucosal lesions are symptoms of malabsorption and/or local immune reactions to gluten exposure characterized by painful inflammation. Lesions carry profound diagnostic importance in CD and may be the only presenting features.[56] Both CD and Sjögrens syndrome (SS) have an autoimmune background and increased risk of oral mucosal and dental abnormalities. Individuals suffering concomitantly from CD and SS could be at a higher risk.[58] Study investigating 128 CD patients on GFD demonstrated intraepithelial T-cells and mast cells were found significantly more frequent in treated CD patients than in controls. Moderate to severe lymphocytic inflammation of the oral mucosa tends to increase with a longer duration of CD with or without treatment. However, lack of strict compliance with a GFD may be related to high prevalence of oral changes and symptoms since raised serum endomysium IgA antibody titres were found in study patients. Even minute amounts of gluten may lead to oral manifestations since ingested food first contacts the oral surfaces. Changes are not associated with mechanical irritation or smoking.[56] Study investigating oral findings in patients with CD and Sjögrens syndrome compared with patients having CD alone and those with SS alone found CD and SS was characterized by higher salivary flow rate and lower inflammatory focus score in the salivary glands than SS. The co-occurrence of CD + SS should be recognized because of its effects on dental and oral mucosal health. A lower salivary gland inflammatory focus score and higher salivary flow rate in CD + SS than in SS suggests that a GFD treatment may alleviate autoimmune inflammation.[58] [M] Marked by oral soreness, burning sensations or xerostoma (dry mouth) seem to be common symptoms in GFD treated CD patients. The tongue is most often affected.[56] [C] Results from CD itself and micronutrient deficiencies induced by CD.[56] [R] CD-related oral mucosal lesions respond to a strict only GFD, but often persist.[56]	Iron, Omega 3-fatty acids, Vitamin B$_1$, Vitamin B$_2$, Vitamin B$_3$, Vitamin B$_6$, Vitamin B$_{12}$, Vitamin C, Vitamin K.

+ (S) = Classic sign/symptom; (AT) = Atypical sign/symptom; (AD) Associated Disorder; (C) = Complication.
++ [P] = Prevalance; [D] = Description; [M] = Sign/symptom; [C] = CD related cause; [R] = Response to gluten Free diet (GFD).

Health Manifestations of Celiac Disease (CD)
Section B: Signs, Symptoms, Associated Disorders and Complications

Affected System	Affected Organ	ID No.	Manifestation	Type[+]	Current Medical Information [++]	Deficient Nutrient
Digestive System	Mouth	78	Tongue - Beefy Red, Smooth, Burning [34,56]	(S)	[P] Common in people with untreated and untreated CD.[56] [D] A beefy, red, smooth, burning tongue is an alteration in tongue tissue characteristic of vitamin B_{12} deficiency.[34] [M] Marked by inflammatory changes advancing to atrophied papillae. [C] Results from vitamin B_{12} deficiency induced by CD. [R] CD-related tongue changes resolve on GFD.	Vitamin B_{12}.
Digestive System	Mouth	79	Tongue - Fiery Red, Smooth, Swollen, Sore [34,56]	(S)	[P] Common in people with untreated and untreated CD.[56] [D] A fiery red, smooth, burning tongue is an alteration in tongue tissue characteristic of pellagra. [M] Marked by tongue soreness preceded by redness of tip and edges. Later, ulceration especially under the tongue may occur. [C] Results from niacin (vitamin B_3) deficiency in CD. [R] CD-related tongue changes resolve on GFD.	Vitamin B_3.
Digestive System	Mouth	80	Tongue - Magenta, Swollen [34,56]	(S)	[P] Common in people with untreated and untreated CD.[56] [D] A magenta, swollen tongue is an alteration in tongue tissue characteristic of riboflavin deficiency.[34] [M] Follows soreness and burning of lips, mouth and tongue, and cheilosis; advances to hypertrophy or atrophy of papillae, showing smooth patches where shrunken. [C] Results from riboflavin (vitamin B2) deficiency in CD. [R] CD-related tongue changes quickly resolve on GFD.	Vitamin B_2.
Digestive System	Mouth	81	Tongue - Pale, Smooth, Burning [34,56]	(S)	[P] Common in people with untreated CD.[56] [D] A pale, smooth, burning tongue is an alteration in tongue tissue characteristic of iron deficiency.[34] [M] Marked by painful tongue with shrunken papillae.[62] [C] Results from iron malabsorption in CD. [R] CD-related tongue changes resolve on GFD.	Iron

+ (S) = Classic sign/symptom; (AT) = Atypical sign/symptom; (AD) Associated Disorder; (C) = Complication.

++ [P] = Prevalance; [D] = Description; [M] = Sign/symptom; [C] = CD related cause; [R] = Response to gluten Free diet (GFD).

Health Manifestations of Celiac Disease (CD)
Section B: Signs, Symptoms, Associated Disorders and Complications

Affected System	Affected Organ	ID No.	Manifestation	Type[+]	Current Medical Information [++]	Deficient Nutrient
Digestive System	Pharnx	82	Cancer of the Pharynx [1,59]	(C)	[P] Increased in frequency in people with CD.[59] [D] Cancer of the pharynx, a malignancy arising in the pharynx, is a major complication of untreated celiac disease.[59] Certain nutritional deficiencies have been shown to increase the potential for cancer, including vitamin E, selenium and omega-3 fatty acids. [M] Marked by difficulty eating and swallowing, with voice changes. [C] Possibly results from cellular damage involving gluten exposure, malnutrition in CD. [R] GFD is protective of CD-related cancer of the pharynx.[59]	Possibly - Omega-3 fatty acids, Selenium, Vitamin E.
Digestive System	Larynx	83	Laryngospasm [23]	(C)	[P] Unusual occurrence is associated with untreated CD.[23] [D] Laryngospasm, or spasm of the laryngeal muscles, is a rare feature of hypocalcemia characterized by severe alteration in nerve conduction and muscle contraction.[23] [M] Marked by dyspnea (difficulty breathing), anxiety, neuromuscular irritability (spasm) and weakness.[23] [C] Results from severe hypocalcemia, also hypomagnesemia from malabsorption of vitamin D, causing the electrolyte imbalance.[23] [R] Good response of CD-related laryngospasm to GFD.[23]	Calcium, Magnesium, Vitamin D.
Digestive System	Larynx	84	Post-Cricoid Carcinoma [1,59]	(C)	[P] Increased in frequency in people with untreated CD.[59] [D] Post-cricoid carcinoma, a malignancy arising in the hypopharynx, is a major complication of CD with early metastasis and poor prognosis.[59] [M] Marked by difficulty swallowing and vague discomfort as initial presenting signs until tumor has grown. [C] Possibly results from cellular damage involving gluten exposure. [R] Studies are inadequate to determine effect of GFD.	Not known.

+ (S) = Classic sign/symptom; (AT) = Atypical sign/symptom; (AD) Associated Disorder; (C) = Complication.

++ [P] = Prevalance; [D] = Description; [M] = Sign/symptom; [C] = CD related cause; [R] = Response to gluten Free diet (GFD).

Health Manifestations of Celiac Disease (CD)
Section B: Signs, Symptoms, Associated Disorders and Complications

Affected System	Affected Organ	ID No.	Manifestation	Type[+]	Current Medical Information [++]	Deficient Nutrient
Digestive System	Esophagus	85	Cancer of the Esophagus [1,59,60]	(C)	[P] Increased risk in CD patients.[60] [D] Cancer of the esophagus, a malignancy arising in the esophagus, is a major complication of untreated celiac disease and may be related to vitamin A deficiency.[59] Morbidity is significantly increased in CD.[60] [M] Marked by feeling of fullness, pressure, indigestion, or substernal burning developing into dysphagia, chest pain usually radiating to the back, and weight loss with metastasis. [C] Possibly results from cellular damage and vitamin A deficiency; associated with GERD and Plummer-Vinson syndrome. [R] Patients who adhere to a GFD are not at increased risk of this cancer.[60]	Iron, Vitamin A.
Digestive System	Esophagus	86	Dysphagia [1,61,62]	(AT)	[P] Common in people with untreated CD.[61] [D] Dysphagia is a functional upper digestive disorder characterized by alteration in swallowing.[61] [M] Marked by difficulty or inability to swallow. [C] Results from gastroesophageal reflux disease (GERD), altered esophageal motility, and iron deficiency in CD. [R] GFD significantly decreases the rate of CD-related dysphagia.[62]	Iron.
Digestive System	Esophagus	87	Esophageal Small Cell Carcinoma [1,60]	(C)	[P] Increased risk in untreated CD.[60] [D] Esophageal small cell carcinoma, a malignancy arising in the esophagus, is a major complication with significant morbidity in CD.[60] Certain nutritional deficiencies have been shown to increase the potential for cancer, including vitamin E, selenium, and omega-3 fatty acids. [M] Marked by feeling of fullness, pressure, burning or indigestion, progressing to difficulty swallowing and weight loss with rapid spread. [C] Possibly results from cellular damage involving gluten exposure, malnutrition, and GERD. [R] Patients who adhere to a strict GFD are not at increased risk.[60]	Possibly - Omega-3 fatty acids, Selenium, Vitamin E.

[+] (S) = Classic sign/symptom; (AT) = Atypical sign/symptom; (AD) Associated Disorder; (C) = Complication.

[++] [P] = Prevalence; [D] = Description; [M] = Sign/symptom; [C] = CD related cause; [R] = Response to gluten Free diet (GFD).

Health Manifestations of Celiac Disease (CD)
Section B: Signs, Symptoms, Associated Disorders and Complications

Affected System	Affected Organ	ID No.	Manifestation	Type+	Current Medical Information ++	Deficient Nutrient
Digestive System	Esophagus	88	Esophageal Motor Abnormalities [61,62]	(AT)	[P] Detected by esophageal manometry and cardiovascular tests in about 50% of untreated patients with CD. Ph-metry abnormal in 30% of study patients, and up to 75% of celiac patients displayed GI motility alterations.[61] [D] Esophageal motor abnormalities involve alterations in motility characterized by impaired esophageal peristalsis and lack of lower esophageal sphincter relaxation. CD patients show a decrease in lower esophageal sphincter pressure.[62] Study investigating upper gut-motor activity in 30 untreated CD patients and exploring the role played by the autonomic nervous system in motility disturbances demonstrated that upper-gut motor abnormalities are frequently present in adult CD. Delayed gastric emptying was documented in about 50% of study patients and was correlated with manometric postprandial hypomotility. Extrinsic motor neuropathy may play a role, although other pathophysiological mechanisms are likely.[61] [M] Marked by dysphagia, possibly regurgitation, chest pain, and nocturnal cough. [C] Results from unclear etiology. [R] Studies are inadequate to determine the effect of a GFD.	Not known.
Digestive System	Esophagus	89	Gastroesophageal Reflux Disease (GERD) [62]	(AT)	[P] Celiac patients have a high prevalence of reflux esophagitis. Retrospective study shows 19% in patients undergoing endoscopy for biopsy.[62] [D] GERD, an upper digestive disorder, is characterized by a decrease in lower esophageal sphincter pressure (LES) allowing reflux of stomach contents into the esophagus. Study evaluating whether untreated celiac patients had an increased prevalence of reflux esophagitis and, if so, to assess whether a GFD exerted any beneficial effect on GERD symptoms demonstrated celiac patients have a high prevalence of reflux esophagitis. That a GFD significantly decreased the relapse rate of GERD symptoms suggests that CD may represent a risk factor for the development of reflux esophagitis.[62] [M] Marked by dysphagia, chest pain and heartburn. [C] Results from gluten exposure and increased abdominal pressure in CD. [R] GFD significantly decreases the relapse rate of CD-related GERD symptoms. [62]	Not applicable.

+ (S) = Classic sign/symptom; (AT) = Atypical sign/symptom; (AD) Associated Disorder; (C) = Complication.

++ [P] = Prevalance; [D] = Description; [M] = Sign/symptom; [C] = CD related cause; [R] = Response to gluten Free diet (GFD).

Health Manifestations of Celiac Disease (CD)
Section B: Signs, Symptoms, Associated Disorders and Complications

Affected System	Affected Organ	ID No.	Manifestation	Type[+]	Current Medical Information [++]	Deficient Nutrient
Digestive System	Esophagus	90	Heartburn [62]	(AT)	[P] Common in people with untreated CD.[62] [D] Heartburn is a functional upper digestive symptom caused by reflux of gastric contents from the stomach into the esophagus. [M] Marked by burning sensation felt in the mid-epigastrium behind the sternum or in the throat. [C] Results from niacin (vitamin B3) deficiency and gastroesophageal reflux disease (GERD). [R] GFD significantly decreases relapse rate of CD-related heartburn.[62]	Vitamin B₃.
Digestive System	Esophagus	91	Plummer-Vinson Syndrome affecting esophagus [1,63]	(AD)	[P] Associated with CD.[63] [D] Plummer-Vinson syndrome, a rare iron deficiency disorder, is characterized by a constellation of postcricoid esophageal webs, iron deficiency anemia, dysphagia and koilonychia, predisposing to esophageal cancer. Webs are thin mucosal membranes growing across the esophageal lumen, causing obstruction. Case report describes unusual clubbing instead of koilonychia and tortuous esophagus in 3 patients diagnosed with CD.[63] [M] Marked by iron deficiency anemia, fatigue, weakness, thin spooning of nails, and difficulty swallowing solid food. [C] Results from iron deficiency due to malabsorption in CD, gastroesophageal reflux disease (GERD). [R] CD-related Plummer-Vinson syndrome resolves on GFD.	Iron.
Digestive System	Stomach	92	Delayed Gastric Emptying [1,61]	(AT)	[P] Frequently present in 50% of patients with untreated CD. Autonomic tests were positive in 45% of study patients.[61] [D] Delayed gastric emptying is a digestive motility disorder characterized by abnormally slow movement of gastric contents into the duodenum. Study investigating upper gut-motor activity in 30 untreated CD patients and exploring the role played by the autonomic nervous system in motility disturbances demonstrated that delayed gastric emptying correlated with manometric post prandial hypomotility.[61] [M] Marked by early fullness after eating, eructation, nausea, vomiting, gas, and abdominal pains that can be temporary or missing in some patients. [C] Results from unclear etiology. Extrinsic motor neuropathy may play a role, although other pathophysiological mechanisms are likely.[61] [R] Studies are inadequate to determine effect of GFD.	Not applicable.

+ (S) = Classic sign/symptom; (AT) = Atypical sign/symptom; (AD) Associated Disorder; (C) = Complication.

++ [P] = Prevalance; [D] = Description; [M] = Sign/symptom; [C] = CD related cause; [R] = Response to gluten Free diet (GFD).

Health Manifestations of Celiac Disease (CD)
Section B: Signs, Symptoms, Associated Disorders and Complications

Affected System	Affected Organ	ID No.	Manifestation	Type[+]	Current Medical Information [++]	Deficient Nutrient
Digestive System	Stomach	93	Gastric Ulcer [1,64]	(C)	[P] 3% occurrence in patients with CD. 7.5% occurrence in celiac patients with anemia.[64] [D] Gastric ulcer is characterized by an excoriated area involving the mucosa lining and deeper muscle layer of the stomach associated with lymphocytic gastritis, and may be accompanied by achlorhydria (poor acid production). [M] Marked by gnawing epigastric pain usually relieved by food or antacids with possible bleeding, resulting in dark stool. [C] Results from disruption in normal tissue repair and defense due to chronic inflammation, gluten exposure, deficiency of niacin (vitamin B_3) and/or iron in CD, and Helicobacter pylori (H. pylori) infection. [R] CD-related gastric ulcer responds to GFD.	Iron, Vitamin B_3.
Digestive System	Stomach	94	Gastric Ulcerations, Multiple [1,65]	(C)	[P] New presentation in CD.[65] [D] Multiple gastric ulcerations are a late complication involving alteration in the superficial gastric mucosa characterized by multilocular peptic ulcers of the gastric antrum. Case report describes a 53 year old woman with diarrhea, epigastric pain and abdominal distention. At upper GI endoscopy, biopsies were taken showing complete atrophy of the villi and colonization of the small bowel mucosa. Uncommon multilocular ulcers were seen in the gastric antrum that proved to be Helicobacter pylori-negative with no evidence of Zollinger-Ellison syndrome. Biopsy showed lymphocytic gastritis with an extensive infiltration of the lamina propria by almost exclusively CD3- and CD45RO positive T-lymphocytes. Intraepithelial T-lymphocytes were found to be increased in the antral as well as the corpus mucosa of the stomach.[65] [M] Marked by diarrhea, epigastric pain, and abdominal distentions.[65] [C] Results from unclear etiology.[65] [R] Studies are inadequate to determine effect of GFD.	Not known.

+ (S) = Classic sign/symptom; (AT) = Atypical sign/symptom; (AD) Associated Disorder; (C) = Complication.

++ [P] = Prevalance; [D] = Description; [M] = Sign/symptom; [C] = CD related cause; [R] = Response to gluten Free diet (GFD).

Section B   *Signs, Symptoms, Associated Disorders & Complications*   133

Health Manifestations of Celiac Disease (CD)
Section B: Signs, Symptoms, Associated Disorders and Complications

Affected System	Affected Organ	ID No.	Manifestation	Type[+]	Current Medical Information [++]	Deficient Nutrient
Digestive System	Stomach	95	Collagenous Gastritis [66]	(C)	[P] New association with untreated CD. [66] [D] Collagenous gastritis, a rarely reported gastric disorder, is characterized in this case report by a thickened (>10 micron) subepithelial collagen band with entrapped capillaries, fibroblasts, and inflammatory cells associated with lymphocytic gastritis. Case report of a 42 year old man describes collagenous gastritis and duodenal mucosa with severe villous atrophy but no subendothelial collagen deposition. No evidence of collagenous or lymphocytic colitis was found in the colon. [66] [M] Marked by stomach pain. [C] Results from unclear etiology and pathogenesis. [66] [R] Reported patient became symptom-free on a GFD and showed partial improvement of histopathologic findings in 3 months. [66]	Not known.
Digestive System	Stomach	96	Gastritis, Lymphocytic [1,67]	(C)	[P] Approximately 50% of children with celiac disease present lymphocytic gastritis. [67] [D] Lymphocytic gastritis (LG), a superficial inflammation of the stomach lining, mainly involves the gastric antrum (bottom of stomach) in children. It is defined by the recognition of >25 intraepithelial lymphocytes (IEL) per 100 surface epithelial cells. Study investigating the intraepithelial population of lymphocytes in children demonstrated that LG associated with CD in children contains a peculiar CD8+ intraepithelial T-lymphocyte population which immunohistochemically lacks perforin and granzyme B, undergoes apoptosis, and is not associated with substantial damage to the epithelial cells. No patient presented with Helicobacter pylori-like organisms at the luminal surface. Findings fit with those reported in adults except for the negative results for granzyme B. [67] [M] Marked by minimal discomfort. [C] Results from gluten exposure in CD. [R] CD-related lymphocytic inflammation disappears after a GFD. [67]	Not applicable.

+ (S) = Classic sign/symptom; (AT) = Atypical sign/symptom; (AD) Associated Disorder; (C) = Complication.

++ [P] = Prevalence; [D] = Description; [M] = Sign/symptom; [C] = CD related cause; [R] = Response to gluten Free diet (GFD).

Health Manifestations of Celiac Disease (CD)
Section B: Signs, Symptoms, Associated Disorders and Complications

Affected System	Affected Organ	ID No.	Manifestation	Type[+]	Current Medical Information [++]	Deficient Nutrient
Digestive System	Stomach	97	Helicobacter Pylori Infection [1,64]	(AD)	[P] 21% prevalence in untreated CD patients of whom 71% had iron deficiency anemia.[64] [D] Helicobacter pylori (H. pylori) is a bacteria that invades the stomach lining. H. pylori infection is characterized by chronic superficial inflammation in 100% of infected patients and ulcerations, causing disruption of normal defense and repair that make mucosa susceptible to injury from acid. H. pylori infection is a factor responsible for iron deficiency in CD patients who are predisposed to iron-deficiency anemia.[64] Study investigating the potential relationship between H. pylori and iron deficiency anemia in 362 patients with CD demonstrated a significant association between H. pylori and iron deficiency anemia. Bacteria impair iron absorption by means of several mechanisms: 1) considerable decrease in the concentration of gastric juice ascorbic acid that is the best promotor of non-heme iron absorption, 2) may significantly increase iron demand because iron is an essential bacteria growth factor, 3) contain a 19.6 kilodalton protein resembling ferritin with a binding activity for heme iron in erythrocytes, and 4) the gastric colonization by H. pylori probably increases increases iron demand. Screening for H. pylori proposed because the infection may worsen the alterations of iron metabolism in patients with CD.[64] [M] Marked by dyspepsia, gastritis, gastric ulcers, peptic ulcers, and iron deficiency anemia in predisposed patients, although most patients remain asymptomatic.[64] [C] Results from invasion of inflamed gastric lining by bacteria enabled by lowered resistance to infection, low gastric acidity, and nutrient deficiencies in CD.[64] [R] Treatment of CD-related H. pylori infection could be associated with a strict GFD.[64]	Iron, Vitamin B₃.
Digestive System	Stomach	98	Vomiting [1]	(S)	[P] Common in people with untreated CD. [D] Vomiting is a well known upper GI sign of CD. [M] Marked by regurgitation of stomach contents into the mouth, especially following ingestion of gluten. [C] Results from gluten exposure in CD and/or vitamin B₃ (niacin) deficiency. [R] Occurrence of CD-related vomiting resolves on a strict GFD.	Vitamin B₃.

[+] (S) = Classic sign/symptom; (AT) = Atypical sign/symptom; (AD) Associated Disorder; (C) = Complication.

[++] [P] = Prevalance; [D] = Description; [M] = Sign/symptom; [C] = CD related cause; [R] = Response to gluten Free diet (GFD).

Health Manifestations of Celiac Disease (CD)
Section B: Signs, Symptoms, Associated Disorders and Complications

Affected System	Affected Organ	ID No.	Manifestation	Type+	Current Medical Information ++	Deficient Nutrient
Digestive System	Biliary tract	99	Autoimmune Cholangitis (Antimitochondrial Antibody-Negative Primary Biliary Cirrhosis)[1,68]	(AD)	[P] New association with CD.[68] [D] Autoimmune cholangitis is a biliary tract disease characterized by progressive inflammation leading to narrowing and destruction of the bile ducts and development of biliary cirrhosis. Case report describes finding CD in a patient with a liver biopsy suggestive of stage 1 primary biliary cirrhosis but negative serum antimitochondrial antibody testing. Resolution of symptoms after initiation of a GFD suggests CD may play a direct role in the development of autoimmune cholangitis. CD should be considered in all patients diagnosed with autoimmune cholangitis.[68] [M] Marked by progressive weakness, iron deficiency anemia, pruritis, and chronic serum liver biochemistry elevations. [C] Results from autoimmune mechanism. [R] Resolution of CD-related iron deficiency anemia, pruritis, and elevated liver biochemistries occurred on a GFD, avoiding the need for immunosuppressive therapy.[68]	Not applicable.
Digestive System	Biliary tract	100	Impaired Gall Bladder Motility[1,69]	(AD)	[P] Increased frequency in people with CD.[69] [D] Impaired gall bladder motility is characterized in CD by reduced secretion of enteric hormones and/or decreased gallbladder sensitivity to them. In particular, untreated CD patients show low postprandial cholecystokinin and increased fasting somatostatin levels.[69] [M] Marked by cramping pain after ingesting fatty foods. [C] Results from effects of gluten sensitive enteropathy.[69] [R] CD-related gall bladder motility improves on GFD.	Not applicable.

+ (S) = Classic sign/symptom; (AT) = Atypical sign/symptom; (AD) Associated Disorder; (C) = Complication.

++ [P] = Prevalance; [D] = Description; [M] = Sign/symptom; [C] = CD related cause; [R] = Response to gluten Free diet (GFD).

Health Manifestations of Celiac Disease (CD)
Section B: Signs, Symptoms, Associated Disorders and Complications

Affected System	Affected Organ	ID No.	Manifestation	Type[+]	Current Medical Information [++]	Deficient Nutrient
Digestive System	Biliary tract	101	Primary Biliary Cirrhosis [1,70,71]	(AD)	[P] 3.4% rate of CD occurs in patients with primary biliary cirrhosis (PBC) and 3.7% rate of PBC occurs in CD patients. [70] [D] Primary biliary cirrhosis (PBC) is a biliary tract disease characterized by chronic cholestasis (stoppage of bile flow) and destruction of intrahepatic bile ducts resulting in back-up of bile in the liver. Study investigating both the prevalence of CD in a series of primary biliary cirrhosis patients and that of antimitochondrial antibodies in a series of adult biopsy proven CD patients demonstrated significant association between PBC and CD. Screening with anti-endomysium antibodies in PBC is justified and screening for antimitochondrial antibodies is advisable in adult CD patients. [70] Study investigating the association between PBC and CD by testing stored sera from 378 patients with PBC demonstrated patients with primary biliary cirrhosis should be considered at high risk for CD. [71] [M] Marked by liver disease, normal liver tests. [71] [C] Results from common immune mechanism. The increased prevalence of celiac-related antibodies in patients with PBC suggests that the two conditions are associated, although the reason for the association remains unclear. [71] [R] Although liver biochemistry does not improve when these patients are fed a GFD, the complications of untreated CD warrant the identification and treatment of the condition in this population. [71]	Not applicable.
Digestive System	Biliary tract	102	Primary Sclerosing Cholangitis [1,72]	(AD)	[P] New association with CD. [72] [D] Primary sclerosing cholangitis is a chronic cholecystatic syndrome characterized by fibrosing inflammation in the intrahepatic and extrahepatic bile ducts leading to narrowing and, eventually, obliteration of the bile ducts. Case report of two patients with primary sclerosing cholangitis (PSC) and ulcerative colitis describes investigation and diagnosis with CD when patients failed to respond to treatment. Review of the literature suggests an increased malignancy potential in these patients. Annual colonoscopic surveillance with early liver and bowel imaging recommended in patients with combination of PSC, ulcerative colitis and CD having clinical deterioration and weight loss. [72] [M] Marked by gradual, progressive fatigue, itching, jaundice, and weight loss. [C] Results most likely from altered immune mechanisms. [R] Studies are inadequate to determine response to GFD.	Not applicable.

[+] (S) = Classic sign/symptom; (AT) = Atypical sign/symptom; (AD) Associated Disorder; (C) = Complication.

[++] [P] = Prevalance; [D] = Description; [M] = Sign/symptom; [C] = CD related cause; [R] = Response to gluten Free diet (GFD).

Health Manifestations of Celiac Disease (CD)
Section B: Signs, Symptoms, Associated Disorders and Complications

Affected System	Affected Organ	ID No.	Manifestation	Type[+]	Current Medical Information [++]	Deficient Nutrient
Digestive System	Small intestine	103	Abdominal Distention, Chronic [1,2,3,73]	(S)	[P] Common in people with untreated CD.[73] [D] Abdominal distention, a classic symptom of CD signifying damage to the small intestine, is characterized by alteration in normal size of abdomen. If accompanied by chronic diarrhea, distention indicates extensive damage to small intestine mucosa.[3] [M] Marked by uncomfortable bloating. [C] Results from effects of bacterial fermentation of malabsorbed macronutrients in the GI tract, dysbiosis, intestinal edema, niacin (vitamin B_3) deficiency, and altered motility in CD. Some associated causes include candida infection, collagenous colitis, duodenal ulcerations, gastric ulcerations, gas, IBS. [R] CD-related abdominal distention resolves on GFD.[73]	Vitamin B_3.
Digestive System	Small intestine	104	Abdominal Pain, Chronic [1,2,73]	(S)	[P] Common in people with untreated CD.[73] [D] Chronic abdominal pain is a classic digestive symptom of CD characterized by an achy, tense sensation increasing after eating and varying in location, intensity, and sharpness. Pain may recur in one area and/or generally throughout the abdomen with gaseousness and spasm, partially relieved by defecation or passing of gas. [M] Marked by abdominal cramping and/or stabbing sensations after eating fatty foods, in diarrhea and small bowel intussusception. Bloating is a feature of candida infection, collagenous colitis, Crohn's disease, intestinal edema, and lymphocytic colitis. Poorly localized pain is a feature of vitamin B_{12} deficiency. [C] Results from gluten sensitive enteropathy and niacin (vitamin B_3) deficiency. [R] CD-related abdominal pain resolves on GFD.[73]	Niacin. Vitamin B_{12}.

[+] (S) = Classic sign/symptom; (AT) = Atypical sign/symptom; (AD) Associated Disorder; (C) = Complication.
[++] [P] = Prevalance; [D] = Description; [M] = Sign/symptom; [C] = CD related cause; [R] = Response to gluten Free diet (GFD).

Health Manifestations of Celiac Disease (CD)
Section B: Signs, Symptoms, Associated Disorders and Complications

Affected System	Affected Organ	ID No.	Manifestation	Type[+]	Current Medical Information[++]	Deficient Nutrient
Digestive System	Small intestine	105	Adenocarcinoma of Small Intestine [1,59,60, 74,75]	(C)	[P] Increased frequency in CD patients.[59] There is a 60 to 80 fold increased risk of small bowel adenocarcinoma in patients with celiac disease.[74] [D] Adenocarcinoma of the small intestine, a malignancy arising in the duodenum, is a major complication of CD. Study investigating prevalence of adenocarcinoma found during esophagogastroduodenoscopy by review of records of 381 patients with biopsy proven celiac disease did not find a significantly increased risk of small bowel adenocarcinoma in CD patients compared to a non-celiac endoscoped population. Conclusion: routine endoscopic examination of the duodenum may not be adequate for screening.[74] Study investigating selenium concentrations in whole blood, plasma, and leukocytes of patients with biopsy confirmed CD, who were clinically well and receiving GFD, demonstrated significantly lower concentrations than controls, probably indicating a decrease in the body content of selenium. A high incidence of malignancy in CD has been reported. As a protective role for selenium against cancer has been postulated, the importance of this unexpected observation of lowered tissue concentrations of selenium requires further investigation.[75] [M] Marked by occult bleeding, bowel changes. [C] May result from cellular damage involving chronic gluten exposure and deficiencies due to malabsorption in CD. [R] GFD is protective against CD-related adenocarcinoma of the small intestine.[60]	Omega-3 fatty acids. Selenium, Vitamin B$_1$, Vitamin B$_3$, Vitamin B$_{12}$.
Digestive System	Small intestine	106	Carbohydrate Malabsorption [1,3]	(S)	[P] Common in people with untreated CD.[3] [D] Carbohydrate malabsorption is a well known symptom of CD characterized by acidic diarrhea and abdominal distention following ingestion of offending carbohydrate(s). Failure to split disaccharides (lactose, sucrose, maltose) allows them to remain in the intestine and osmotically retain fluid, causing diarrhea, urgency, and distention. Resulting bacterial fermentation of undigested carbohydrates produces gaseous, acidic stool with pH below 6. There is a poor temporal relationship of carbohydrate consumption to symptoms. Symptoms result 1- 8 hours after ingesting offending carbohydrate. [M] Marked by digestive symptoms including abdominal cramps, bloating, borborygmi (loud bowel sounds), gas, urgency and diarrhea. Neurologic symptoms include hypoglycemia and fatigue and metabolic symptoms include failure to gain weight in a child. [C] Results secondarily from diffuse villous injury in CD. [R] CD-related carbohydrate malabsorption resolves on GFD.	Not applicable.

[+] (S) = Classic sign/symptom; (AT) = Atypical sign/symptom; (AD) Associated Disorder; (C) = Complication.

[++] [P] = Prevalance; [D] = Description; [M] = Sign/symptom; [C] = CD related cause; [R] = Response to gluten Free diet (GFD).

Health Manifestations of Celiac Disease (CD)
Section B: Signs, Symptoms, Associated Disorders and Complications

Affected System	Affected Organ	ID No.	Manifestation	Type[+]	Current Medical Information [++]	Deficient Nutrient
Digestive System	Small intestine	107	Candida Albicans Mucosal Infection [76]	(AD)	[P] Increased frequency in untreated CD patients.[76] [D] Candida albicans is a yeast that invades the mucosal lining of the digestive tract. Candida albicans mucosal infection is characterized by superficial, irregular white patches and possible invasion of the bloodstream. Organism appears to be a trigger in the onset of CD. The virulence factor of C. albicans hyphal wall protein 1 (HWP1) contains amino acid sequences that are identical or highly homologous to known CD-related alpha-gliadin and gamma-gliadin T-cell epitopes. HWP1 is a transglutaminase substrate, and is used by C albicans to adhere to the intestinal epithelium. Furthermore, tissue transglutaminase and endomysium components could become covalently linked to the yeast. Subsequently, C albicans might function as an adjuvant that stimulates antibody formation against HWP1 and gluten, and formation of autoreactive antibodies against tissue transglutaminase and endomysium.[76] [M] Marked by bloating abdominal pain and distention. [C] Results from disruption of normal flora, lowered resistance to infection, local inflammation, and malnutrition in CD. [R] Studies are inadequate to determine effect of GFD.	Iron, Omega-3 fatty acids, Vitamin A, Vitamin C.
Digestive System	Small intestine	108	Diarrhea, Acute [34,77,78]	(AT)	[P] Acute severe onset of CD is very uncommon in adults.[77] [D] Acute diarrhea, also called celiac crisis, is characterized by excessively rapid movement of intestinal contents through the small intestine with excessive loss of fluid and electrolytes that leads rapidly to a life threatening hypokalemia and acidosis (so-called celiac crisis).[77] Acute diarrhea that resists medical treatment must evoke the hypothesis of CD and lead to gastroscopy with duodenal biopsies not only to obtain rapid disappearance of the clinical signs after introduction of a GFD, but also to avoid an increased risk of small bowel malignancies.[78] Celiac crisis, described mainly in children younger than two years of age, has become very rare due to earlier diagnosis and effective therapy of the disease. It should be considered in the differential diagnosis, even in adults suffering from acute diarrhea and acidosis.[77] [M] Marked by passage of fluid or unformed non-bloody stools, acidosis, and hypokalemia (low potassium).[78] [C] Results from osmotic action of undigested solutes in the colon, fermentation, altered intestinal motility, and zinc deficiency in CD. [R] CD-related acute diarrhea disappears on GFD. [78]	Zinc.[34]

+ (S) = Classic sign/symptom; (AT) = Atypical sign/symptom; (AD) Associated Disorder; (C) = Complication.

++ [P] = Prevalance; [D] = Description; [M] = Sign/symptom; [C] = CD related cause; [R] = Response to gluten Free diet (GFD).

Health Manifestations of Celiac Disease (CD)
Section B: Signs, Symptoms, Associated Disorders and Complications

Affected System	Affected Organ	ID No.	Manifestation	Type[+]	Current Medical Information [++]	Deficient Nutrient
Digestive System	Small intestine	109	Diarrhea, Chronic [1,2,3,5,34,73,79, 80,81]	(S)	[P] Most frequent symptom of people with untreated CD.[73] 79% of patients experienced diarrhea before treatment, and 17% had chronic diarrhea (of lesser severity) after treatment.[79] [D] Chronic diarrhea is a classic symptom of malabsorption in CD characterized by alteration in stool formation and quantity indicating extensive damage to small intestinal mucosa.[3] Loss of potassium alters bowel motility, encourages anorexia, and can introduce a cycle of bowel distress.[34] Diarrhea is one of the clinical manifestations of zinc deficiency and has been isolated in infants with CD and diarrhea.[80] Chronic diarrhea interferes with normal carbohydrate salvage by colonic bacteria (reclaiming energy, generating short-chain fatty acids, and stimulating sodium and fluid absorption), production of butyrate and proprionate for nourishing the colonocytes, and production of acetate for the liver. Study demonstrated that after treatment with a GFD, chronic diarrhea persists in a substantial percentage of patients. Athough ongoing gluten ingestion is one possible cause, other causes may be more frequent. Other causes include microscopic colitis, steatorrhea secondary to pancreatic insufficiency, dietary lactose malabsorption, anal sphincter dysfunction causing fecal incontinence, and the irritable bowel syndrome. Therefore, a diagnostic evaluation of diarrhea in CD after treatment seems warranted.[79] Study investigating the effect of a GFD on GI symptoms revealed that steatorrhea occurred in only 1/5th of CD patients.[73] Study measuring IgG and IgA isotypes and IgG subclasses observed that a significantly higher proportion of patients with positive IgA gliadin antibodies reported unexplained diarrhea attacks.[5] [M] Marked by passage of bulky, frequent fluid or unformed stool, and gas. [C] Results from osmotic action of undigested nutrients in the small intestine, dysbiosis, altered intestinal motility, and deficiencies of zinc, vitamin A, and vitamin B12 in CD. [R] CD-related chronic diarrhea responds to GFD within days for most patients.[73] Correction of low vitamin A and zinc is important.[81]	Vitamin A, Vitamin B12, Zinc.

[+] (S) = Classic sign/symptom; (AT) = Atypical sign/symptom; (AD) Associated Disorder; (C) = Complication.

[++] [P] = Prevalance; [D] = Description; [M] = Sign/symptom; [C] = CD related cause; [R] = Response to gluten Free diet (GFD).

Health Manifestations of Celiac Disease (CD)
Section B: Signs, Symptoms, Associated Disorders and Complications

Affected System	Affected Organ	ID No.	Manifestation	Type[+]	Current Medical Information [++]	Deficient Nutrient
Digestive System	Small intestine	110	Duodenal Erosions in the Second Part of the Duodenum [82]	(C)	[P] New presentation representing 7% of patients with untreated CD.[82] [D] Duodenal erosions in the second part of the duodenum is specific for villous atrophy, although sensitivity is low. Erosions are accompanied by edema and spasm. The second part of the duodenum consists of the descending duodenum, where bile from the liver and secretions from the pancreas enter the small intestine. Study observing incidence of duodenal erosions in the second part of the duodenum as an abnormality associated with villous atrophy in CD patients at endoscopy demonstrated that 5 patients out of 1,200 over the course of 2 years showed erosions were multiple, superficial, and present in the second half of the duodenum but not the duodenal bulb. Of the 5 patients, 4 had at least one other endoscopic marker: scalloped duodenal folds (3), fold loss (2), or mosaic pattern mucosa (2). Finding should be added to the list of endoscopic markers of CD because this pattern of erosions is not found in patients without CD.[82] [M] Marked by typical findings of CD (iron deficiency anemia, osteopenia/osteoporosis).[82] Erosions show as blood in vomitus (red) and stool (dark, tarry), heartburn, indigestion, nausea, and possible epigastric pain. [C] Results from chronic gluten exposure. Resulting deficiencies of omega-3 fatty acids, folic acid, and iron may exacerbate inflammation. [R] Studies are inadequate to determine effect of GFD	Folic acid, Omega-3 fatty acids, Iron may exacerbate.
Digestive System	Small intestine	111	Edema, Intestinal [3,83]	(S)	[P] Common in active CD.[3] [D] Intestinal edema is characterized by fluid accumulation in intestinal mucosa and can be demonstrated by contrast radiography and sonography showing abnormal appearance of the small bowel wall structure.[83] [M] Marked by abdominal bloating pain and distention. [C] Results from inflammation of the mucosa in response to gluten exposure. [R] CD-related intestinal edema resolves on GFD.	Not applicable.

[+] (S) = Classic sign/symptom; (AT) = Atypical sign/symptom; (AD) Associated Disorder; (C) = Complication.

[++] [P] = Prevalance; [D] = Description; [M] = Sign/symptom; [C] = CD related cause; [R] = Response to gluten Free diet (GFD).

Recognizing Celiac Disease Signs, Symptoms, Associated Disorders & Complications

Health Manifestations of Celiac Disease (CD)
Section B: Signs, Symptoms, Associated Disorders and Complications

Affected System	Affected Organ	ID No.	Manifestation	Type[+]	Current Medical Information [++]	Deficient Nutrient
Digestive System	Small intestine	112	Food Allergy, IgE and Non IgE [84,85]	(AD)	[P] New association with CD. [D] Food allergy (FA) is characterized by an abnormal immunologic reactivity to food proteins. The GI tract serves not only a nutritive function but also is a major immunologic organ. Although previously thought to be triggered primarily by an IgE-mediated mechanism of injury, considerable evidence now suggests that non-IgE mechanisms may also be involved in the pathogenesis of food allergy.[85] There is little known about the initial event that triggers FA. Hyperpermeability of the intestinal barrier is believed to contribute to the pathogenesis of food allergy.[84] Alteration in mucosal permeability is a secondary phenomenon, possibly caused by hypersensitivity reactions in the intestinal mucosa.[84] Enteropathy is similiar to a GI virus response. Heiner's syndrome marks a lung response. Review of research data allows construction of the following hypothesis for a new classification of FA: the clinical manifestations of food allergy, expressed in target organs, may be the result of immunologic injury mediated by interaction of food antigens with contiguous elements of mucosal associated lymphoid tissue. These appear to be modulated by relative imbalances of the Th1/Th2 paradigm, which may be the ultimate determinant governing the expression of food allergy as IgEmediated, non-IgE-mediated, or mixed forms of IgE/non-IgE mechanisms in food allergy.[85] [M] Marked by eczema, sudden hives, angioedema, asthma, rhinitis, and anaphylaxis in IgE reactions. Non-GI reactions involve a delay of 2 hours and include enterocolitis with vomiting, lethargy, bloody stools, edema, abdominal cramps and distention. [C] Results from unclear etiology. [R] GFD appears to have little effect on food allergy occurrence.	Not applicable.

+ (S) = Classic sign/symptom; (AT) = Atypical sign/symptom; (AD) Associated Disorder; (C) = Complication.

++ [P] = Prevalance; [D] = Description; [M] = Sign/symptom; [C] = CD related cause; [R] = Response to gluten Free diet (GFD).

Health Manifestations of Celiac Disease (CD)
Section B: Signs, Symptoms, Associated Disorders and Complications

Affected System	Affected Organ	ID No.	Manifestation	Type[+]	Current Medical Information [++]	Deficient Nutrient [++]
Digestive System	Small intestine	113	Gluten Sensitive Enteritis [2,3,84,85,86]	(S)	[P] Present in all patients with active CD.[3] [D] Gluten sensitive enteritis is characterized by inflammation of the small intestinal mucosa that results from a genetically based immunologic intolerance to ingested gluten. The inflammation causes damage to villi with progressive atrophy and elongation of crypts, increased round cells in the lamina propria, and cuboidal epithelial cells with few, irregular microvilli. The inflammatory sequence depends on a competent cellular immune response in the small intestine. It also likely affects the structural support and microcirculation of the villus, leading to collapse of the villus. The thickening of the crypt is not so much a response to loss of surface enterocytes but represents inflammation of the mucosa. This damage is most intense in the proximal small intestine and decreases caudally. The extent of the damage to the intestine determines the malabsorptive consequences of the disease.[3] Both gastric and small intestinal permeability is disrupted in patients with CD.[84] There is a clear association between degree of mucosal damage and the intestinal-permeability ratio, and a normal ratio generally implies near-normal small intestinal morphology. A raised intestinal permeability of the mucosal lining could predispose to a high absorption of gluten and exacerbate an existing lesion and hence convert a latent to an overt enteropathy.[86] [M] Marked by GI distress including abdominal pain and distention, diarrhea and/or constipation, steatorrhea, gas, weight loss or failure to thrive; resulting deficiencies of carbohydrate, protein, fat and fat-soluble vitamins (D, E, A, and K), iron, zinc, folic acid, and calcium are common. A wide spectrum of both pathophysiologic changes in the intestines and clinical syndromes may develop.[3] [C] Results from immune response to dietary gluten exposure. [R] Functional recovery occurs early on a GFD and precedes small intestinal morphometric recovery which is often incomplete.[85]	Not applicable.

[+] (S) = Classic sign/symptom; (AT) = Atypical sign/symptom; (AD) Associated Disorder; (C) = Complication.

[++] [P] = Prevalance; [D] = Description; [M] = Sign/symptom; [C] = CD related cause; [R] = Response to gluten Free diet (GFD).

Health Manifestations of Celiac Disease (CD)
Section B: Signs, Symptoms, Associated Disorders and Complications

Affected System	Affected Organ	ID No.	Manifestation	Type[+]	Current Medical Information [++]	Deficient Nutrient
Digestive System	Small intestine	114	Increased Intestinal Permeability [84,86, 87,88]	(AD)	[P] Common in patients with either CD or gluten sensitivity without CD. [85,86,87] [D] Increased intestinal permeability is characterized by greater than normal intestinal permeability allowing for the penetration of harmful entities into the circulation from the gut. Both gastric and small intestinal permeability is disrupted in patients with CD. Intestinal permeability is determined by interactions among several barrier components including the unstirred water layer, mucosal surface hydrophobicity, the surface mucous coat, epithelial factors (especially tight junctions) and endothelial factors. Each of these components has a different permeability property, but the epithelium has been the most intensively studied. Hyperpermeability of this barrier is believed to contribute to the pathogenesis of CD. [84] Permeation of disaccharides into the small intestine is by the paracellular route and thus it correlates with degree of "leakiness" of the intestine, whereas monosaccharides are absorbed via the transcellular route so their absorption correlates with mucosal surface area. There is a clear association between degree of mucosal damage and the intestinal-permeability ratio, and a normal ratio generally implies near-normal small intestinal morphology. A raised intestinal permeability of the mucosal lining could predispose to a high absorption of gluten and exacerbate an existing lesion and hence convert a latent to an overt enteropathy. Since timing of the histological response to a GFD is so variable, a sugar permeability test is an appropriate assessment, particularly within the first 6 months of treatment. [86] It is important to test gastric and intestinal permeability simultaneously in CD, such as a gas chromatographic method to estimate rhamose, lactulose, and sucrose in urine. [87] Study comparing changes in intestinal permeability (lactulose/rhamose absorption as an indicator of microvilli recovery) with changes in intestinal biopsy (villus area, crypt length, and mitotic count per crypt) at diagnosis and various intervals after commencing a GFD to assess small bowel recovery in adults with CD demonstrated intestinal permeability improves within 2 months after starting a GFD, but measurable intestinal biopsy improvement requires ingestion of a GFD for at least 3-6 months, and even then remains incomplete. [88] [M] Marked by positivity to a sugar-permeability test. [86,87,88] [C] Results from action of an agent that affects the cell junctures including foods (eg, lactose, cayenne pepper), organisms, and toxins in addition to gluten. [86] [R] Intestinal permeability improves within 2 months after starting a GFD. [88]	Not applicable.

+ (S) = Classic sign/symptom; (AT) = Atypical sign/symptom; (AD) Associated Disorder; (C) = Complication.

++ [P] = Prevalence; [D] = Description; [M] = Sign/symptom; [C] = CD related cause; [R] = Response to gluten Free diet (GFD).

Affected System	Affected Organ	ID No.	Manifestation	Type[+]	Current Medical Information [++]	Deficient Nutrient
Digestive System	Small intestine	115	Jejunitis, Chronic Ulcerative [1,59]	(C)	[P] May be present in patients with active CD.[59] [D] Chronic ulcerative jejunitis is a severe complication. It arises in the setting of CD and most cases are probably part of the evolution of reactive intra-epithelial lymphocytes through a low grade lymphocytic neoplasm to a high-grade tumor. If the ulceration occurs at a time when the neoplastic T-cells are of a low grade, morphological recognition of tumor cells in the ulcers may be impossible.[59] [M] Marked by bowel changes, abdominal distention and pain, chronic occult bleeding and possible signs of anemia (weakness, easy fatigability, pallor). [C] Results from chronic gluten exposure in CD. [R] May respond to a strict GFD.	Not applicable.
Digestive System	Small intestine	116	Lactose Intolerance [3,34,55,84]	(S)	[P] Affects about 50% of untreated celiacs.[3] [D] Lactose intolerance is a well known symptom of carbohydrate malabsorption characterized by inability to properly digest lactose, the sugar in milk, due to low brush border lactase activity. Undigested lactose acts osmotically to draw water into the intestine. Colonic bacteria ferment the lactose, generating short-chain fatty acids and hydrogen gas resulting in the classic symptoms.[34] Lactose increases intestinal permeability.[84] Positive response to a breath hydrogen test (BHT), involving 1 - 3 hours of time post ingestion of lactose test dose, signifies malabsorption in the small intestine and fermentation in the colon. If BHT is positive before 60 minutes, the result implies bacteria is abnormally present in the small intestine, causing fermentation there. Endoscopy is used to measure activity of lactase in a tissue sample. Study investigating the clinical manifestations of CD related to malnutrition and analyzing the associations between CD and other diagnoses confirmed the known association of CD with lactase deficiency.[55] [M] Marked by diarrhea, bloating, flatulence (gas), and cramping abdominal pain/distention. [C] Results secondarily in CD from lactase deficiency due to diffuse villous atrophy. [R] CD-related lactose intolerance should improve in 90% of newly diagnosed celiacs.[3]	Not applicable.

[+] (S) = Classic sign/symptom; (AT) = Atypical sign/symptom; (AD) Associated Disorder; (C) = Complication.

[++] [P] = Prevalance; [D] = Description; [M] = Sign/symptom; [C] = CD related cause; [R] = Response to gluten Free diet (GFD).

Health Manifestations of Celiac Disease (CD)
Section B: Signs, Symptoms, Associated Disorders and Complications

Affected System	Affected Organ	ID No.	Manifestation	Type[+]	Current Medical Information [++]	Deficient Nutrient
Digestive System	Small intestine	117	Maltose Intoleance [3,34]	(S)	[P] Common in people with untreated CD.[3] [D] Maltose, the sugar in starch, intolerance is a well known symptom characterized by inability to properly digest maltose due to low brush border maltase activity. Undigested maltose acts osmotically to draw water into the intestine, and colonic bacteria ferment the maltose, generating short-chain fatty acids and hydrogen gas resulting in the classic symptoms.[34] Positive response to a breath hydrogen test (BHT), involving 1 - 3 hours of time post ingestion of maltose test dose, signifies malabsorption in the small intestine and fermentation in the colon. If BHT is positive before 60 minutes, the result implies bacteria is abnormally present in the small intestine, causing fermentation there. [M] Marked by diarrhea, bloating, flatulence, and cramping abdominal pain/distention. [C] Results secondarily from maltase deficiency due to diffuse villous atrophy in CD. [R] CD-related maltose intolerance improves in most newly diagnosed patients on GFD.	Not applicable.

Digestive System	Small intestine	118	Milk Intolerance (Bovine Beta Casein Enteropathy) [89,90]	(AD)	[P] CD occurs in 12% of patients with cow's milk intolerance.[89]
					
					[D] Bovine beta casein enteropathy is characterized by raised serum IgA antibodies to bovine beta casein and damage to the mucosa of the jejunum.
					    Study investigating 54 infants with malabsorption syndrome and cow's milk intolerance demonstrated high incidence of CD 2 years after bovine beta casein enteropathy diagnosis in infants on a gluten containing diet. CD regarded as the primary disorder.[89]
					    Study investigating the antibody response to bovine-casein to establish whether such an antibody response is specific to Type 1 diabetes demonstrated that significantly raised antibodies to beta-casein were found in patients with Type 1 diabetes, latent autoimmune diabetes in adults (LADA), and CD. Highest response to beta-casein in Type 1 diabetic patients and in patients with CD could reflect the gut mucosal immune disorder common to Type 1 diabetes and CD. Furthermore, the elevated beta-casein antibody levels found in LADA patients suggest that the antibody response to this protein may be relevant in autoimmune diabetes.[90]
					
					[M] Marked by diarrhea, failure to thrive, vomiting, atopic eczema, and recurrent respiratory infections.[89]
					
					[C] Results from immune mechanism.
					
					[R] CD-related bovine beta-casein enteropathy responds to a casein-free GFD.
						Not applicable.

+ (S) = Classic sign/symptom; (AT) = Atypical sign/symptom; (AD) Associated Disorder; (C) = Complication.

++ [P] = Prevalance; [D] = Description; [M] = Sign/symptom; [C] = CD related cause; [R] = Response to gluten Free diet (GFD).

Health Manifestations of Celiac Disease (CD)
Section B: Signs, Symptoms, Associated Disorders and Complications

Affected System	Affected Organ	ID No.	Manifestation	Type[+]	Current Medical Information[++]	Deficient Nutrient
Digestive System	Small intestine	119	Postbulbar Duodenal Ulceration and Stenosis [1,91]	(C)	[P] More common complication of CD than previously thought.[91] [D] Postbulbar duodenal ulceration and stenosis is a chronic duodenal disorder characterized by thickening with excoriation penetrating the muscularis mucosae associated with villous atrophy. Case histories of 5 patients with CD and postbulbar duodenal ulceration and stenosis describe unexpected finding until endoscopic biopsy revealed villous atrophy. It may precede the clinical diagnosis of CD or occur when there are minimal symptoms and nonspecific radiographic findings for the disease.[91] [M] Marked by bloating, abdominal distention, nausea and localized pain relieved by food. [C] Results from gluten exposure in CD. [R] CD-related duodenal ulcerations resolve on GFD.	Not applicable.
Digestive System	Small intestine	120	Small Bowel Intussusception [1,92, 93,94]	(C)	[P] CD in intussusception is rare.[92] 16% of CD patients showed intussusception.[93] [D] Small bowel intussusception, a bowel derangement, is characterized by the slipping of one section of intestine into another, leading to obstruction. Intussusception associated with CD often presents in an atypical way: elementary forms, spontaneously resolvent and recidivious.[92] Study investigating results of barium meal with flow-through examinations of the small intestine in CD patients demonstrated one or more images of invagination present in 4 of 25 cases. In 15 of 25 CD patients there were one or more central or marginal lacunar images probably due in varying degrees to disorder of intestinal motility in hypotonic loops with edematous walls.[93] Concomitant failure to thrive and cramping abdominal pain should prompt investigation for CD and small bowel intussusception.[94] Case report of diagnosis of CD in a 9 month old infant with bowel intussusception appears to be earliest described.[92] [M] Marked by weight loss, denutrition symptoms, concomitant cramping abdominal pain and severe failure to thrive in children.[94] [C] Results from disorders of motility in CD as indirect cause.[92,93] [R] GFD allows evolution and prevents recurrence of intussusception.[92]	Not applicable.

[+] (S) = Classic sign/symptom; (AT) = Atypical sign/symptom; (AD) Associated Disorder; (C) = Complication.

[++] [P] = Prevalance; [D] = Description; [M] = Sign/symptom; [C] = CD related cause; [R] = Response to gluten Free diet (GFD).

Health Manifestations of Celiac Disease (CD)
Section B: Signs, Symptoms, Associated Disorders and Complications

Affected System	Affected Organ	ID No.	Manifestation	Type[+]	Current Medical Information [++]	Deficient Nutrient
Digestive System	Small intestine	121	Sucrose Intolerance and Sucrosemia [5,34,95,96]	(S)	[P] Sucrose intolerance is common in CD.[95] 100% of patients with untreated CD and 75% of first-degree relatives showed sucrosemia.[96] [D] Sucrose intolerance, a well known symptom of CD, is characterized by inability to properly digest sucrose due to low brush border sucrase activity. Undigested sucrose acts osmotically to draw water into the intestine, and colonic bacteria ferment the sucrose generating short-chain fatty acids and hydrogen gas resulting in the classic symptoms.[34] Positive response to a breath hydrogen test (BHT), involving 1 - 3 hours of time post ingestion of sucrose test dose, signifies malabsorption in the small intestine and fermentation in the colon. If BHT is positive before 60 minutes, the result implies bacteria is abnormally present in the small intestine, causing fermentation there. Endoscopy is used to measure sucrase activity in tissue sample. Sucrosemia is characterized by the abnormal presence of sucrose molecules in the bloodstream and is shown to affect all patients with CD. Study to develop serum tests of small intestinal permeability demonstrated sucrose in the blood of all untreated celiacs who were IgA endomysial antibody negative. Brush border sucrase activity was low.[95] Study investigating intestinal permeability demonstrated the presence of sucrose in sera of all untreated patients with CD after an 8-g or 50-g challenge compared to none of the treated CD patients having small intestinal mucosal atrophy.[96] [M] Marked by diarrhea, abdominal pain/distention, bloating, flatulence and cramps..[95] [C] Results secondarily from sucrase deficiency due to diffuse villous atrophy in CD. [R] CD-related sucrose intolerance improves on GFDand sucrosemia resolves.[95]	Not applicable.
Digestive System	Large intestine	122	Colonic Volvulus and Ulcerative Jejunoileitis [1,97]	(C)	[P] Rare complication of CD.[97] [D] Colonic volvulus, or twisting of the bowel on itself, is described in a case report of a patient diagnosed with CD post-operatively and subsequently following his poor course after elected surgery for hernia repair. A cecal volvulus and an ulcerative jejunoileitis developed that required extensive intestinal resection. Patient had a long-standing history of diarrhea and abdominal distension with a diagnosis of IBS.[97] [M] Marked by development of short bowel syndrome with poor course after reinstatement of oral diet.[97] [C] Results from gluten sensitive enteropathy. [R] Patient improved on a GFD after diagnosis of CD.[97]	Not applicable.

+ (S) = Classic sign/symptom; (AT) = Atypical sign/symptom; (AD) Associated Disorder; (C) = Complication.

++ [P] = Prevalance; [D] = Description; [M] = Sign/symptom; [C] = CD related cause; [R] = Response to gluten Free diet (GFD).

Health Manifestations of Celiac Disease (CD)
Section B: Signs, Symptoms, Associated Disorders and Complications

Affected System	Affected Organ	ID No.	Manifestation	Type[+]	Current Medical Information [++]	Deficient Nutrient
Digestive System	Large intestine	123	Colitis, Collagenous [1,98,99,100]	(C)	[P] CD is found in 20% of patients with collagenous colitis (CC),[98] and may be the presenting manifestation of CD.[99] [D] Collagenous colitis is characterized by microscopic inflammation of the large intestine consisting predominantly of lymphocytic infiltration and a thickened subepithelial collagen band. Endoscopic and radiological examinations are usually normal.[100] Study investigating the clinical features of CC and lymphocytic colitis (LC) demonstrated that CC and LC are largely similar but the differences in the occurrence of autoimmune conditions and bronchial asthma suggest that they differ in immunopathogenesis. Concomittent autoimmune diseases were present in 53% of patients with CC.[98] Study investigating the presence of CD in patients with chronic diarrhea and the initial finding of collagenous colitis demonstrated that CC may be the presenting clinical and pathologic feature of CD. All patients found to have CD had severely abnormal small bowel biopsy changes characteristic of untreated CD. In some patients lymphocytic or collagenous gastritis were also detected with or without CD. Diagnosis of CC should lead the clinician to consider exclusion of underlying occult CD.[99] [M] Marked by diarrhea, with or without cramping, bloating, abdominal distention, weight loss, and lactose intolerance.[98] [C] Results from unclear mechanisms involved in the pathogenesis.[100] [R] Diarrhea resolved in all patients with collagenous colitis and CD on a GFD; collagen deposits persisted in more than half of patients.[99]	Omega-3 fatty acids, Vitamin A may exacerbate.
Digestive System	Large intestine	124	Colitis, Lymphocytic [1,98,100]	(C)	(C) [P] CD is common, occurring in 14.8% of patients with lymphocytic colitis.[98] [D] Lymphocytic colitis (LC) is a microscopic inflammation with lymphocytic infiltration of the large intestine mucosa characterized by secretory diarrhea. Up to 10% of adults undergoing colonoscopy for investigation of chronic diarrhea and having endoscopically normal appearing mucosa may have LC.[100] Study investigating the clinical features of collagenous colitis (CC) and lymphocytic colitis demonstrated CC and LC are largely similar but the differences in the occurrence of autoimmune conditions and bronchial asthma suggest that they differ in immunopathogenesis. Hypolactasia (lactase deficiency) is common, affecting 54% of patients with LC. Concomitant autoimmune diseases are common (25.9%) as is bronchial asthma (25.9%).[98] [M] Marked by diarrhea, with or without cramping, bloating, abdominal distention, weight loss, and lactose intolerance.[98] [C] Results from unclear immunopathogenesis.[98] [R] CD-related diarrhea improves on GFD.	Omega-3 fatty acid, Vitamin A deficiencies may exacerbate.[34]

[+] (S) = Classic sign/symptom; (AT) = Atypical sign/symptom; (AD) Associated Disorder; (C) = Complication.

[++] [P] = Prevalance; [D] = Description; [M] = Sign/symptom; [C] = CD related cause; [R] = Response to gluten Free diet (GFD).

Health Manifestations of Celiac Disease (CD)
Section B: Signs, Symptoms, Associated Disorders and Complications

Affected System	Affected Organ	ID No.	Manifestation	Type+	Current Medical Information ++	Deficient Nutrient
Digestive System	Large intestine	125	Colitis, Ulcerative [1,34,101]	(AD)	[P] Significantly increased prevalence of familial ulcerative colitis in patients with CD.[101] [D] Ulcerative colitis is an inflammatory disorder of the colon characterized by continuous inflammation of the mucosa and submucosa, usually with small ulcers, extending from the rectum and typically involving the distal colon, rectum, and anus and producing bloody diarrhea. Iron deficiency anemia often develops. Case control study evaluating the familial occurrence of inflammatory bowel disease in 600 first degree relatives of 111 consecutive patients with CD revealed 10 cases of IBD of whom 7 cases were ulcerative colitis and 3 cases were Crohn's disease.[101] [M] Marked by rectal bleeding, frequent diarrhea with outpouring of blood, mucous, and pus increasing fecal content, pain with the passage of stools, and probable weight loss, anemia, and nutritional deficits. [C] Results from unclear mechanism. [R] GFD prevents increased morbidity from malnutrition and malignancy in untreated CD.	Omega-3 fatty acid, Vitamin A deficiencies may exacerbate.[34]
Digestive System	Large intestine	126	Constipation [1,73]	(AT)	[P] About 20% of people with celiac disease have constipation instead of diarrhea.[73] [D] Constipation is a chronic digestive symptom of CD characterized by alteration in stool formation, consistency, and evacuation. [M] Marked by decrease in frequency of bowel movements with difficult or incomplete passage of stool and/or passage of excessively dry, hard stool or soft pasty stool, flatulence, gas, bloating and cramping. [C] Results from abnormal bowel motility, dysbiosis, and malabsorption in CD. [R] CD-related constipation responds to GFD.[73]	Magnesium, Vitamin B$_1$. Vitamin B$_{12}$.
Digestive System	Large intestine	127	Constipation Alternating with Diarrhea [1,73]	(AT)	[P] Common in people with untreated CD.[73] [D] Constipation alternating with diarrhea is a chronic digestive symptom of CD characterized by alteration in stool formation, consistency, and evacuation. [M] Marked by passage of excessively dry, hard stool and loose stool in the same movement or at different times, gas and flatulence. [C] Results from abnormal bowel motility, dysbiosis, and malabsorption in CD. [R] CD-related constipation alternating with diarrhea responds to GFD.[73]	Magnesium, Vitamin B$_1$.

+ (S) = Classic sign/symptom; (AT) = Atypical sign/symptom; (AD) Associated Disorder; (C) = Complication.

++ [P] = Prevalance; [D] = Description; [M] = Sign/symptom; [C] = CD related cause; [R] = Response to gluten Free diet (GFD).

Health Manifestations of Celiac Disease (CD)
Section B: Signs, Symptoms, Associated Disorders and Complications

Affected System	Affected Organ	ID No.	Manifestation	Type+	Current Medical Information ++	Deficient Nutrient
Digestive System	Large intestine	128	Crohn's Disease [1,55,80,102]	(AD)	[P] Association with CD is statistically significant.[55] [D] Crohn's disease is an inflammatory bowel disease characterized by patchy inflamed areas involving the full thickness of the intestinal wall occurring anywhere in the intestinal tract in addition to mucosal disease. Some of the symptoms of Crohn's disease, like retarded growth and hypogonadism, have been related to hypozinchemia (low blood zinc level).[80] Study investigating the clinical manifestations of CD related to malnutrition and analyzing the associations between CD and other diagnoses revealed a statistically significant association of CD with Crohn's disease.[55] Study investigating whether there were anti-Saccharomyces cerevisiae antibodies (ASCA) in biopsy-confirmed CD patients and patients with inflammatory bowel diseases demonstrated ASCA positivity not only in Crohn's disease but also in CD. It is conceivable that ASCA positivity correlates with the autoimmune inflammation of the small intestines and it is a specific marker of Crohn's disease.[102] [M] Marked by non-bloody diarrhea, abdominal pain, bloating, steatorrhea, and weight loss. Complications include abcess, fistulas, and strictures. [C] Results from unknown pathological mechanism. [R] GFD can normalize zinc levels and prevent increased morbidity from malnutrition and malignancy from untreated CD.	Omega-3 fatty acid, Zinc deficiencies may exacerbate.[34]
Digestive System	Large intestine	129	Gas, Excessive [73,103]	(S)	[P] Common, presenting complaint in 50% of patients with untreated CD.[103] [D] Excessive gas is a well known symptom of CD characterized by production of mainly hydrogen and carbon dioxide gas in the lumen due to bacterial metabolism of undigested fermentable food entering the colon, altered motility, and dysbiosis. [M] Marked by abdominal pain, bloating, distention, and lingering stink after passing foul-smelling gas. [C] Results from spasm and maldigestion in CD and niacin (vitamin B_3) deficiency. [R] CD-related gas resolves on GFD.[73]	Niacin.
Digestive System	Large intestine	130	Gastrointestinal Bleeding, Occult [1]	(C)	[P] Increased occurrence in people with untreated CD. [D] Occult gastrointestinal (GI) bleeding is characterized by unseen or minute quantities of blood in stool. [M] Marked by positivity to fecal occult blood test. [C] Results from vitamin K and/or vitamin C deficiency, chronic GI inflammation in CD. [R] CD-related GI bleeding resolves on GFD.	Vitamin C, Vitamin K.

+ (S) = Classic sign/symptom; (AT) = Atypical sign/symptom; (AD) Associated Disorder; (C) = Complication.

++ [P] = Prevalance; [D] = Description; [M] = Sign/symptom; [C] = CD related cause; [R] = Response to gluten Free diet (GFD).

Health Manifestations of Celiac Disease (CD)
Section B: Signs, Symptoms, Associated Disorders and Complications

Affected System	Affected Organ	ID No.	Manifestation	Type[+]	Current Medical Information [++]	Deficient Nutrient
Digestive System	Large intestine	131	Irritable Bowel Syndrome (IBS) [104,105,106, 107,108]	(AT)	[P] Prevalence of CD is 3.3% in irritable bowel syndrome (IBS) patients. [104] [D] Irritable bowel syndrome is a motility disorder without anatomic cause involving the entire GI tract characterized by 1) abdominal pain usually relieved by defecation or passing of gas, 2) disturbance of evacuation, 3) bloating and abdominal distention, and 4) mucus in the stool. There is an overlap of IBS symptoms with those of CD, and selected patients should be tested for the latter disease. [105] Study involving 2000 volunteers recruited from primary care practices to establish prevalence of CD in the general population and in specific conditions such as IBS, iron deficiency anemia, fatigue, and other CDrelated conditions demonstrated a prevalence of 3.3% CD in participants with IBS. [104] Study demonstrated that testing for CD in patients with suspected IBS is likely to be cost-effective even at a relatively low CD prevalence and with small improvements in qualtiy of life with a GFD. [106] Study assessing the association of CD with IBS in patients fulfilling Rome II criteria demonstrated that a panel of immunological tests including IgG antigliadin, IgA antigliadin, and EMA should be mandatory in assessment of patients who fulfill diagnostic criteria for IBS when referred to secondary care. The implications of missed diagnoses are the potential complications for osteoporosis, infertility, and an increased risk of malignant disease. [107] Screening of patients with the common symptoms of IBS is becoming accepted standard of practice. [108] [M] Marked by constipation, gas, intestinal spasm and pain with diarrhea, or alternating constipation gas and diarrhea. [C] Results from unclear etiology. [R] CD-related IBS responds to GFD with improvements in quality of life. [106]	Not applicable.

[+] (S) = Classic sign/symptom; (AT) = Atypical sign/symptom; (AD) Associated Disorder; (C) = Complication.

[++] [P] = Prevalance; [D] = Description; [M] = Sign/symptom; [C] = CD related cause; [R] = Response to gluten Free diet (GFD).

Health Manifestations of Celiac Disease (CD)
Section B: Signs, Symptoms, Associated Disorders and Complications

Affected System	Affected Organ	ID No.	Manifestation	Type[+]	Current Medical Information [++]	Deficient Nutrient
Glandular System	Adrenal	132	Addison's Disease [1,109]	(AD)	[P] Prevalence of CD is 7.9% in patients with Addison's disease. [109] [D] Addison's Disease is an immunologically mediated insidious adrenal disease characterized by adrenocortical failure. CD is often asymptomatic or associated with unspecific symptoms. Study demonstrated high prevalence of CD in patients with Addison's disease. All patients with CD carried the CD-associated HLA haplotype DR3-DQ2. Risk of CD seems to be higher than can be explained by the common DR3-DQ2 association alone. Addison's patients should be screened for CD on a regular basis. [109] [M] Marked in early stages by weakness and fatigue, progressing to hyperpigmentation of skin and mucous membranes, dark freckles, vitiligo, bluish-black discoloration of areolas and mucous membranes, nausea, vomiting, anorexia, diarrhea, decreased tolerance to cold with hypometabolism; dizziness and fainting may occur. Late stage includes weight loss, small heart size, orthostatic hypotension, hypoglycemia following fasting, hyperkalemia and elevated blood urea nitrogen (BUN). [C] Results from autoimmune mechanism. [R] CD-related Addison's disease responds to GFD.	Not applicable.
Glandular System	Liver	133	Autoimmune Hepatitis [1,110,111]	(AD)	[P] Presence of CD in autoimmune hepatitis is high (at least one in 36 patients) [110] [D] Autoimmune hepatitis is an immunologically mediated disorder characterized by chronic liver disease. Because CD may be a cause of unexplained elevated liver enzymes levels, a high index of suspicion is required. [111] Study investigating the frequency of CD in autoimmune hepatitis, demonstrated presence of CD is high and predominantly asymptomatic. Subtotal villous atrophy was present in all patients undergoing duodenal biopsy. Screening with anti-endomysial and anti-gliadin antibodies should be performed and results confirmed with intestinal biopsy. [110] [M] Predominantly asymptomatic. [110,111] [C] Results from autoimmune mechanism. [110] [R] In majority of patients, CD-related elevated liver enzyme levels will normalize on GFD. [111]	Not applicable.

[+] (S) = Classic sign/symptom; (AT) = Atypical sign/symptom; (AD) Associated Disorder; (C) = Complication.

[++] [P] = Prevalance; [D] = Description; [M] = Sign/symptom; [C] = CD related cause; [R] = Response to gluten Free diet (GFD).

Health Manifestations of Celiac Disease (CD)
Section B: Signs, Symptoms, Associated Disorders and Complications

Affected System	Affected Organ	ID No.	Manifestation	Type+	Current Medical Information ++	Deficient Nutrient
Glandular System	Liver	134	Non-Alcoholic Fatty Liver Disease [1,55,111,112,113]	(C)	[P] Statistically significantly associated fatty liver disease in CD.[55] Prevalence of silent CD is 3.4% in patients with non-alcoholic fatty liver disease.[112] [D] Non-alcoholic fatty liver is a non-inflammatory hepatic disorder characterized by degenerative changes in the liver secondary to excessive accumulation of lipid in hepatocytes. Because most patients do not have overt GI symptoms, a high index of suspicion for CD is required.[111] Serology Study demonstrated high prevalence of CD in patients with fatty liver disease. Serology screening for CD should include tests for anti-endomysium antibodies in addition to anti-transglutaminase antibodies, since positivity for tissue transglutaminase antibodies in the absence of confirmatory anti-endomysium antibodies is not sufficient to perform diagnostic endoscopy.[112] Case report of a 25 year old woman with swelling of the lower limbs documents development of serious diffuse large droplet steatosis as a result of malnutrition due to unrecognized CD, later confirmed by small bowel biopsy finding of total villous atrophy. Albumin, prothrombin time, and trace elements normalized with gradual improvement in amino transferase levels on GFD.[113] [M] Marked by non-tender, diffuse hepatomegaly, elevated liver enzymes, and hypoproteinemia. [C] Results from malnutrition, especially protein in CD.[113] [R] After 6 months on GFD, liver enzymes normalized in study patients.[112]	Omega-6 fatty acids, Protein, Vitamin K.
Glandular System	Liver	135	Hepatic Granulomatous Disease [1,45]	(AD)	[P] New association with CD.[45] [D] Hepatic granulomatous disease is an immunologically mediated infiltrative chronic liver disorder characterized by growth of small granulomas. Liver biopsy is essential for diagnosis. Case study of a patient with CD in whom idiopathic thrombocytopenic purpura and associated hepatic granulomatous disease developed is described. The three processes appear linked through autoimmune mechanisms.[45] [M] Marked by minor liver enlargement, mild change in liver enzymes, and possible fever. [C] Results from unclear etiology involving host attempt to protect against irritants; autoimmune mechanism appears to be involved. [R] GFD does not appear to reverse granuloma formation but will prevent increased morbidity from malnutrition and malignancy from untreated CD.	Not applicable.

+ (S) = Classic sign/symptom; (AT) = Atypical sign/symptom; (AD) Associated Disorder; (C) = Complication.

++ [P] = Prevalance; [D] = Description; [M] = Sign/symptom; [C] = CD related cause; [R] = Response to gluten Free diet (GFD).

Health Manifestations of Celiac Disease (CD)
Section B: Signs, Symptoms, Associated Disorders and Complications

Affected System	Affected Organ	ID No.	Manifestation	Type+	Current Medical Information ++	Deficient Nutrient
Glandular System	Pancreas	136	Diabetes Mellitus, Type 1[1,114,115,116,117,118,119]	(AD)	[P] Prevalence of silent CD is 5.7% among diabetic patients and 1.9% among their first-degree relatives.[114] Prevalence of CD in children with type 1 diabetes mellitus (also called juvenile diabetes mellitus) in Wisconsin is at least 4.6% which is comparable to European and Canadian studies.[115] [D] Type 1 diabetes mellitus (type 1 DM) is a pancreatic disorder characterized by lack of insulin production. CD antibodies may be present before, at the same time as, or several years after diagnosis of type I DM. One third of diabetics with the CD associated HLA DQ genotype tested serologically positive for CD compared with less than 2% of patients lacking DQ2.[116] Type 1A DM has become one of the most intensively studied autoimmune disorders. It is now possible to predict its development, beginning with HLA-encoded genetic susceptibility, followed by the development of a series of anti-islet autoantibodies. Patients with type 1A DM and their relatives inherit susceptibility to express multiple autoantibodies including CD.[117] Study investigating silent CD in type 1 DM confirmed high prevalence of undiagnosed CD among 491 diabetic patients and their relatives and that other autoimmune disorders are significantly more prevalent in diabetic patients with CD than in those without CD. Newly diagnosed patients showed excellent compliance with GFD.[114] Study confirmed that CD is prevalent in adults with type 1 DM in Tunisia and serological screening for CD in type 1 DM is important because many patients are asymptomatic and most are detected by the screening.[118] Study evaluating the role of autoantibody tests for autoimmune diseases in children with newly diagnosed type 1 DM demonstrated that the most accurate test for CD is the IgA anti-endomysium. If an enzyme linked immunoassay test is required, the IGA tissue transglutaminase is accurate for screening.[119] [M] Marked by inability to control blood sugar and use in the body. [C] Results from immune mediated, selective destruction of more than 90% of insulin secreting beta cells, sharing the same high-risk HLA DQ2 genotype as CD.[116] [R] GFD improves management of DM and reduces or eliminates risk of associated diseases.[116]	Not applicable.

+ (S) = Classic sign/symptom; (AT) = Atypical sign/symptom; (AD) Associated Disorder; (C) = Complication.

++ [P] = Prevalance; [D] = Description; [M] = Sign/symptom; [C] = CD related cause; [R] = Response to gluten Free diet (GFD).

Health Manifestations of Celiac Disease (CD)
Section B: Signs, Symptoms, Associated Disorders and Complications

Affected System	Affected Organ	ID No.	Manifestation	Type[+]	Current Medical Information [++]	Deficient Nutrient
Glandular System	Pancreas	137	Diabetic Instability [1,3,116]	(AD)	[P] Increased frequency in patients with untreated CD.[116] [D] Diabetic instability is a non-gastrointestinal presentation of gluten sensitive enteropathy characterized by fluctuation in blood glucose level.[3] Absorption of nutrients could be variable or overt malabsorption could occur, altering insulin requirements and affecting diabetic control. Improvement in diabetic control and a decrease in hypoglycemic episodes have been demonstrated in children with CD and type 1 DM after institution of a GFD.[116] [M] Marked by difficulty controlling blood glucose level. [C] Results from malabsorption in CD.[116] [R] CD-related diabetic instability responds to GFD.	Carbohydrate, Chromium, Fat, Protein.
Glandular System	Pancreas	138	Gastrointestinal Complications in Type I Diabetes Mellitus [120]	(AD)	[P] Associated with CD.[120] [D] Gastrointestinal complications in type I diabetes mellitus are functional or organic changes resulting from diabetes affecting every organ of the GI tract. Impaired function of individual organs in diabetes can significantly influence level of diabetes compensation and vice versa. On the other side, unsatisfactory diabetes compensation can result in manifestation of digestive problems. The most frequent (55 to 75%) and the most serious clinical complication is diabetic gastroparesis characterized by impaired evacuation and motility of the stomach and small intestine. Another possible connection between diabetes mellitus and the GI tract can be CD.[120] [M] Marked by early fullness, eructation, nausea, vomiting, and abdominal pains that can be temporary or missing in some patients.[120] [C] Results from gastric autonomous neuropathy, impaired sensory innervation, and a direct effect of chronic hyperglycemia.[120] [R] Insufficient studies available to determine effect of GFD.	Not applicable.
Glandular System	Pancreas	139	Pancreatic Insufficiency [1,55]	(AD)	[P] Statistically significantly associated at diagnosis.[55] [D] Pancreatic insufficiency is characterized by insufficient exocrine production of pancreatic enzymes for normal digestion of fats, proteins, and carbohydrates. Study investigating the clinical manifestations of CD related to malnutrition and analyzing the associations between CD and other diagnoses, revealed statistically significant occurrence of pancreatic insufficiency.[55] [M] Marked by maldigestion, bulky, foul-smelling oily stools. [C] Results from inflammation in CD. [R] CD-related pancreatic insufficiency improves on GFD.	Not applicable.

[+] = (S) = Classic sign/symptom; (AT) = Atypical sign/symptom; (AD) Associated Disorder; (C) = Complication.

[++] = [P] = Prevalance; [D] = Description; [M] = Sign/symptom; [C] = CD related cause; [R] = Response to gluten Free diet (GFD).

Health Manifestations of Celiac Disease (CD)
Section B: Signs, Symptoms, Associated Disorders and Complications

Affected System	ID No.	Manifestation	Type+	Current Medical Information ++	Deficient Nutrient
Glandular System	140	Steatorrhea [1,3,50,73]	(S)	[P] Common in patients with untreated CD, occurring in one fifth of patients with diarrhea. [73] [D] Steatorrhea, the formation of fatty stools, is a classic presentation of CD characterized by alteration in stool character and consistency due to high undigested fat content. [3] [M] Marked by bulky, pale, foul-smelling stool that stick to the toilet and are hard to flush. [50] [C] Results from malabsorption of fat in CD. [R] Rapid and substantial improvement of CD-related steatorrhea with GFD. [73]	Not applicable.
Glandular System	141	Hyperparathyroidism, Primary [1,121]	(AD)	[P] New association with CD. [121] [D] Primary hyperparathyroidism is a parathyroid disorder characterized by excessive secretion of parathyroid hormone by one or more parathyroid glands for more than 6 months. It is seldom associated with autoimmune disorders. Case report of a 34 year old woman with severe bone deformities, severe muscle weakness and weight loss, describes finding CD subsequent to revealed Grave's disease and hypophosphatemia, normal plasma calcium levels, very low urinary calcium, and low 25-hydroxy vitamin D level. The patient underwent a near-total thyroidectomy, with removal of a parathyroid adenoma. The presence of normocalcemia in primary hyperparathyroidism should prompt the physician to look for vitamin D deficiency and to rule out intestinal malabsorption. [121] [M] Marked by anorexia, nausea, constipation and weight loss, muscle weakness, fatigue, confusion, osteopenia and osteomalacia. [121] [C] Results from adenoma in most cases and vitamin D malabsorption in CD. [R] CD-related primary hyperparathyroidism responds to GFD. [121]	Vitamin D.

+ (S) = Classic sign/symptom; (AT) = Atypical sign/symptom; (AD) Associated Disorder; (C) = Complication.

++ [P] = Prevalance; [D] = Description; [M] = Sign/symptom; [C] = CD related cause; [R] = Response to gluten Free diet (GFD).

Health Manifestations of Celiac Disease (CD)
Section B: Signs, Symptoms, Associated Disorders and Complications

Affected System	Affected Organ	ID No.	Manifestation	Type[+]	Current Medical Information [++]	Deficient Nutrient
Glandular System	Parathyroid	142	Hyperparathyroidism, Secondary [1,10,20,22,122]	(C)	[P] Common in untreated CD. 55.5% prevalence in CD women (18-68 years) at diagnosis.[20] [D] Secondary hyperparathyroidism is a parathyroid disorder resulting from calcium malabsorption in CD characterized by excessive levels of parathyroid hormone (PTH) that is refractory in untreated CD. It is associated with decreased bone mineral density in CD patients. Case report of a patient describes isolated hypocalcemia with hypocalciuria, and secondary hyperparathyroidism as initial manifestations of CD. Vitamin D was normal. Correction was demonstrated after dietary gluten withdrawal.[22] Study investigating whether PTH remained elevated and whether abnormalities of parathyroid function were still present in CD patients after treatment with GFD demonstrated higher basal 1-PTH values with normal parathyroid function in treated CD. Normal parathyroid function in treated patients suggests a lack of previous severe secondary hypoparathyroidism and/or complete adaptation to prior changes in parathyroid function.[122] [M] Marked by hypocalcemia, hypophosphatemia, and bone pain. [C] Results from calcium deficiency in CD.[20] [R] Parathyroid function normalizes in treated patients.[20] Normal parathyroid function with increased bone mass density (BMD) is suggestive of continuing long term benefit of gluten withdrawal on bone metabolism in CD patients.[10]	Calcium.
Glandular System	Parathyroid	143	Idiopathic Hypoparathyroidism [1,123]	(AT) (AD)	[P] New documentation shows it occurs in CD, but is rare.[123] [D] Idiopathic hypoparathyroidism, a condition in which the parathyroid glands atrophy, is characterized by insufficient or absent secretion of parathormone. Coexisting CD is one of the mechanisms responsible for the malabsorption associated with idiopathic hypoparathyroidism. CD is relatively common and this association could occur by coincidence. Alternately, there may be shared determinants of susceptibility or perhaps a direct immunological relationship. In such patients, both GFD and correction of the hypoparathyroid state may be necessary to correct malabsorption. Importance of intestinal biopsy in evaluating malabsorption is emphasized.[123] [M] Marked by hypocalcemia and hypophosphatemia often with chronic tetany, carpalpedal spasms, muscle cramps, wheezing, mood changes, urinary frequency, and lassitude. [C] Results from calcium and phosphorus malabsorption in CD.[123] [R] CD-related malabsorption in idiopathic hypoparathyroidism responds to GFD. Correction of the hypoparathyroid state may be necessary.	Calcium, Phosphorus.

[+] (S) = Classic sign/symptom; (AT) = Atypical sign/symptom; (AD) Associated Disorder; (C) = Complication.
[++] [P] = Prevalance; [D] = Description; [M] = Sign/symptom; [C] = CD related cause; [R] = Response to gluten Free diet (GFD).

Health Manifestations of Celiac Disease (CD)
Section B: Signs, Symptoms, Associated Disorders and Complications

Affected System	Affected Organ	ID No.	Manifestation	Type[+]	Current Medical Information [++]	Deficient Nutrient
Glandular System	Parathyroid	144	Parathyroid Carcinoma [1,124]	(C)	[P] New association of CD occurring with rare parathyroid carcinoma.[124] [D] Parathyroid carcinoma is a malignancy involving overactive parathyroid glands characterized by asymptomatic hypercalcemia in most patients, suppressed serum PTH levels, and renal failure in some. Case report describes parathyroid carcinoma associated with CD in a patient with review of natural history of the disease and proposes that there is malignant transformation of benign parathyroid hyperplastic tissue in these cases.[124] [M] Marked by hypercalcemia, renal calculi, and osteopenia. [C] May result from prolonged hyperplasia of parathyroid tissue.[124] [R] Insufficient studies to determine effect of GFD.	Not applicable.
Glandular System	Thyroid	145	Autoimmune Thyroiditis (Hypothyroidism) [1,125,126]	(AD)	[P] Reported prevalence of CD in autoimmune thyroiditis is 2%.[125] A 10 year study found auto-immune thyroid disease in 4.3% of patients with DH and 6.0% with CD.[126] [D] Autoimmune thyroiditis is an immunologically mediated thyroid disease characterized by insufficient thyroid hormone circulating in the body due to autoimmune destruction of thyroid tissue. Study evaluating the presence of CD in 100 patients with autoimmune thyroid disease demonstrated that serologic markers became undetectable 6 months after beginning GFD, but thyroid autoantibodies did not positively correlate with GFD.[125] Study investigating the occurrence of associated diseases in a cohort of 305 patients with dermatitis herpetiformis (DH) followed for a mean of 10 years compared with results from a cohort of 385 patients with CD demonstrated auto-immune thyroid disease in 4.3% of DH patients and 6.0% CD patients.[126] [M] Marked by lowered basal metabolism, slow pulse, paresthesias, intolerance of cold, fatigue, mental apathy, sluggishness, constipation, muscle aches, dry skin and hair, brittle nails, periorbital edema and facial puffiness. [C] Results from common immunopathogenesis with CD. [R] CD-related autoimmune thyroiditis responds to GFD.[125]	Not applicable.

[+] (S) = Classic sign/symptom; (AT) = Atypical sign/symptom; (AD) Associated Disorder; (C) = Complication.

[++] [P] = Prevalence; [D] = Description; [M] = Sign/symptom; [C] = CD related cause; [R] = Response to gluten Free diet (GFD).

Health Manifestations of Celiac Disease (CD)
Section B: Signs, Symptoms, Associated Disorders and Complications

Affected System	Affected Organ	ID No.	Manifestation	Type[+]	Current Medical Information [++]	Deficient Nutrient
Glandular System	Thyroid	146	Grave's Disease (Hyperthyroidism) [1,127]	(AD)	[P] Prevalence of CD in patients with Grave's disease is 4.5% compared with 0.9% in matched healthy controls.[127] [D] Grave's Disease, or hyperthyroidism, is an immunologically mediated thyroid disease characterized by diffuse nontender goiter, elevated thyroxine levels, suppressed thyrotropin (TSH), and presence of thyroid receptor antibodies. Study investigating the prevalence of CD in patients with Grave's disease and evaluating the role of screening for CD prospectively demonstrated that routine screening for CD should be considered. Screening of 111 consecutive patients with Grave's hyperthyroidism revealed anti-gliadin antibodies in 14%, anti-tissue transglutaminase antibodies in 2% and IgA deficiency in 3%.[127] [M] Marked by proptosis and pretibial myxedema in most patients, including rapid pulse, staring, increased blood pressure, palpitations, nervousness, depression, anxiety, heat intolerance, weight loss, proximal weakness (thigh and upper arms), brisk tendon reflexes, cardiac abnormalities, and oligomenorrhea. [C] Results from autoimmune attack on the thyroid gland. [R] GFD treatment of thyroid and CD is successful.	Not applicable.
Immune System	Antibodies	147	Allergic Rhinitis [128]	(AD)	[P] Associated with CD.[128] [D] Allergic rhinitis is an immune disorder characterized by inflammation of the nasal mucosa by IgE antibody reaction. An increase in T gamma-delta intraepithelial lymphocytes (IEL), a subset of T-cells located in the respiratory mucosa with pro-inflammatory functions, is implicated. An increase in the intestinal IEL gammadelta population is involved in CD, but its significance is not well known.[128] [M] Marked by acute nasal congestion. [C] Results from immune mechanism.[128] Exacerbated by omega-3 fatty acid deficiency. [R] Insufficient studies to determine effect of GFD.	Unknown.

[+] (S) = Classic sign/symptom; (AT) = Atypical sign/symptom; (AD) Associated Disorder; (C) = Complication.

[++] [P] = Prevalance; [D] = Description; [M] = Sign/symptom; [C] = CD related cause; [R] = Response to gluten Free diet (GFD).

Section B   Signs, Symptoms, Associated Disorders & Complications

161

Health Manifestations of Celiac Disease (CD)
Section B: Signs, Symptoms, Associated Disorders and Complications

Affected System	Affected Organ	ID No.	Manifestation	Type[+]	Current Medical Information [++]	Deficient Nutrient
Immune System	Antibodies	148	Antiphospholipid Syndrome [129]	(AD)	[P] 14% of patients with antiphospholipid syndrome (APS) found to have EMA (endomysium) antibodies compared to 1.1% of controls.[129] [D] Antiphospholipid Syndrome (APS) is an autoimmune disease characterized by defined clinical (vascular thrombosis and/or complications of pregnancy) and laboratory criteria (anticardiolipin and/or lupus anti-coagulant antibodies). APS is associated with autoantibodies directed against negatively charged phospholipids, and B2-glycoprotein-I has been found as a major target antigen for antiphospholipid antibodies. CD and APS share common clinical features including hypercoagulability, thrombotic phenomena, and various neurological manifestations, as well as recurrent abortions and lower birth weight.[129] Study investigating the prevalence of CD antibodies in patients with APS demonstrated that the presence of EMA-ELISA antibodies is associated with high prevalence of antibodies recognizing certain B2-glycoprotein epitopes and with cutaneous manifestations of APS. Vasculitic skin lesions were significantly more common in EMA positive patients than controls (62.5 vs. 2%) and there was a higher prevalence of superficial cutaneous necrosis (37.5 vs. 2%). CD and APS share common clinical features, but the relationship between skin manifestations of APS and CD needs to be explored.[129] [M] Marked by superficial necrosis, ulcerations, livedo reticularis, digital gangrene, and unusually high proportion of pregnancy losses after 10th week of gestation.[129] [C] Results from autoimmune mechanism. Evidence suggests that tTG (tissue transglutaminase) tissue expression may be enhanced during tissue injury in APS, and in predisposed individuals may lead to the manifestations of CD antibodies and potentially to CD. On the other hand, in patients with CD, tTG may be involved in the pathogenesis of APS.[129] [R] Studies are inadequate to determine how GFD could delay or mitigate the course of APS.[129]	Copper, Vitamin B$_{12}$.

[+] (S) = Classic sign/symptom; (AT) = Atypical sign/symptom; (AD) Associated Disorder; (C) = Complication.

[++] [P] = Prevalance; [D] = Description; [M] = Sign/symptom; [C] = CD related cause; [R] = Response to gluten Free diet (GFD).

Health Manifestations of Celiac Disease (CD)
Section B: Signs, Symptoms, Associated Disorders and Complications

Affected System	Affected Organ	ID No.	Manifestation	Type[+]	Current Medical Information [++]	Deficient Nutrient
Immune System	Antibodies	149	Asthma [130]	(AD)	[P] Prevalence of asthma found in children with CD is 24.6% vs. 3.4% in controls.[130] [D] Asthma is an inherited immunologically mediated respiratory disorder characterized by narrowing and inflammation of the lung airways as a response to gluten as trigger in CD. Asthma is generally regarded as a disease with strong T(H)2-type cytokine expression, whereas in CD T(H) 1-type expression is seen.[130] Study investigating whether asthma could coexist in children with T(H)1-type diseases such as CD demonstrated that T(H)1 and T(H)2 cytokine expression can coexist. An increase in T gamma-delta lymphocytes, a subset of T-cells located in the repiratory mucosa, is implicated. The cumulative incidence of asthma is significantly higher in children with CD than in children without CD.[130] [M] Marked by wheezing and shortness of breath. Exacerbated by omega-3 fatty acid deficiency. [C] Results from a common environmental denominator in susceptible patients.[130] [R] Studies are inadequate to determine effect of GFD.	Not applicable.

+ (S) = Classic sign/symptom; (AT) = Atypical sign/symptom; (AD) Associated Disorder; (C) = Complication.

++ [P] = Prevalance; [D] = Description; [M] = Sign/symptom; [C] = CD related cause; [R] = Response to gluten Free diet (GFD).

Health Manifestations of Celiac Disease (CD)
Section B: Signs, Symptoms, Associated Disorders and Complications

Affected System	Affected Organ	ID No.	Manifestation	Type[+]	Current Medical Information [++]	Deficient Nutrient
Immune System	Antibodies	150	Autoimmune Disorders in CD [1,7,126,131,132,133,134]	(AD)	[P] 21% of patients with CD had associated autoimmune disorders.[131] Concomitant endocrine and connective tissue disorder associations were found in 19.1% of patients with CD over a mean of 10 years.[126] 4.8% of first degree relatives of children with CD had autoimmune disorders.[132] [D] Development of autoimmune disorders in CD is clearly related to the duration of exposure to gluten.[7] To think early of the possibility of intolerance to gluten is to give the means of a very easy diagnosis.[133] Study assessing the prevalence of organ-specific autoantibodies in celiac patients and evaluating whether their finding is an expression of associated autoimmune diseases demonstrated that the finding of organ specific autoantibodies in celiac patients discloses the coexistence of a wide spectrum of immunological diseases.[131] Study investigating the occurrence of associated diseases in a cohort of 305 patients with DH demonstrated that patients with DH are similar to patients with CD in that many have associated endocrine or connective tissue disorders. The following associations were found: auto-immune thyroid disease (4.3% of DH patients and 6.0% of CD patients), 5.5% CD), lupus erythematosus (1.3% DH and 0.3% CD), Sjögren's syndrome (1.0% DH and 2.9% CD), sarcoidosis (1.3% DH and 1.8% CD).[126] Study investigating the prevalence of autoimmune disorders in first degree relatives of patients with CD demonstrated that increased prevalence is most likely connected with unrecognized subclinical or silent forms of CD. 82% of first degree relatives with silent or subclinical forms of CD had flat mucosa on intestinal biopsy.[132] [M] Marked by increased risk of developing associated autoimmune disorders with increased diagnostic delay. [C] Results from gluten exposure, associated autoimmune mechanism.[134] [R] Early elimination of gluten food will make various manifestations disappear.[133]	Not applicable.

[+] (S) = Classic sign/symptom; (AT) = Atypical sign/symptom; (AD) Associated Disorder; (C) = Complication.

[++] [P] = Prevalance; [D] = Description; [M] = Sign/symptom; [C] = CD related cause; [R] = Response to gluten Free diet (GFD).

Health Manifestations of Celiac Disease (CD)
Section B: Signs, Symptoms, Associated Disorders and Complications

Affected System	Affected Organ	ID No.	Manifestation	Type[+]	Current Medical Information [++]	Deficient Nutrient
Immune System	Antibodies	151	Autoimmune Disorders in Dermatitis Herpetiformis [126]	(AD)	[P] Concomitant endocrine and connective tissue disorders associations were found in 9.5% of patients with DH over a mean of 10 years.[126] [D] Development of autoimmune disorders in DH is similar to those with CD. Study investigating the occurrence of associated diseases in a cohort of 305 patients with DH demonstrated that patients with DH are similar to patients with CD in that many have associated endocrine or connective tissue disorders. The following associations were found: auto-immune thyroid disease (4.3% of DH patients and 6.0% of CD patients), type 1 diabetes mellitus (1.0% DH and 5.5% CD), lupus erythematosus (1.3% DH and 0.3% CD), Sjögren's syndrome (1.0% DH and 2.9% CD), sarcoidosis (1.3% DH and 1.8% CD), and vitiligo or alopecia areata (1.6% DH and 0% CD). Most of these diseases began before DH had been diagnosed.[126] [M] Marked by increased risk of developing associated autoimmune disorders with increased diagnostic delay. [C] Results from gluten exposure, related autoimmune mechanism. [R] Patients already on a GFD are not at special risk of contracting endocrine and connective tissue disorders.[126]	Not applicable.
Immune System	Antibodies	152	Autoimmune Polyglandular Syndromes [134,135,136]	(AD)	[P] Patients with CD are at great risk for developing autoimmune polyglandular syndromes.[134] [D] Autoimmune polyglandular syndromes are characterized by association of two or more endocrine and non-endocrine auto-immune disorders. Type1 DM is one of the most frequent components of autoimmune polyglandular syndrome and is often its first symptom. First degree relatives have an increased incidence of latent or manifest autoimmune pathology.[135] Autoim-mune polyglandular syndromes seem to be related to gluten exposure. Growth, bone metabo-lism, and fertility can be affected in patients with CD, especially if they are not on a GFD.[134] Gluten could represent a starting or a maintenance factor of autoimmune processes and the risk is proportional to the duration of exposure to gluten. Screening for a quick singling out of autoimmune pathologies is suggested for type1 DM patients, their first relatives and for subjects affected by other autoimmune diseases or CD.[135] Case report of patient with diagnosed biliary cirrhosis, Sjögren's syndrome, and renal tubular acidosis who developed diarrhea and weight loss, describes subsequent diagnosis of CD. She went on to develop autoimmune hyperthyroidism despite a GFD.[136] [M] Marked by symptoms distinguishing involved antibodies. [C] Results from common autoimmune mechanisms, genetic susceptibility and favorable environ-mental factors commonly shared by the [associated] diseases.[136] [R] Studies are inadequate to determine how a GFD could delay or mitigate the course of type 1 DM and other autoimmune pathologies in genetically predisposed subjects.[135]	Not applicable.

[+] (S) = Classic sign/symptom; (AT) = Atypical sign/symptom; (AD) Associated Disorder; (C) = Complication.

[++] [P] = Prevalance; [D] = Description; [M] = Sign/symptom; [C] = CD related cause; [R] = Response to gluten Free diet (GFD).

Health Manifestations of Celiac Disease (CD)
Section B: Signs, Symptoms, Associated Disorders and Complications

Affected System	Affected Organ	ID No.	Manifestation	Type[+]	Current Medical Information [++]	Deficient Nutrient
Immune System	Antibodies	153	Common Variable Immunodeficiency [137,138]	(AD)	[P] Frequently associated with subtotal villous atrophy of CD and the association should not be considered fortuitous.[137] [D] Common variable immunodeficiency (CVID) is an immunodeficiency disease characterized by the onset of recurrent bacterial infections resulting from markedly decreased Ig and antibody levels. CVID patients with associated CD may develop neurological disease including sensory loss, ataxia, and retinitis pigmentosa due to free radical mediated neuronal damage induced by vitamin E deficiency.[138] All CVID patients with evidence of enteropathy should be screened for vitamin E deficiency, as early detection and consequent treatment may prevent, halt or reverse the neurological sequelae.[138] Clinicians should be aware of the low sensitivity of serologic testing in CVID.[137] [M] Marked by recurrent bacterial infections. [C] Results from vitamin E deficiency in CD. [R] CD-related CVID is unchanged by GFD.[137]	Vitamin E.
Immune System	Antibodies	154	IgA Deficiency [1,139,140]	(AD)	[P] Frequently associated with CD.[139] [D] IgA deficiency (IgAD) is an immunodeficiency disease characterized by the presence of high IgG antibody levels but with marked absence of IgA antibodies to endomysium, transglutaminase, and gliadin. IgA deficiency may be a potential source of false-negative results on tests for IgA antibodies. IgA-deficient CD patients (CD-IgAD) are not identified by IgA serology.[140] Study investigating both type 1 and type 2 plasma cytokine levels in CD and in CD-IgAD demonstrated that CD and especially CD-IgAD patients display persistently higher pro-inflammatory cytokine levels, suggesting a persistent state of activation of pro-phlogistic signals in CD, particularly when IgAD coexists. IL-10 had significantly higher plasma levels in CD-IgAD but not in CD with a significant decrease after a GFD. Serial measurement of serum IL-10 may be an adjunctive evaluating criterion in the follow-up of CD-IgAD patients.[139] Study investigating the utility of IgG-tTG for the detection of untreated CD in IgA-deficient patients demonstrated that IgG-tTG detection with recombinant human tTG is a good alternative to IgG-EMA detection, and the addition of IgG-tTG assessment to the present screening methods may improve the ability to identify IgA-deficient patients with CD. The overall concordance of the positive and negative results between IgG-tTG and IgG-EMA was 97%, and the IgG-tTG assay discriminated between IgG-EMA- positive and -negative subjects with IgA-deficiency at a rate of 100%.[140] [M] Marked by recurrent infections, chronic diarrhea, allergy or autoimmune disease, although most patients are asymptomatic. [C] Results from same genetic background as CD.[139] [R] Of plasma cytokine levels, only IL-10 shows a significant decrease after GFD.[139]	Not applicable.

[+] (S) = Classic sign/symptom; (AT) = Atypical sign/symptom; (AD) Associated Disorder; (C) = Complication.

[++] [P] = Prevalance; [D] = Description; [M] = Sign/symptom; [C] = CD related cause; [R] = Response to gluten Free diet (GFD).

Health Manifestations of Celiac Disease (CD)
Section B: Signs, Symptoms, Associated Disorders and Complications

Affected System	Affected Organ	ID No.	Manifestation	Type[+]	Current Medical Information[++]	Deficient Nutrient[++]
Immune System	Antibodies	155	Sarcoidosis [1,126,141,142]	(AD)	[P] Report of 4% CD occurrence in patients with sarcoidosis,[141] and sarcoidosis occurrence in 1.3% of patients with DH and 1.8% in CD.[126] [D] Sarcoidosis is an autoimmune multisystem granulomatous disease characterized by hard granulomas and inflammation of the alveoli occurring in 80% of patients. Study investigating the prevalence of CD in patients with sarcoidosis demonstrated moderate increase and susceptibility to sarcoidosis and CD is linked to HLA-DR3, DQ2. Estimation of EMA is recommended and should be restricted to those with susceptible haplotypes.[141] Study investigating the occurrence of associated diseases in a cohort of 305 patients with dermatitis herpetiformis (DH) followed for a mean of 10 years compared with results from a cohort of patients with CD demonstrated sarcoidosis in 1.3% of DH patients and 1.8% of CD patients.[126] Case report of a patient describes improvement of dermatological lesions while on a GFD and relapse each time diet stopped. Report refers to same reaction to GFD in a patient with lung involvement.[142] [M] Marked by fatigue, shortness of breath, non-productive cough, night sweats, anorexia, and weight loss with death from heart and lung failure. [C] Results from shared autoimmune mechanism with CD, but relationship is unclear.[142] [R] Sarcoidosis responds to GFD.	Not applicable.
Immune System	Antibodies	156	Sjögren's Syndrome [1,126,143]	(AD)	[P] Prevalence of Sjögren's syndrome (SS) is reported in 1.0% of patients with DH and 2.9% with CD.[126] CD occurs in 12% of patients with SS.[143] [D] Sjögren's syndrome is a systemic autoimmune disease affecting the lacrimal glands of the eye and the salivary glands of the mouth characterized by dryness of mucosa. Study investigating the occurrence of associated diseases in a cohort of 305 patients with dermatitis herpetiformis (DH) followed for a mean of 10 years compared with results from a cohort of 383 patients with CD demonstrated Sjögren's syndrome in 1.0% of DH patients and 2.9% of CD patients.[126] Study evaluating the prevalence of IgA-anti-tissue transglutaminase antibody (Anti-tTG ELISA) in patients with SS demonstrated that anti-tTG ELISA is a reliable method to indicate a coexisting diagnosis of CD in patients with Sjögren's syndrome. Anti-tTG is more prevalent in SS than in other systemic rheumatic diseases. It may be used as a screening test to identify patients with SS who are at risk and require further evaluation for the presence of CD.[143] [M] Marked by dry eye and dry mouth resulting in dental decay, difficulty chewing and swallowing, gingivitis, and distorted sense of taste. [C] Results from immune mechanism. [R] Studies are inadequate to determine effect of GFD.	Not applicable.

[+] (S) = Classic sign/symptom; (AT) = Atypical sign/symptom; (AD) Associated Disorder; (C) = Complication.

[++] [P] = Prevalance; [D] = Description; [M] = Sign/symptom; [C] = CD related cause; [R] = Response to gluten Free diet (GFD).

Health Manifestations of Celiac Disease (CD)
Section B: Signs, Symptoms, Associated Disorders and Complications

Affected System	Affected Organ	ID No.	Manifestation	Type[+]	Current Medical Information [++]	Deficient Nutrient
Immune System	Antibodies	157	Systemic Lupus Erythematosus [1,1,126, 129,144]	(AD)	[P] Systemic lupus erythematosus (SLE) is reported in 1.3% of patients with DH and 0.3% in patients with CD.[126] [D] SLE, an immunologically mediated chronic inflammatory disease, is characterized by involvement of multiple organs with acute flare-ups. Reports give conflicting results regarding association with CD. There is a high rate of false-positive serology results for CD in SLE. In one study that examined 103 patients with SLE, none had either antiendomysial antibodies or a mucosal lesion, but 23.3% had anti-gliadin antibodies. Nevertheless, the association of CD and SLE may shed light on the pathogenesis of autoimmune disorders in patients with CD since anti-DNA antibodies from a patient with CD induced experimental SLE in a mouse model.[129] In five cases of SLE with villous atrophy on duodenal biopsy, only four had positive serological tests and only three had abdominal symptoms.[144] Study investigating the occurrence of associated diseases in a cohort of 305 patients with dermatitis herpetiformis (DH) followed for a mean of 10 years compared with results from a cohort of 383 patients with CD demonstrated SLE in 1.3% of DH patients and 0.3% of CD patients.[126] [M] Marked by any of four disorders including erythematous rash over the nose and cheeks, raised scaly discoid skin lesions, antinuclear antibodies, autoantibodies, pleuritis or pericarditis, arthritis, anemia, lymphopenia. [C] Results from autoimmune mechanism. [R] Studies are inadequate to determine effect of GFD.	Not applicable.

+ (S) = Classic sign/symptom; (AT) = Atypical sign/symptom; (AD) Associated Disorder; (C) = Complication.

++ [P] = Prevalance; [D] = Description; [M] = Sign/symptom; [C] = CD related cause; [R] = Response to gluten Free diet (GFD).

Health Manifestations of Celiac Disease (CD)
Section B: Signs, Symptoms, Associated Disorders and Complications

Affected System	Affected Organ	ID No.	Manifestation	Type[+]	Current Medical Information [++]	Deficient Nutrient
Immune System	Antibodies	158	Urticaria, Chronic - Hives [1,145, 146,147]	(AD)	[P] Increased prevalence in patients with untreated CD, occurring in 1 in 53 patients.[145] [D] Chronic urticaria is an immunologically mediated cutaneous disorder characterized by multiple areas of well-demarcated edematous, intensely pruritic plaques that may be small or reach the diameter of many centimeters with surrounding erythema each lasting less than 24 hours.[146] Lesions are manifestations of vasoactive mediators derived from mast cells and other sources, usually involving an immunoglobulin E antibody reaction. Urticaria as a presenting manifestation may provide an early clue to diagnosis of CD in patients with minor or absent GI symptoms.[147] Inflammation in the GI tract may have an important role in the etiology of chronic urticaria.[145] Study investigating 107 patients with chronic urticaria demonstrated a diagnosis of CD in 2 patients and anti-gliadin antibodies in 4 patients.[145] Case report of patient with skin manifestation unresponsive to treatment with astemizole for one month describes hospitalization for worsening generalized urticaria. Patient tested positive for antibodies for CD but not IgE to wheat. CD was confirmed by intestinal biopsy. The alcohol soluble prolamin fraction of gluten (gliadin in wheat, secalin in rye, avenin identified as the offending substance. No significant difference in total serum IgE level measurement was observed during the course of the disease. It is possible that immune-complex-dependent sequelae might cause urticarial lesions also when concomitant CD occurs. Consequently, the restoration of mucosal integrity after a GFD may explain the improvement of urticaria.[146] [M] Marked by raised wheals on skin and mucosa. [C] Results from immune mechanism, GI inflammation in CD, and increased intestinal permeability facilitating the passage of antigens. [R] Urticaria improved after one month and totally disappeared after 3 months GFD.[146]	Not applicable.

[+] (S) = Classic sign/symptom; (AT) = Atypical sign/symptom; (AD) Associated Disorder; (C) = Complication.

[++] [P] = Prevalance; [D] = Description; [DI] = Description; [M] = Sign/symptom; [C] = CD related cause; [R] = Response to gluten Free diet (GFD).

Health Manifestations of Celiac Disease (CD)
Section B: Signs, Symptoms, Associated Disorders and Complications

Affected System	Affected Organ	ID No.	Manifestation	Type+	Current Medical Information ++	Deficient Nutrient
Integumentary System	Hair	159	Alopecia Areata [1,126,147,148]	(AD)	[P] Increased frequency in patients with CD.[147] Rate is 1.6% in patients with DH.[126] [D] Alopecia areata is an immunologically mediated cutaneous condition characterized by sudden hair loss involving scalp or beard although any hairy area may be affected. All body hair may be lost (alopecia universalis). In a substantial proportion of patients with untreated CD, GI symptoms are minor or absent, and alopecia areata may provide an early clue to diagnosis.[147] Case report of two children with alopecia areata, age 13 years and 29 months, describes diagnosis of CD. Both children had raised IgA endomysium antibodies, IgG antigliadin antibodies, and subtotal villous atrophy on jejunal biopsy. Administration of GFD resulted in complete hair growth.[148] Study investigating the occurrence of associated diseases in a cohort of 305 patients with dermatitis herpetiformis (DH) followed for a mean of 10 years compared with results from a cohort of 383 patients with CD demonstrated alopecia areata in 1.6% of DH patients.[126] [M] Marked by sharply defined areas of hair loss. [C] Results from immune mechanism with zinc deficiency. [R] CD-related hair loss resolves on GFD.[147,148]	Zinc.
Integumentary System	Hair	160	Alopecia, Diffuse [147,149]	(S)	[P] Increased frequency in patients with untreated CD.[147] [D] Diffuse alopecia, a cutaneous manifestation of zinc deficiency, is now recognized as a clinical feature of zinc deficient CD subjects characterized by hair thinning. Serum zinc levels should be included in the work-up of patients with diffuse alopecia. In the setting of hypozincemia with adequate nutritional intake, a malabsorption syndrome should be suspected, and serological testing for CD should be performed. A GFD normalizes zinc levels persistently low on supplementation. Alopecia is also a common dermatological manifestation of iron deficiency which may be attributable to undiagnosed CD.[147] Case report describes diffuse alopecia that developed in 3 children. In one child alopecia developed after 4 years nonadherance to a GFD; the other 2 children presented with alopecia. Administration of a GFD resulted in partial regrowth of hair in the first child and complete hair growth in the other two children.[149] [M] Marked by balding. [C] Results from iron and/or zinc malabsorption in CD, biotin and essential fatty acids. [R] CD-related diffuse alopecia reponds to GFD.[147]	Biotin, Iron, Omega-3 fatty acids, Omega-6 fatty acids, Zinc.

+ (S) = Classic sign/symptom; (AT) = Atypical sign/symptom; (AD) Associated Disorder; (C) = Complication.

++ [P] = Prevalance; [D] = Description; [M] = Sign/symptom; [C]= CD related cause; [R] = Response to gluten Free diet (GFD).

Health Manifestations of Celiac Disease (CD)
Section B: Signs, Symptoms, Associated Disorders and Complications

Affected System	ID No.	Manifestation	Type[+]	Current Medical Information[++]	Deficient Nutrient
Integumentary System	161	Hair Diameter Lower and Cuticolar Erosion Scores Higher [1,150]	(S)	[P] New association in patients with untreated CD.[150] [D] Significantly lower hair diameter and higher erosion scores determined by scanning electron microscopy are abnormal hair shaft features characterizing patients with CD not on a GFD from those following a GFD. Proton-induced X-ray emission showed significantly lower zinc content of the hair shaft in the group with acute CD and after a short term GFD, which approached the normal range only after a year long GFD. Genotyping found significant positive association with CD. Significant hyperprolactinemia, elevated erythrocyte glutathione content, and significantly decreased glutathione disulfide level was found in children consuming gluten.[150] [M] Marked by thinness of individual hair with abnormal outside covering.[150] [C] Results from autoimmune mechanism, zinc deficiency in CD.[150] [R] Responds to the GFD with near normal range after a year long diet.[150]	Zinc.
Integumentary System	162	Dry and Brittle Nails that Chip, Peel, Crack or Break Easily [34]	(S)	[P] Common in people with untreated CD. [D] Nail abnormalities, a feature of multiple deficiencies, is characterized by poor nail structure of both fingernails and toenails. External causes such as detergents and cleaners would only affect fingernails. Nails that are dry and brittle result from vitamin A and calcium deficiencies. Nails that chip, peel, crack or break easily result from protein, calcium, and omega-3 fatty acid deficiencies. [M] Marked by unhealthy condition of nails. [C] Results from malabsorption in gluten sensitive enteropathy and dehydration. [R] CD-related nail abnormalities respond to GFD.	Calcium, Omega-3 fatty acids, Protein, Vitamin A, Water.[34]

[+] (S) = Classic sign/symptom; (AT) = Atypical sign/symptom; (AD) Associated Disorder; (C) = Complication.

[++] [P] = Prevalance; [D] = Description; [M] = Sign/symptom; [C] = CD related cause; [R] = Response to gluten Free diet (GFD).

Health Manifestations of Celiac Disease (CD)
Section B: Signs, Symptoms, Associated Disorders and Complications

Affected System	Affected Organ	ID No.	Manifestation	Type+	Current Medical Information ++	Deficient Nutrient
Integumentary System	Nails	163	Horizontal & vertical ridges; fragile nails	(S)	[P] Common in people with untreated CD. [D] Ridges and fragile nails are features of multiple deficiencies characterized by abnormal nail structure. [M] Marked by poor health and malnutrition. Iron deficiency is indicated by vertical ridges. Severe stress with vitamin B depletion/malabsorption is indicated by horizontal ridges. [C] Results from malabsorption in CD. [R] CD-related nail abnormalities respond to GFD.	B vitamins, Iron.
Integumentary System	Nails	164	Koilonychia [147]	(S)	[P] Increased frequency in people with untreated CD. [D] Koilonychia is a feature of an iron deficiency state characterized by spoon shaped nails and vertical ridges. [M] Marked by thin nails and depression in the center with raised edges. [C] Results from iron deficiency in CD and/or achlorhydria. [147] [R] Nail health responds to GFD. Usually requires iron supplementation.	Iron.
Integumentary System	Nails	165	Subungual Splinter Hemorrhages [34]	(S)	[P] Increased frequency in people with untreated CD. [D] Subungual splinter hemorrhages, a feature of vitamin C deficiency, is characterized by fragility of the underlying capillaries resulting in bleeding under the nail. [34] [M] Marked by small dark red streaks under nail. [C] Results from malabsorption in CD. [R] Resolves on GFD.	Vitamin C.
Integumentary System	Nails	166	Nails Rounded with Curved Ends, Dark and Excessively Dry	(S)	[P] Increased frequency in people with untreated CD. [D] Rounded, curved, dark and dry nails is a well known feature of vitamin B_{12} deficiency in CD. [M] Marked by likeness to animal claw. [C] Results from vitamin B_{12} deficiency induced by CD. [R] Responds to GFD.	Vitamin B_{12}.

+ (S) = Classic sign/symptom; (AT) = Atypical sign/symptom; (AD) Associated Disorder; (C) = Complication.

++ [P] = Prevalance; [D] = Description; [M] = Sign/symptom; [C] = CD related cause; [R] = Response to gluten Free diet (GFD).

Health Manifestations of Celiac Disease (CD)
Section B: Signs, Symptoms, Associated Disorders and Complications

Affected System	Affected Organ	ID No.	Manifestation	Type[+]	Current Medical Information [++]	Deficient Nutrient
Integumentary System	Nails	167	White Spots and White Bands in Nails	(S)	[P] Increased frequency in patients with untreated CD. [D] White spots in the nails is a feature of zinc deficiency and white bands signify protein deficiency characterized by abnormal appearance anywhere in one or more nails. [M] Marked by lesions that vary in size and whiteness according to severity of deficiency. [C] Results from deficiency of zinc and/or protein induced by CD. [R] Responds to GFD.	Omega-3 fatty acids, Zinc.
Integumentary System	Skin	168	Cutaneous Vasculitis [147,151]	(AD)	[P] Increased frequency in patients with untreated CD.[147] [D] Cutaneous vasculitis is an immunologically mediated disorder characterized by segmental inflammation of cutaneous blood vessels resulting in necrosis and scarring. Sores develop in the skin overlying sections of inflamed blood vessels. 　　Case report presenting rare complication of cutaneous vasculitis and nephritis in a patient describes how exogenous or endogenous antigens permeate the abnormal bowel mucosa leading to formation of circulating complexes. Subsequent tissue deposition of these complexes result in vasculitis and in this case, nephritis.[151] [M] Marked by skin lesions and kidney lesions.[151] [C] Results from gluten exposure and increased intestinal permeability in CD.[151] [R] Skin lesions cleared completely after treatment with a strict GFD.[151]	Not applicable.

[+] (S) = Classic sign/symptom; (AT) = Atypical sign/symptom; (AD) Associated Disorder; (C) = Complication.

[++] [P] = Prevalence; [D] = Description; [M] = Sign/symptom; [C] = CD related cause; [R] = Response to gluten Free diet (GFD).

Health Manifestations of Celiac Disease (CD)
Section B: Signs, Symptoms, Associated Disorders and Complications

Affected System	Affected Organ	ID No.	Manifestation	Type[+]	Current Medical Information [++]	Deficient Nutrient

Integumentary System	Skin	169	Cutis Laxa, Generalized Acquired [1,152]	(AT)	[P] Uncommon disorder associated with CD.[152]
					 [D] Generalized acquired cutis laxa (GACL) is an uncommon elastolytic disorder characterized by abnormal reduction and degeneration of elastic fibers of the skin.
					     Case report of a 35 year old man with generalized acquired cutis laxa associated with a persistent papular erythematous eruption that histopathologically showed some resemblence to dermatitis herpetiformis describes investigation and subsequent diagnosis of CD. A marked reduction and degeneration of dermal elastic fibers was noted in biopsies from loose hanging skin. Direct immunofluorescence from non-inflammatory loose skin revealed granular IgA deposits at the basement membrane zone and fibrillar IgA deposits in the dermal papillae. Immunoelectron microscopy of an erythematous papule revealed IgA deposits around dermal elastic fibers. Antigliadin, anti-reticulin, and antiendomysium antibodies were present and jejunal biopsy positive for CD. A possible IgA-mediated immune mechanism for the development of GACL is suggested.[152]
					 [M] Marked by thick, loose and sagging skin.
					 [C] Results from possible immune mechanism although unclear.[152]
					     Involves nutritional deficiencies including copper, vitamin A, and C.
					 [R] Studies are inadequate to determine response to GFD.
						Copper, Vitamin A, Vitamin C.

[+] (S) = Classic sign/symptom; (AT) = Atypical sign/symptom; (AD) Associated Disorder; (C) = Complication.

[++] [P] = Prevalance; [D] = Description; [M] = Sign/symptom; [C] = CD related cause; [R] = Response to gluten Free diet (GFD).

Health Manifestations of Celiac Disease (CD)

Section B: Signs, Symptoms, Associated Disorders and Complications

Affected System	Affected Organ	ID No.	Manifestation	Type+	Current Medical Information++	Deficient Nutrient
Integumentary System	Skin	170	Dermatitis Herpetiformis 1,3,127, 153,154,155,156	(S)	[P] Affects 25% of patients with CD.[153] [D] Dermatitis herpetiformis (DH) is a cutaneous manifestation of CD developing in those patients with mild CD who produce epidermal transglutaminase autoantibodies of high avidity and affinity. It is characterized by granular IgA deposits in the papillary dermis.[154] Tissue transglutaminase seems to be the predominent autoantigen both in the intestine and the skin.[153] Serum IgA in DH has been found to bind epidermal transglutaminase, an enzyme not previously detected in the papillary region of normal skin.[154] The enteropathic damage in the intestine may be asymptomatic when the skin rash appears, but is indistinguishable from that seen in CD.[3] Both conditions can appear in the same family and are closely linked to HLA class II locus in chromosome 6. 90% of patients have HLA DQ2 and almost all the remainder have HLA DQ8. Oral dapsone is usually needed in newly detected DH in order to alleviate symptoms.[153] Study investigating the occurrence of lymphoma in a large series of patients consecutively diagnosed with DH during 1969 to 2001 and their first degree relatives demonstrated that patients with DH can have both B- and T-cell lymphoma. The DH patients with lymphoma (1%) had not adhered as strictly to the GFD as had the control patients without lymphoma. The occurrence of lymphoma in the first-degree relatives was lower (0.2%) than in the patients with DH.[155] Study investigating both intestinal permeability and serum zonulin levels in patients with DH demonstrated that abnormally increased intestinal permeability and zonulin up-regulation are common and concomitant findings among patients with DH, likely involved in pathogenesis. Patients with more severe enteropathy had significantly greater permeability. Increased permeability can be observed even in patients with no evidence of histologic damage in biopsy specimens.[156] A 10 year study revealed that diseases associated with DH include autoimmune thyroid (4.3%), type 1 DM (1.0%), SLE (1.3%), Sjögren's syndrome (1.0%), sarcoidosis (1.3%), and alopecia areata or vitiligo (1.6%).[127] [M] Marked by an extremely itchy, bullous skin rash affecting the extensor surfaces of the limbs, trunk, and scalp. All patients with DH have at least some degree of mucosal inflammation consistent with CD.[153] [C] Results from an etiology not fully understood involving exposure to gluten; immune complex basis is most likely.[154] [R] GFD is essential and skin lesions resolve on a strict GFD.[153]	Not applicable.

+ (S) = Classic sign/symptom; (AT) = Atypical sign/symptom; (AD) Associated Disorder; (C) = Complication.

++ [P] = Prevalance; [D] = Description; [M] = Sign/symptom; [C] = CD related cause; [R] = Response to gluten Free diet (GFD).

Health Manifestations of Celiac Disease (CD)
Section B: Signs, Symptoms, Associated Disorders and Complications

Affected System	Affected Organ	ID No.	Manifestation	Type[+]	Current Medical Information [++]	Deficient Nutrient
Integumentary System	Skin	171	Dermatomyositis [1,157]	(AD)	[P] New uncommon association of CD in dermatomyositis. [157] [D] Dermatomyositis (DM), an immunologically mediated systemic disease of the connective tissue, is characterized by inflammatory and degenerative changes in the muscles and in the skin. Case report of a patient with malabsorption after a 2 year history of DM describes subsequent diagnosis of CD. CD should be suspected in patients with DM exhibiting malabsorption syndrome. Evaluation for CD, including anti-gliadin antibodies, anti-endomysium antibodies, and tissue transglutaminase antibodies should be considered in DM patients presenting with unusual and unexplained GI features. [157] [M] Marked by edema, itchy rash, weakness, muscle pain, inflammation and wasting of skeletal muscles, especially of the shoulder and pelvic girdles. Sores appear in mouth and skin. [C] Results from possible immune mechanism. [R] GFD will prevent increased morbidity from malnutrition and malignancy related to misdiagnosed CD. [157]	Not applicable.
Integumentary System	Skin	172	Edema [34,35]	(S)	[P] Common in patients with untreated CD. [35] [D] Edema is characterized by excess extracellular fluid volume. Reduction in plasma proteins and malnutrition in CD cause edema by failing to provide colloid osmotic pressure sufficient to prevent loss of plasma from capillaries into tissues. Significant or borderline significant associations with intestinal damage were found for plasma albumin in patients at diagnosis of CD and at follow-up in patients with noncontrolled CD. [35] Scurvy is a cause of lower limb edema. [34] Study reporting data on long-term control of CD and its correlates demonstrated that CD is often poorly controlled in the majority of patients on long-term treatment with a GFD due to lack of adherence to strict GFD. Intestinal damage at follow-up was absent in only 43.6% and EMA were present in the serum of 24.9%. In patients with noncontrolled CD, albumin level in long-term treatment was low and/or lower than pretreatment and correlated with the presence of intestinal damage. [35] [M] Marked by weight gain, coarsening of facial features, thickening of subcutaneous skin, and swelling of lower extremities. [C] Results from low plasma proteins, multiple micronutrient deficiencies, and vitamin C in lower limb edema. [R] CD-related edema resolves on a GFD.	Copper, EPA, Protein, Vitamin B$_1$, Vitamin C, Vitamin K.

[+] (S) = Classic sign/symptom; (AT) = Atypical sign/symptom; (AD) Associated Disorder; (C) = Complication.

[++] [P] = Prevalance; [D] = Description; [M] = Sign/symptom; [C] = CD related cause; [R] = Response to gluten Free diet (GFD).

Health Manifestations of Celiac Disease (CD)
Section B: Signs, Symptoms, Associated Disorders and Complications

Affected System	Affected Organ	ID No.	Manifestation	Type+	Current Medical Information ++	Deficient Nutrient
Integumentary System	Skin	173	Eczema [34]	(AD)	[P] Increased frequency in people with untreated CD. [D] Eczema, a feature of multiple nutritional deficiencies, is an inflammatory skin disorder characterized by failure to hold moisture, becoming dry then inflammed. [M] Marked by an itchy red rash that initially weeps or oozes serous fluid and may become crusted, thickened or scaly. [C] Results from deficiencies of nutrients including zinc, calcium, and EPA (omega-3 fatty acid) induced by CD. [R] CD-related eczema responds to a GFD.	Calcium, Omega-3 fatty acids, Zinc.
Integumentary System	Skin	174	Erythema Elevatum Diutinum (EED) [1,147,158]	(AT) (AD)	[P] New association with CD.[158] [D] Erythema elevatum diutinum (EED) is an immunologically mediated cutaneous disease recognized in the setting of CD.[147] Case report of a female presenting with EED describes subsequent diagnosis of CD based on duodenal biopsy revealing total villous atrophy. Appearance of EED lesions was preceded by widespread joint pain. In lesional skin, granular deposits of IgA and C3 were seen at the dermo-epidermal junction. In extensive laboratory tests, the only abnormal findings were an elevated erythrocyte sedimentation rate (ESR) and decreased hemoglobin and folic acid levels. Dapsone was partly effective, but complete healing of the EED lesions was achieved only after the introduction of a strict GFD.[158] [M] Marked by yellow papules or nodules changing to red, purple or brown. [C] Results from immune mechanism involving gluten exposure. [R] CD-related lesions disappeared on a strict GFD.[158]	Not applicable.

+ (S) = Classic sign/symptom; (AT) = Atypical sign/symptom; (AD) Associated Disorder; (C) = Complication.

++ [P] = Prevalance; [D] = Description; [M] = Sign/symptom; [C] = CD related cause; [R] = Response to gluten Free diet (GFD).

Health Manifestations of Celiac Disease (CD)
Section B: Signs, Symptoms, Associated Disorders and Complications

Affected System	Affected Organ	ID No.	Manifestation	Type[+]	Current Medical Information [++]	Deficient Nutrient
Integumentary System	Skin	175	Erythema Nodosum [159]	(AD)	[P] New association with CD.[159] [D] Erythema nodosum is an inflammatory disease of the deep dermis and subcutaneous fat. It is the most common form of panniculitis characterized by inflammation of the fat septa. It is most commonly found in young adults. Case report of girl age 16 with a 4 year history of chronic persistent erythema nodosum involving 2-3cm painful, bright red to brown subcutaneous nodules on the extensor surfaces below both knees describes course and subsequent diagnosis of CD, suggested by low serum iron levels. Within a month of starting a strict GFD, the development of new nodules ceased and the old lesions resolved. After an approximately 3 month symptom-free period, she was unintentionally exposed to gluten. Two erythematous, infiltrated nodules appeared on her legs, which regressed spontaneously.[159] [M] Marked by recurrent or persistent multiple, painful red to brown nodules in the pretibia area below knees of both legs.[159] [C] Results from increased intestinal permeability to exogenous antigens and the hypersensitivity reactions or the formation of immune complexes involving gluten exposure in CD.[159] [R] CD-related erythema nodosum responds to a strict GFD.[159]	Not applicable.
Integumentary System	Hair	176	Follicular Hyperkeratosis [34]	(S)	[P] Increased frequency in people with untreated CD. [D] Follicular hyperkeratosis is a clinical feature of vitamin C and/or vitamin A deficiency characterized by disordered overgrowth of the horny layer of the epidermis with horny plugs filling the orifices of hair follicles. Coiled hairs appear in scurvy (vitamin C deficiency).[34] [M] Marked by dry, scaly, rough skin having "goose flesh" appearance mainly on the lateral aspects of the upper arms, thighs and buttocks. Facial lesions may occur, especially in children. [C] Results from malabsorption in CD. [R] CD-related follicular hyperkeratosis resolves on GFD.	Vitamin A, Vitamin C.

[+] (S) = Classic sign/symptom; (AT) = Atypical sign/symptom; (AD) Associated Disorder; (C) = Complication.

[++] [P] = Prevalance; [D] = Description; [M] = Sign/symptom; [C] = CD related cause; [R] = Response to gluten Free diet (GFD).

Health Manifestations of Celiac Disease (CD)
Section B: Signs, Symptoms, Associated Disorders and Complications

Affected System	Affected Organ	ID No.	Manifestation	Type+	Current Medical Information ++	Deficient Nutrient
Integumentary System	Skin	177	Hangnail	(S)	[P] Increased frequency in people with untreated CD. [D] Hangnail, a feature of multiple deficiencies, is characterized by broken epidermis at root or lateral edge of fingernail or toenail. [M] Marked by partly detached piece of skin. [C] Results from malabsorption in CD involving protein, folic acid, and vitamin C. [R] CD-related occurrence of hangnail responds quickly to GFD.	Folic acid, Protein, Vitamin C.
Integumentary System	Skin	178	Ichthyosis, Acquired [1,160]	(AD)	[P] New association with CD.[160] [D] Acquired ichthyosis is a disorder of cornification (the epidermis changes to horny tissue) characterized by dry scaliness of the epidermis layer of skin. Case report of a 29 year old woman presenting a lamellar desquamation (scaling and peeling of skin) on the abdomen, submammary folds, and on the limbs, but without GI symptoms or dryness of skin, describes diagnosis and treatment of CD. Lab tests revealed high values of parathormone and a high level of anti-endomysial antibodies. Duodenal biopsy showed atrophy of the villi. Skin biopsy revealed an acquired ichthyosis mimicking an ichthyosis vulgaris. The total bone mineral density was about 78% of normal values. Remarkable improvement of cutaneous symptoms was obtained in 6 months on a GFD with folic acid and vitamin D supplements, after regression of secondary hyperthyroidism.[160] [M] Marked by scaling and peeling of skin on the abdomen, submammary folds and on the limbs.[160] [C] Results from malabsorption in CD involving zinc, folic acid, vitamin D, EPA (omega-3 fatty acid). [R] CD-related ichthyosis responds to GFD.[160]	EPA, Folic acid, Vitamin D, Zinc.
Integumentary System	Skin	179	Melanoma [60]	(C)	[P] Significantly increased risk in CD.[60] [D] Melanoma is a cutaneous malignancy with rapid invasion and metastasis characterized by growth from melanocytes appearing as a new mole or enlarging from an exisiting mole, changing shape, size or color. [M] Marked by changing or enlarging nevus on skin and/or mucous membranes that is usually dark but may have normal color and may ooze or bleed. [C] Results from unclear mechanism. Multiple nutrient malabsorption may predispose. [R] Patients who adhere to strict GFD are not at increased risk of melanoma.[60]	Antioxidant minerals and vitamins, Iron, Omega-3 fatty acids, Protein.

+ (S) = Classic sign/symptom; (AT) = Atypical sign/symptom; (AD) = Associated Disorder; (C) = Complication.

++ [P] = Prevalance; [D] = Description; [M] = Sign/symptom; [C] = CD related cause; [R] = Response to gluten Free diet (GFD).

Health Manifestations of Celiac Disease (CD)
Section B: Signs, Symptoms, Associated Disorders and Complications

Affected System	Affected Organ	ID No.	Manifestation	Type[+]	Current Medical Information [++]	Deficient Nutrient
Integumentary System	Skin	180	Pityriasis Rubra Pilaris [161]	(AD)	[P] New association with CD.[161] [D] Pityriasis rubra pilaris is a chronic generalized exfoliative dermatitis characterized by erythema, scaling and keratoderma development, often associated with anemia and low serum albumin. Case report describes palmar-plantar keratoderma and follicular keratosis in a young man diagnosed with CD and his response to high dose vitamin A therapy (500,000 IU orally per day for 14 days) and GFD. There was complete exfoliation of the palmar-plantar keratoderma and a decrease in the peeling and follicular keratosis. After 7 months on a GFD and 100,000 IU of vitamin A per day, patient had persistent erythema but minimal hyperkeratosis.[161] [M] Marked by generalized reddening of the skin surface with thickening and scaling between areas of normal skin. Lesions of the palms, soles and scalp may be severe. [C] Results from unclear etiology involving vitamin A malabsorption and often iron and protein in CD. [R] Pityriasis rubra pilaris responds to GFD with vitamin A supplementation.[161]	Vitamin A, Often Iron and Protein.
Integumentary System	Skin	181	Prurigo Nodularis (Hyde's Prurigo) [1,162]	(AT)	[P] New association with CD.[162] [D] Prurigo nodularis is a chronic dermatitis characterized by hard, dry, deep seated, intensely itchy papules. Case report describes prurigo beginning in a patient 15 years before the diagnosis of CD and effect of compliance with GFD.[162] [M] Marked by recurring itchy sores that scar after scratching. [C] Results from malabsorption in CD involving vitamin A and omega-3 fatty acids. [R] CD-related prurigo responds to a GFD.[162]	Omega-3 fatty acids, Vitamin A.
Integumentary System	Skin	182	Pruritic Skin Rash [1,147]	(S)	[P] Common in people with untreated CD.[147] [D] Pruritic skin rash, a cutaneous change associated with nutritional deficiency states, is a symptom of a primary disease, cutaneous or systemic. [M] Marked by itchiness that induces scratching. [C] Results from malabsorption in CD involving iron.[147] [R] CD-related itchy skin resolves on GFD.	Iron.

+ (S) = Classic sign/symptom; (AT) = Atypical sign/symptom; (AD) Associated Disorder; (C) = Complication.
++ [P] = Prevalance; [D] = Description; [M] = Sign/symptom; [C] = CD related cause; [R] = Response to gluten Free diet (GFD).

Health Manifestations of Celiac Disease (CD)
Section B: Signs, Symptoms, Associated Disorders and Complications

Affected System	Affected Organ	ID No.	Manifestation	Type+	Current Medical Information ++	Deficient Nutrient
Integumentary System	Skin	183	Psoriasis [1,163,164]	(AD)	[P] High prevalence of CD in psoriasis. [163] [D] Psoriasis is a chronic relapsing dermatosis characterized by scaling, erythema, and less commonly pustulation. [164] Psoriatic arthritis may develop. Case report describes dramatic and rapid regression of significant and widespread psoriatic skin lesions of 22 year duration in a patient after a short time on a strict GFD without pharmacologic support. Patient had not previously responded to pharmacological therapy. He had mild peripheral edema, iron deficiency anemia with microcytosis, low serum levels of folate, vitamin B_{12}, vitamin D, and leukocytosis with neutrophilia. Antiendomysial antibodies were absent, IgA and IgG antibodies to gliadin serum levels were not raised, whereas total immunoglobulin IgA were increased. Duodenal biopsy showed total atrophy of intestinal villi and intra-epithelial inflammatory infiltrate. Steatorrhea was present and a severe degree of osteoporosis. [164] [M] Marked by gradual onset of red, scaly plaques with sharply defined borders appearing on scalp, knees, shins, elbows, umbilicus, lower back, buttocks, ears, and along hairline with possible pitting of nails. [C] Results from T-cell mediated immune mechanism not clearly understood, and the relationship with CD remains controversial. A further hypothesis is that psoriatic lesions in CD patients may be partly due to vitamin D deficiency and a GFD could ameliorate psoriatic skin lesions by restoring normal absorption and vitamin D levels. [164] Zinc deficiency has been implicated. [R] CD-related psoriasis can be improved by a GFD. [164]	EPA, Vitamin D, Zinc.
Integumentary System	Skin	184	Scleroderma [1,165]	(AD)	[P] Associated with high prevalence of gluten sensitivity. [D] Scleroderma is a chronic skin manifestation of progressive systemic sclerosis characterized by generalized thickened, edematous skin firmly bound to subcutaneous tissue, causing limited movement. CD may account for malabsorption in scleroderma even when tests suggest bacterial overgrowth. A small bowel biopsy is essential. [165] [M] Marked by taut, firm, shiny skin, and hyperpigmented with development of mask-like appearance of face. [C] Results from an immune mechanism; the mechanism between scleroderma and CD is unclear. [R] Studies are inadequate to determine effect of GFD. GFD prevents increased morbidity from malnutrition and malignancy from failed diagnosis of CD.	Not applicable.

+ (S) = Classic sign/symptom; (AT) = Atypical sign/symptom; (AD) = Associated Disorder; (C) = Complication.

++ [P] = Prevalance; [D] = Description; [M] = Sign/symptom; [C] = CD related cause; [R] = Response to gluten Free diet (GFD).

Health Manifestations of Celiac Disease (CD)
Section B: Signs, Symptoms, Associated Disorders and Complications

Affected System	ID No.	Manifestation	Type⁺	Current Medical Information ⁺⁺	Deficient Nutrient
Integumentary System	185	Seborrhea [34]	(AD)	[P] Increased in people with untreated CD. [D] Seborrhea is a disorder of the sebaceous glands characterized by scaly patches of skin, often with bumps. [M] Marked by patches, most often affecting the scalp, face and chest, that appear yellowish and may be dry and flaky or greasy. [C] Results from inflammation caused by body's reaction to Pityrosporum yeast that naturally inhabits the scalp, and may be linked to nutritional deficiencies, especially vitamin A and biotin. [34] [R] CD-related seborrhea responds to GFD.	Biotin, Omega-3 fatty acids, Omega-6 fatty acids, Vitamin B₆, Vitamin B₂, Vitamin A.
Integumentary System	186	Vitiligo [1,126]	(AD)	[P] Occurrence is 1.3% in dermatitis herpetiformis (DH). [126] [D] Vitiligo is a hypopigmentation disorder characterized by permanent loss of melanocytes and in some patients, antibodies to melanin. [M] Marked by unpigmented flat, white patches of varying size surrounded by normal pigmented skin. [C] Results from unclear etiology. Immune mechanism postulated. [R] Studies are inadequate. GFD has no effect on restoring depigmented areas.	Not applicable.

⁺ (S) = Classic sign/symptom; (AT) = Atypical sign/symptom; (AD) Associated Disorder; (C) = Complication.

⁺⁺ [P] = Prevalance; [D] = Description; [M] = Sign/symptom; [C] = CD related cause; [R] = Response to gluten Free diet (GFD).

Health Manifestations of Celiac Disease (CD)
Section B: Signs, Symptoms, Associated Disorders and Complications

Affected System	Affected Organ	ID No.	Manifestation	Type+	Current Medical Information ++	Deficient Nutrient
Lymphatic System	Lymphocytes	187	B-cell non-Hodgkin Lymphoma (NHL) [60,155,166]	(C)	[P] Significant increased risk for B-cell non-Hodgkin's lymphoma (NHL) in CD patients with 9% rate for intestinal B-cell NHL and 20% for non-intestinal B cell NHL of total incident malignant lymphomas. [166] [D] B-cell non-Hodgkin's lymphoma is a malignant, monoclonal proliferation of lymphocytes preceded by lymphadenopathy and characterized by varying, less predictable spread than Hodgkin's disease. 80% to 85% of NHLs arise from B cells. Study investigating the distribution and risk of lymphoma subtypes in 11,650 patients hospitalized with CD demonstrated that most lymphomas complicating CD are related to the disease and are not of the enteropathy-type T-cell lymphoma (ETTL). 44% of patients with B-cell NHL had a history of other autoimmune/inflammatory diseases. Significantly increased risks were observed for B-cell NHL. [166] Study investigating the occurrence of lymphoma in a large series of patients consecutively diagnosed with dermatitis herpetiformis (DH) during 1969 to 2001, and their first degree relatives, demonstrated that patients with DH can have both B- and T-cell lymphoma. The DH patients with lymphoma (1%) had not adhered as strictly to the GFD as the control patients without lymphoma. Of eleven cases, eight patients had B-cell lymphoma. [155] [M] Marked by asymptomatic lymphadenopathy, anemia in many, and in some, night sweats, fever, and weight loss. [C] Results from gluten sensitive enteropathy. Multiple nutrient deficiencies may predispose. [R] The risk of non-Hodgkin's lymphoma persists despite a GFD. [60]	Omega-3 fatty acids, Protein, Selenium, Vitamin A, Vitamin E, deficiencies may predispose.
Lymphatic System	Lymphocytes	188	Cryptic Intestinal T-cell Lymphoma (Refractory Sprue) [3,167,168]	(C)	[P] Rare occurrence in a subgroup of CD patients. [167] [D] Refractory celiac disease is a severe complication characterized by persistence of symptoms and intestinal inflammation despite GFD. [3] Refractory sprue may occur after an initial response to GFD or without any evidence of preexisting CD. The presence of an aberrant clonal intraepithelial T-cell population has led to the designation of refractory sprue with this population as a Cryptic Intestinal T-cell Lymphoma. Cryptic Intestinal T-cell Lymphoma is characterized by frequent dissemination to the blood and the entire GI epithelium. [168] In a subgroup of patients with enteropathy-associated T-cell lymphoma (EATL) there is progressive deterioration of a refractory form of CD. [167] The prognosis is poor, although some patients respond to corticosteroids and immunosuppressive agents. [168] [M] Marked by intractable diarrhea, villous atrophy causing wasting malnutrition, constant fatigue, and weight loss. [C] Results from gluten exposure. Malnutrition may predispose. [R] Refractory sprue is poorly responsive to GFD. [168]	Omega-3 fatty acids, Protein, Selenium, Vitamin A, Vitamin E, deficiencies may predispose.

+ (S) = Classic sign/symptom; (AT) = Atypical sign/symptom; (AD) Associated Disorder; (C) = Complication.

++ [P] = Prevalance; [D] = Description; [M] = Sign/symptom; [C] = CD related cause; [R] = Response to gluten Free diet (GFD).

Health Manifestations of Celiac Disease (CD)
Section B: Signs, Symptoms, Associated Disorders and Complications

Affected System	Affected Organ	ID No.	Manifestation	Type[+]	Current Medical Information [++]	Deficient Nutrient
Lymphatic System	Lymphocytes	189	Enteropathy-Associated T cell Lymphoma (EATL) [1], [59,60,166,167,169,170]	(C)	[P] Most common neoplasm in CD.[59] The risk of enteropathy-associated T-cell lymphoma (EATL) is markedly increased in CD.[166] [D] Enteropathy-associated T cell lymphoma (EATL), a severe complication of CD, is a rare form of high grade T-cell non-Hodgkins lymphoma (NHL) of the upper small intestine, specifically associated with CD.[59] EATL is often disseminated at diagnosis.[167] This tumor usually affects the jejunum and grossly presents as multiple circumferential ulcers without the formation of definite tumor masses. Mesenteric lymph nodes are commonly involved.[169] EATL is often multifocal with ulcerative lesions, which explains the high perforation rate at presentation or during chemotherapy.[170] Molecular, biological and immunohistochemical studies have shown that the intestinal mucosa distant from the tumor contains clonal populations of small T cells, often of the same clone as the high grade T-cell lymphoma. These findings suggest that EATL arises in the setting of CD and evolves from reactive intraepithelial lymphocytes through a low-grade lymphocytic neoplasm to a high grade tumor, which is usually the cause of the presenting symptoms. Most cases of chronic ulcerative enteropathy are probably part of the same disease. Patients have the celiac associated HLA DQA1*0501, DQB1*0201 phenotype.[59] EATLs can present in 20% of patients as extra-small-bowel T-cell lymphomas such as panniculitis-like lymphoma. The majority present as large cell lymphoma CD 3 +, CD 8 -, CD 8 +, CD 30. Work-up of EATL must include immunohistology, T-cell flow cytometry, T-cell rearrangement and adequate imaging with CT and PET scanning. There is no satisfactory treatment for EATL.[170] Case report describes a 60 year old male diagnosed with EATL after segmental small bowel resection, who presented with recurrent GI bleeding. The clinical course of EATL is very unfavorable and the prognosis is poor.[169] [M] Marked by localized abdominal pain, diarrhea, and weight loss. Some patients may manifest with nonspecific symptoms for a period of years or an acute emergency of perforation, obstruction, or hemorrhage.[169] [C] Results from chronic gluten exposure in CD. Refractory CD with abberant T cells carries a high risk of development of EATL.[170] Multiple nutrient deficiencies may predispose. [R] Strict adherence to the GFD seems to be the only possibility of preventing this subset of rare but very aggressive forms of cancer.[167]	Omega-3 fatty acids, Protein, Selenium, Vitamin A, Vitamin E, deficiencies may predispose.

+ (S) = Classic sign/symptom; (AT) = Atypical sign/symptom; (AD) Associated Disorder; (C) = Complication.

++ [P] = Prevalance; [D] = Description; [M] = Sign/symptom; [C] = CD related cause; [R] = Response to gluten Free diet (GFD).

Health Manifestations of Celiac Disease (CD)
Section B: Signs, Symptoms, Associated Disorders and Complications

Affected System	Affected Organ	ID No.	Manifestation	Type+	Current Medical Information ++	Deficient Nutrient
Lymphatic System	Lymphocytes	190	Extraintestinal Lymphomas [1,60,166]	(C)	[P] Significantly increased risk for lymphoma of non-intestinal origin observed for patients with CD.[166] [D] Extraintestinal lymphomas are malignancies that arise in lymphatic tissue outside the intestinal tract. Study investigating the distribution and risk of lymphoma subtypes in CD demonstrated that most lymphomas complicating CD are indeed related to the disease and are not of the enteropathy-type T cell lymphoma. Extraintestinal lymphomas comprised 47% of lymphomas in study of CD patients.[166] [M] Marked by painless lymphadenopathy, unexplained fever, night sweats, constant fatigue, and weight loss. [C] Results from chronic gluten exposure.[166] Multiple nutrient deficiencies may predispose. [R] The risk of non-Hodgkin's lymphoma persists despite GFD.[60]	Omega-3 fatty acids, Protein, Selenium, Vitamin A, Vitamin E, deficiencies may predispose.
Lymphatic System	Lymphocytes	191	Intraepithelial Lymphocytosis in Small Bowel Samples [171]	(C)	[P] Can be the initial presentation of CD in 10% of cases.[171] [D] Intraepithelial lymphocytosis is characterized by increase in intraepithelial lymphocytes (IELs) in the small intestinal mucosa. Study investigating the specificity of increase in IELs for diagnosis of gluten sensitivity (GS) in an otherwise normal small bowel biopsy concluded it is somewhat non-specific for GS but, because of the prevalence of GS, all patients with this finding should be investigated for GS. Increased IELs may also be associated with autoimmune disorders and non-steroidal anti-inflammatory drugs (NSAID).[171] [M] Asymptomatic. [C] Results from unclear etiology. [R] Favorable response to GFD.	Not applicable.
Lymphatic System	Lymph nodes	192	Lymphadenopathy [1,55]	(C)	[P] Increased frequency in untreated CD. [D] Lymphadenopathy is characterized by enlargement of lymph nodes greater than 1.5 cm caused by proliferation of lymphocytes within the node. Study investigating the clinical manifestations of CD related to malnutrition and analyzing the associations between CD and other diagnoses confirmed the known associations of CD with enlarged lymph nodes.[55] [M] Marked by swollen nodes, with or without tenderness. [C] Results from unclear etiology. [R] Studies inadequate to determine effect of GFD.	Not applicable.

+ (S) = Classic sign/symptom; (AT) = Atypical sign/symptom; (AD) Associated Disorder; (C) = Complication.

++ [P] = Prevalance; [D] = Description; [M] = Sign/symptom; [C] = CD related cause; [R] = Response to gluten Free diet (GFD).

Affected System	Affected Organ	ID No.	Manifestation	Type+	Current Medical Information ++	Deficient Nutrient
Lymphatic System	Lymph node/spleen	193	Mesenteric Lymph Node Cavitation and Hyposplenism [172]	(C)	[P] New association with CD.[172] [D] Mesenteric lymph node cavitation and hyposplenism combination is a rare lymphatic entity related to CD. It is characterized by involution of a mesenteric lymph node and absence of functional splenic tissue presenting with small bowel mucosal atrophy. Case reports of 5 patients all show peculiar cavitation of mesenteric lymph nodes. Clinically, 3 presented with abdominal symptoms, a mass or obstruction warranting laparotomy. Two patients showed cavitating lymph nodes at autopsy. Lymph nodes were enlarged with central, partly cystic degeneration; milky fluid exuded from the cut surface. In each case, investigation showed intestinal villous atrophy and splenic atrophy. Three patients died, 2 from cachexia and the other from pneumonia; the other two are alive and well one year and 6 years after presentation. Mortality rate is 50%.[172] [M] Marked by abdominal mass, persistent diarrhea, and weight loss with small bowel atrophy.[172] [C] Results from unknown pathogenesis.[172] [R] Response varies after treatment on GFD.	Not applicable.

+ (S) = Classic sign/symptom; (AT) = Atypical sign/symptom; (AD) Associated Disorder; (C) = Complication.

++ [P] = Prevalance; [D] = Description; [M] = Sign/symptom; [C]= CD related cause; [R] = Response to gluten Free diet (GFD).

Health Manifestations of Celiac Disease (CD)
Section B: Signs, Symptoms, Associated Disorders and Complications

Affected System	Affected Organ	ID No.	Manifestation	Type[+]	Current Medical Information [++]	Deficient Nutrient
Lymphatic System	Spleen	194	Hyposplenism [1,59,173,174]	(C)	[P] Common complication of adult CD. 82.4% of CD patients had hyposplenic changes at diagnosis.[173] [D] Hyposplenism secondary to CD is characterized by low lymphocyte count and presence of Howell-Jolly bodies in red blood cells (may not be present in mild cases). CD, with or without dermatitis herpetiformis, is one of two most common causes of hyposplenism.[174] Splenic atrophy is related to the severity of the disease and degree of dietary control. Splenic atrophy predisposes to infection with encapsulated bacteria, although mortality studies indicate that infection with these organisms is not a major cause of death in patients with CD.[59] Children are especially at risk because they often have lower levels of specific antibodies against encapsulated organisms.[174] Splenic macrophages have a major role in phagocytosing bacteria and aging blood cells from the circulation. The spleen is also the major producer of antibodies. Unimmunized patients who have functional hyposplenism should be immunized as soon as their conditions are identified. Sporadic cases of pneumococcal and other vaccine failures have been reported in appropriately immunized persons. For this reason, a vaccination program, by itself, should not confer a false sense of security.[174] [M] Marked by lifelong susceptibility to serious infections.[174] [C] Results from CD with or without dermatitis herpetiformis. [R] Non-significant tendency to improve morphologic changes on strict GFD.[173]	Not applicable.

+ (S) = Classic sign/symptom; (AT) = Atypical sign/symptom; (AD) Associated Disorder; (C) = Complication.
++ [P] = Prevalance; [D] = Description; [M] = Sign/symptom; [C] = CD related cause; [R] = Response to gluten Free diet (GFD).

Health Manifestations of Celiac Disease (CD)
Section B: Signs, Symptoms, Associated Disorders and Complications

Affected System	Affected Organ	ID No.	Manifestation	Type+	Current Medical Information ++	Deficient Nutrient
Muscular System	Muscles	195	Hypokalemic Rhabdomyolysis in Celiac Disease and Dermatitis Herpetiformis [1,26,175,176]	(AD)	[P] New association with CD[26,175] and DH.[176] [D] Hypokalemic rhabdomyolysis, an acute and sometimes fatal disease, is characterized by the accumulation of by-products of skeletal muscle destruction in the renal tubules and producing acute kidney failure caused by rapid potassium loss. Case report describes hypokalemic rhabdomyolysis in a 12 year old girl with atrophy of the lower extremity muscles, sudden weakness of upper and lower extremities, and inability to walk with chronic diarrhea, fatigue, and failure to thrive. Case represents the earliest reported case in CD.[175] Case report describes rare occurrence of hypokalemic rhabdomyolysis in a 22 year old woman with CD and DH. Diarrhea and emesis resolved and myopathy ceased on potassium supplementation on a GFD.[176] Case report describes hypokalemic rhabdomyolysis in a 63 year old man with diarrhea and steatorrhea. CD should be considered a cause of malabsorption induced hypokalemic rhabdomyolysis.[26] [M] Marked by sudden weakness of extremities and inability to walk associated with diarrhea and/or vomiting.[175] [C] Results from rapid loss of potassium in association with diarrhea and emesis in CD.[176] [R] GFD resolves weakness and diarrhea.[26] Potassium supplementation indicated.	Potassium.

+ (S) = Classic sign/symptom; (AT) = Atypical sign/symptom; (AD) Associated Disorder; (C) = Complication.

++ [P] = Prevalence; [D] = Description; [M] = Sign/symptom; [C] = CD related cause; [R] = Response to gluten Free diet (GFD).

Health Manifestations of Celiac Disease (CD)
Section B: Signs, Symptoms, Associated Disorders and Complications

Affected System	Affected Organ	ID No.	Manifestation	Type+	Current Medical Information ++	Deficient Nutrient
Muscular System	Muscles	196	Muscle Pain and Tenderness [34]	(S)	[P] Common in people with untreated CD. [D] Muscle pain and tenderness are well-recognized features of multiple vitamin and mineral deficiencies. [M] Marked by painful sensation when pressed, and while using muscle or at rest; more pronounced after exercise. [C] Results from deficiency of nutrients, including thiamin, vitamin C, vitamin E, vitamin K, niacin, pyridoxine, vitamin B_{12}, magnesium or selenium. [34] [R] CD-related muscle pain and tenderness responds to nutritious GFD. Supplementation may be needed.	Magnesium, Selenium, Vitamin B_1, Vitamin C, Vitamin E, Vitamin K, Vitamin B_3, Vitamin B_6, Vitamin B_{12}. [34]
Muscular System	Muscles	197	Muscle Spasm and Muscle Cramps [34]	(S)	[P] Common in people with untreated CD. [D] Muscle spasm and muscle cramps are well-recognized features of multiple vitamin and mineral deficiencies is a feature of idiopathic hypoparathyroidism. [M] Marked by painful involuntary contraction of a skeletal muscle. Cramps are stronger and more painful than spasms, occurring while the muscle is in its most shortened state. [C] Results from deficiency of electrolytes and magnesium, calcium (occurring in legs and feet usually at night), thiamin (affecting calves) and vitamin E in CD. [34] [R] CD-related muscle spasms/cramps resolve on GFD. Supplementation may be needed.	Calcium, Chlorides, Magnesium, Potassium, Sodium, Vitamin B_1, Vitamin E.
Muscular System	Muscles	198	Muscle Wasting [1,34]	(S)	[P] Increased frequency in untreated CD. [D] Muscle wasting is a well-recognized feature of multiple vitamin deficiencies. [34] [M] Marked by decrease in muscle size, fatigue on using them, loss of power, and difficulty walking. [C] Results from deficiencies of protein, thiamin and vitamin C due to malabsorption in CD. [R] CD-related muscle wasting responds to a GFD. Supplementation may be needed.	Vitamin B_1, Vitamin C, Protein.
Muscular System	Muscles	199	Muscle Weakness [34]	(S)	[P] Increased frequency in untreated CD. [D] Muscle weakness is a well-recognized feature of multiple deficiencies. [34] [M] Marked by decreased muscle strength and inability to perform normal work. [C] Results from deficiencies of thiamin, vitamin C, and selenium due to malabsorption in CD. [R] CD-related muscle weakness resolves on GFD. Supplementation may be needed.	Selenium, Vitamin B_1, Vitamin C.

+ (S) = Classic sign/symptom; (AT) = Atypical sign/symptom; (AD) Associated Disorder; (C) = Complication.

++ [P] = Prevalance; [D] = Description; [M] = Sign/symptom; [C] = CD related cause; [R] = Response to gluten Free diet (GFD).

Health Manifestations of Celiac Disease (CD)
Section B: Signs, Symptoms, Associated Disorders and Complications

Affected System	Affected Organ	ID No.	Manifestation	Type[+]	Current Medical Information [++]	Deficient Nutrient
Muscular System	Muscles	200	Osteomalacic Myopathy [29]	(AD)	[P] Newly recognized presentation of CD.[29] [D] Osteomalacic myopathy is a feature of osteomalacia characterized by painful proximal muscle weakness and hyperreflexia. Case report describes how recognition of increased level of serum alkaline phosphatase and hypophosphatemia led to diagnosis of osteomalacia in a 45 year old woman with thigh pain followed within a year by proximal muscle weakness. Identification of iron deficiency anemia and hypocholesterolemia implicated previously unrecognized CD with associated vitamin D malabsorption as the cause of osteomalacia.[29] [M] Marked by thigh pain followed by proximal muscle weakness and brisk reflexes.[29] [C] Results from vitamin D and phosphorus malabsorption in CD.[29] [R] CD-related osteomalacic myopathy responds to GFD. Supplementation may be needed.	Phosphorus, Vitamin D.
Muscular System	Muscles	201	Polymyositis [1,157]	(AD)	[P] New association with CD.[157] [D] Polymyositis is an immunologically mediated body-wide connective tissue disease characterized by inflammatory and degeneratory changes in skeletal muscles. CD should be suspected in patients with polymyositis exhibiting malabsorption syndrome.[157] [M] Marked by weakness and wasting of the proximal muscles of the limbs, elevated muscle enzymes in the blood, and muscle necrosis (destruction). [C] Results from immune mechanism. [R] GFD will prevent increased morbidity from malnutrition and malignancy.[157]	Not applicable.

[+] (S) = Classic sign/symptom; (AT) = Atypical sign/symptom; (AD) Associated Disorder; (C) = Complication.

[++] [PJ] = Prevalance; [D] = Description; [M] = Sign/symptom; [C] = CD related cause; [R] = Response to gluten Free diet (GFD).

Health Manifestations of Celiac Disease (CD)
Section B: Signs, Symptoms, Associated Disorders and Complications

Affected System	Affected Organ	ID No.	Manifestation	Type+	Current Medical Information++	Deficient Nutrient
Muscular System	Muscles	202	Tetany [1,177,178,179]	(S)	[P] Rare form of presentation in CD.[177] [D] Tetany, a feature of multiple deficiencies involving muscles of the extremities, is characterized by paroxysmal intermittent tonic spasm. Case report describes origin of tetany in 3 patients who were subsequently diagnosed with CD as severe hypocalcemia and hypomagnesemia. After treatment with intravenous calcium and GFD with supplements, clinical remission was achieved. In the presence of isolated tetany, CD must be disclosed.[177] Case report describes severe tetany secondary to hypocalcemia causing bilateral fractures of the femoral necks. Severe muscle pains, an organic mental syndrome, and personality changes are rare complications of CD and are reversible on GFD.[178] Case report describes hypocalcemic tetany with hypovitaminosis D in an 8 month old baby subsequently diagnosed with CD.[179] [M] Marked by nervousness, irritability, and apprehension with numbness and tingling of the extremities and painful muscle spasms, especially hands and feet. [C] Results from malabsorption of magnesium and calcium due to lack of vitamin D in gluten sensitive enteropathy, and steatorrhea, if present. [R] Tetany resolves on GFD.[177,178,179] Supplementation may be needed.	Calcium, Magnesium, Vitamin D.

+ (S) = Classic sign/symptom; (AT) = Atypical sign/symptom; (AD) = Associated Disorder; (C) = Complication.

++ [P] = Prevalance; [D] = Description; [M] = Sign/symptom; [C] = CD related cause; [R] = Response to gluten Free diet (GFD).

Health Manifestations of Celiac Disease (CD)
Section B: Signs, Symptoms, Associated Disorders and Complications

Affected System	ID No.	Manifestation	Affected Organ	Type+	Current Medical Information ++	Deficient Nutrient
Nervous System	203	Nervous System Disorders [1,180,181,182]	Brain, spinal cord, and peripheral nerves	(AT) (AD) (C)	[P] Neurologic disorders were found in 51.4% of CD patients. [180] Hard neurologic disorders were found in 10% of patients with CD. [181] Perfusion abnormalities were found in 71% of patients with CD. [182] [D] Nervous system disorders include both hard and soft disorders. Hard neurological disorders in CD include epilepsy, ataxia, myoclonus, internuclear ophthalmoplegia, multifocal leukoencephalopathy, dementia, and peripheral neuropathies. [181] Study screening children and young adults suggests that the variability of neurologic disorders that occur in CD is broader than previously reported and includes "softer" and more common neurologic disorders. Strong association in soft disorders includes hypotonia, developmental delay, learning disorders and ADHD, headache, and cerebellar ataxia. In most cases no significant increase in liability to develop soft neurologic disorders between patients with infantile-onset GI symptoms and patients with the late onset or asymptomatic CD could be shown. This differs from the trend to regard CD as gluten sensitivity, found in patients with neurologic disorder and atypical or subclinical CD. [180] Study investigating the incidence of brain perfusion abnormalities, and whether gluten intake and associated autoimmune diseases may be considered risk factors in causing cerebral impairment, demonstrated that brain perfusion abnormalities seem common in CD. [182] [M] Marked by neurological dysfunction. [C] Results from obscure mechanism but may be immunological or related to trace vitamin deficiencies. [181] [R] CD-related hard disorders respond poorly to gluten restriction except peripheral neuropathies. [181] Brain perfusion may be improved by a GFD. Soft disorders improve or resolve on a GFD.	B complex vitamins, Calcium, Copper, Folic acid, Iron, Magnesium, Omega-3 fatty acids, Potassium, Protein, Vitamin C, Vitamin E.
Nervous System	204	Ataxia, Gait Disturbance [1,49,183,184]	Brain: cerebellum	(AD)	[P] Common neurological presentation in CD patients. [183] [D] Gait ataxia is a cerebellar disorder characterized by defective muscular coordination of skeletal muscles used for locomotion. Manifestations can be a consequence of vitamin B[12], vitamin B[1], nicotinamide, vitamin D, or vitamin E deficiency. [184] Study investigating the prevalence of gluten sensitivity in a large cohort of patients with various causes of ataxia demonstrated 100% of patients with gluten ataxia had gait ataxia. [183] Study investigating the role of oxidative stress in CD demonstrated the level of markers for vitamin E were significantly lower in CD than in contols. [49] [M] Marked by unsteady staggering walking movements and use of a wide base of support. [C] Results from vitamin E deficiency in CD. [R] Symptoms usually persist, but a GFD prevents further deterioration.	Vitamin B[1], Vitamin B[3], Vitamin B[12], Vitamin E, Vitamin D.

+ (S) = Classic sign/symptom; (AT) = Atypical sign/symptom; (AD) Associated Disorder; (C) = Complication.

++ [P] = Prevalance; [D] = Description; [M] = Sign/symptom; [C] = CD related cause; [R] = Response to gluten Free diet (GFD).

Health Manifestations of Celiac Disease (CD)
Section B: Signs, Symptoms, Associated Disorders and Complications

Affected System	Affected Organ	ID No.	Manifestation	Type[+]	Current Medical Information [++]	Deficient Nutrient
Nervous System	Brain: cerebellum	205	Ataxia, Gluten [1,49,183,185,186]	(AD)	[P] CD found in 24% of patients with gluten ataxia.[183] Ataxia is the most common neurological complication of gluten sensitivity.[183] As high as 68% of patients with idiopathic ataxia.[185] [D] Gluten ataxia is a cerebellar degeneration characterized by motor abnormalities (intentional movements). The duration of immunological activity resulting in Purkinje cell damage, a finding commonly encountered in cerebellar degeneration, correlates with the severity and the presence of cerebellar atrophy.[185] Most patients have negligible GI symptoms.[183,185] Ataxia may be the sole presentation in latent CD. Therefore, antigliadin antibody testing for CD is essential at first presentation of patients with sporadic idiopathic ataxia.[185] Study investigating CD in patients with various ataxia demonstrated the following clinical characteristics for gluten ataxia: ocular signs in 84%, dysarthria in 66%, upper limb in 75%, lower limb in 90%, and gait ataxia in 100%; atrophy of cerebellum in 79%, white matter hyperintensities in 19%; and sensorimotor axonal neuropathy in 45%. GI symptoms were present in only 13%, CD in 24%, and HLA DQ2 in 72% of patients.[183] Study investigating gluten sensitivity in patients with sporadic ataxia demonstrated susceptibility of both the central and peripheral nervous system to the immune response triggered by sensitivity to gluten. Necropsy in two patients showed lymphocytic infiltration of the cerebellum, damage to the posterior columns of the spinal cord, and sparse infiltration of those peripheral nerves. Antibodies to endomysium may be useful in the identification of those patients with cryptic CD, but may not be found in patients with gluten sensitivity and histologically normal mucosa.[185] Study investigating the humoral response in patients with gluten ataxia demonstrated antibodies against Purkinje cells.[186] Study investigating the role of oxidative stress in CD demonstrated the level of markers for vitamin E were significantly lower in CD than in controls.[49] [M] Marked by lack of coordination in movement and walking. [C] Results from unclear relation between gluten sensitivity, malabsorption, nutritional deficiencies, and ataxia.[185] Immunologically mediated neural damage implies an autoimmune mechanism from exposure to gluten.[185,186] [R] Symptoms may persist, but GFD prevents further deterioration. Prompt diagnosis of gluten ataxia affords complete resolution of symptoms after strict adherence to a GFD.[185]	Vitamin E.

+ (S) = Classic sign/symptom; (AT) = Atypical sign/symptom; (AD) Associated Disorder; (C) = Complication.

++ [P] = Prevalance; [D] = Description; [M] = Sign/symptom; [C] = CD related cause; [R] = Response to gluten Free diet (GFD).

Health Manifestations of Celiac Disease (CD)
Section B: Signs, Symptoms, Associated Disorders and Complications

Affected System	Affected Organ	ID No.	Manifestation	Type[+]	Current Medical Information[++]	Deficient Nutrient
Nervous System	Brain: cerebellum	206	Ataxia, Progressive Myoclonic [1,49,181,183,187,188]	(AD)	[P] Increased frequency in CD.[183] New association with CD.[187,188] [D] Progressive myoclonic ataxia is a movement disorder characterized by defective muscular coordination of cortical origin. The pathology is in the cerebellum.[188] Case report describes asymptomatic CD associated with stimulus induced myoclonus, stiff gait, and abnormalities of eye movement. 31 year old female experienced jerks triggered by sudden sound or touch since her childhood, and recurrent episodes of nausea and vomiting. She had spasticity in all four limbs, brisk deep tendon reflexes with bilateral Achilles clonus, and flexor plantar reflexes. CT showed mild cortical cerebral atrophy. Serum anti-endomysium antibodies were negative, serum antigliadin antibodies IgA and IgG were positive. Small bowel biopsy revealed subtotal villus atrophy. CD has to be considered in the differential diagnosis of patients presenting with neurologic symptoms of unknown origin, even in the absence of GI symptoms. Nausea and vomiting and stimulus-sensitive myoclonus responded well to a GFD but not the general neurologic condition.[187] Case report describes onset of a neurological syndrome dominated by action and stimulus sensitive myoclonus of cortical origin with mild ataxia and infrequent seizures. Condition progressed in 2 older patients without overt features of CD or nutritional deficiency on a strict GFD. Post-mortum examination of the brain in one case showed selective symmetrical atrophy of the cerebellar hemispheres with Purkinje cell loss and Bergmann astrocytosis, and with preservation of the cerebral hemispheres and brainstem. CD should be considered in the differential diagnosis of all patients presenting with a progressive myoclonic ataxic syndrome.[188] Study investigating the role of oxidative stress in CD demonstrated the level of markers for vitamin E were significantly lower in CD than in controls.[49] [M] Marked by brief, rapid contraction of a muscle or a group of muscles. [C] Thought to result from vitamin E deficiency and gluten exposure with immune mechanism. Mechanism is unresolved and requires a more rigorous approach to examine the role of disordered metabolism secondary to trace vitamin deficiency as well as immunological dysfunction.[181] [R] Response to GFD varies.	Vitamin E.

[+] (S) = Classic sign/symptom; (AT) = Atypical sign/symptom; (AD) Associated Disorder; (C) = Complication.

[++] [P] = Prevalance; [D] = Description; [M] = Sign/symptom; [C] = CD related cause; [R] = Response to gluten Free diet (GFD).

Health Manifestations of Celiac Disease (CD)
Section B: Signs, Symptoms, Associated Disorders and Complications

Affected System	Affected Organ	ID No.	Manifestation	Type+	Current Medical Information ++	Deficient Nutrient
Nervous System	Brain: cerebellum	207	Chorea [189]	(AD)	[P] New association with CD.[189] [D] Chorea is a movement disorder characterized by brief, purposeless involuntary movements of the distal limbs and face. Case report describes 4 patients average age 61 years old with CD and chorea. GFD produced notable improvement in the motor symptoms of all 4 patients.[189] [M] Marked by writhing of the limbs or facial muscles. [C] Results from exposure to gluten, but mechanism is unclear as yet. [R] CD-related chorea improves on GFD.	Unknown.
Nervous System	Brain: cerebellum	208	Tremors [34]	(AD)	[P] Increased frequency in untreated CD. [D] Tremors are characterized by repetitive patterns of involuntary muscle contraction and relaxation. [M] Marked by rhythmic, alternating, oscillatory movements. [C] Results from magnesium deficiency due to malabsorption in CD.[34] [R] CD-related tremors resolves on GFD.	Magnesium.

+ (S) = Classic sign/symptom; (AT) = Atypical sign/symptom; (AD) Associated Disorder; (C) = Complication.

++ [P] = Prevalance; [D] = Description; [M] = Sign/symptom; [C] = CD related cause; [R] = Response to gluten Free diet (GFD).

Health Manifestations of Celiac Disease (CD)
Section B: Signs, Symptoms, Associated Disorders and Complications

Affected System	Affected Organ	ID No.	Manifestation	Type[+]	Current Medical Information [++]	Deficient Nutrient
Nervous System	Brain: cerebrum	209	Brain Atrophy [181,188,190,191]	(C)	[P] New association with CD.[190] Diffuse cerebral atrophy evident in 80% of patients with CD and late onset epilepsy.[191] [D] Brain atrophy is characterized by loss of brain tissue. Case report describes diffuse cerebral or cerebellar atrophy, with intellectual deterioration ranging from moderate to severe, found on brain CT scan in 5 patients subsequently diagnosed with CD in whom GI symptoms were mild. One of 5 patients responded to a GFD.[190] Case report describes selective symmetrical atrophy of the cerebellar hemispheres with Purkinje cell loss and Bergmann astrocytosis and with preservation of the cerebral hemispheres and brainstem at necropsy in a patient with progressive myoclonic ataxia. Onset followed years after the development of CD or dermatitis herpetiformis, and brain imaging was either normal or showed mild cerebral and cerebellar atrophy. Syndrome progressed on GFD when started late in life.[188] Study investigating the occurrence CD in living patients with epilepsy of unknown etiology demonstrated the prevalence of CD was increased among patients with epilepsy of unknown etiology and of them 80% had supratentorial brain atrophy vs. 26% of controls. Screening of CD seems warranted in patients with epilepsy of unknown etiology, particularly when there is co-existent cerebral atrophy of unknown etiology.[191] [M] Marked by neurologic dysfunction or impairment including moderate to severe intellectual deterioration, mild ataxia and infrequent seizures. [C] Results from obscure pathogenetic mechanisms, and immunologic mechanisms are implicated.[190] The role of trace vitamin deficiencies involving niacin, pyridoxine and thiamin or disordered biopterin synthesis has not been investigated in detail.[181] [R] Response to GFD varies.	DHA, Vitamin B_1, Vitamin B_3, Vitamin B_6.

[+] (S) = Classic sign/symptom; (AT) = Atypical sign/symptom; (AD) Associated Disorder; (C) = Complication.

[++] [P] = Prevalance; [D] = Description; [M] = Sign/symptom; [C] = CD related cause; [R] = Response to gluten Free diet (GFD).

Recognizing Celiac Disease *Signs, Symptoms, Associated Disorders & Complications*

Health Manifestations of Celiac Disease (CD)
Section B: Signs, Symptoms, Associated Disorders and Complications

Affected System	Affected Organ	ID No.	Manifestation	Type[+]	Current Medical Information [++]	Deficient Nutrient
Nervous System	Brain: cerebrum	210	Cerebral Perfusion Abnormalities [182]	(S)	[P] Common phenomenon, occurring in 71% of patients with untreated CD.[182] [D] Cerebral perfusion abnormalities, evaluated by brain single-photon emission computed tomography (CT), are characterized by cerebral impairment. Study investigating whether gluten intake and associated autoimmune diseases may be considered risk factors in causing cerebral impairment demonstrated that the more significant abnormalities were localized in frontal regions, and were significantly different from controls only in CD patients on an unrestricted diet. The prevalence of single-photon emission CT abnormalities was similar in CD patients, 74% with associated autoimmune disease and 69% without associated autoimmune disease. This phenomenon is similar to that previously described in other autoimmune diseases, but does not appear to be related to associated autoimmunity and, at least in the frontal region, may be improved by a GFD.[182] [M] Marked by neurological and psychiatric disorders. [C] Results from exposure to gluten.[182] [R] CD-related perfusion abnormalities normalize on a GFD.[182]	Not applicable.
Nervous System	Brain: cerebrum	211	Cortical Calcifying Angiomatosis [1,181, 192, 193]	(AD)	[P] New association with CD.[192,193] [D] Cortical calcifying angiomatosis, a cortical vascular abnormality, is characterized by calcification related to underlying folate deficiency and is usually present in the parietal or occipital cortical and subcortical regions.[181] Case report describes pathological changes in the syndrome of CD, folate deficiency, bilateral occipital calcifications, and intractable epilepsy. A child with this disorder had a field defect correlating with active lateralized epileptic discharges and asymmetrical lesions. A cortical vascular abnormality with patchy pial angiomatosis, fibrosed veins, and large jagged microcalcifications was found on resection of the right occipital lobe.[192] Case report describes a patient with ophthalmic migraine found to have bilateral cerebellar and cerebral calcifications. She progressively developed severe intracranial hypertension, with swelling of the brain and downward transtentorial and tonsillar herniation. Resection of the right occipital pole demonstrated meningo-cortical calcifying angiomatosis. Subtle signs of malabsorption led to diagnosis of CD.[193] [M] Marked by neurological abnormalities including seizures, migraine, intracranial hypertension. [C] Results from folate deficiency in CD. [R] Seizures may be stabilized by gluten restriction and folate supplementation.[181]	Folic acid.

+ (S) = Classic sign/symptom; (AT) = Atypical sign/symptom; (AD) Associated Disorder; (C) = Complication.

++ [P] = Prevalance; [D] = Description; [M] = Sign/symptom; [C] = CD related cause; [R] = Response to gluten Free diet (GFD).

Health Manifestations of Celiac Disease (CD)
Section B: Signs, Symptoms, Associated Disorders and Complications

Affected System	Affected Organ	ID No.	Manifestation	Type+	Current Medical Information++	Deficient Nutrient
Nervous System	Brain: cerebrum	212	Dementia 3,181,190	(C)	[P] New association with CD.[190] [D] Dementia is a non-gastrointestinal presentation of gluten sensitive enteropathy.[3] Progressive deterioration in intellectual function is characterized by memory and cognitive impairment involving deficits in reasoning, judgment, abstract thought, comprehension, learning, use of language, and task execution. Case report describes 5 patients before age 60 with dementia subsequently found to have CD. Intellectual deterioration ranged from moderate to severe, and diffuse cerebral or cerebellar atrophy was found on brain CT. GI symptoms were mild. A GFD improved the neurologic disability in one out of 5 patients. CD may play a role in some cases of pre-senile dementia.[190] [M] Marked by significant interference with ability to perform activities of daily living, to interact socially, and to think and reason. [C] Results from unclear pathogenetic mechanism.[190] The role of trace vitamin deficiencies involving niacin, pyridoxine, and thiamin or disordered biopterin synthesis has not been investigated in detail. Speculation that immune dysfunction is causal has not been proved.[181] [R] Response to GFD varies with cause of dementia.	Copper, Folic acid, Omega-3 fatty acids, Omega-6 fatty acids, Iron, Vitamin B$_1$, Vitamin B$_{12}$, Vitamin B$_3$,

Nervous System	Brain: cerebrum	213	Emicrania 1,39,180,194	(AT)	[P] Significantly higher occurrence of headache in patients with untreated CD than controls.[194] Prevalence of headache in CD is migraine (45.1%), tension-psychogenic (19.4%), and non-specific (35.5%).[180]
					
					[D] Emicrania is a headache resulting from stimulation of, or traction of, or pressure on any of the pain sensitive structures of the head characterized by pain felt anywhere in the head.
					    Study measuring IgG and IgA isotypes and IgG subclasses demonstrated significantly higher proportion of persistent or recurrent headache in patients with positive IgA gliadin antibodies.[39]
					    Study assessing the occurrence of neurological signs and symptoms in adult patients with CD revealed that headache is associated with CD and can be ameliorated by a GFD.[194]
					
					[M] Marked by pain felt in the head, eyes, jaw, or neck.
					
					[C] Results from malabsorption in CD and gluten exposure.
					
					[R] CD-related headaches can be ameliorated by a strict GFD[194,180]
						Magnesium.

+ (S) = Classic sign/symptom; (AT) = Atypical sign/symptom; (AD) Associated Disorder; (C) = Complication.

++ [P] = Prevalance; [D] = Description; [M] = Sign/symptom; [C] = CD related cause; [R] = Response to gluten Free diet (GFD).

Health Manifestations of Celiac Disease (CD)
Section B: Signs, Symptoms, Associated Disorders and Complications

Affected System	Affected Organ	ID No.	Manifestation	Type+	Current Medical Information ++	Deficient Nutrient
Nervous System	Brain: cerebrum	214	Epilepsy [181,191,195,196]	(AD)	[P] Prevalence of epilepsy is 5.5% in CD patients. Prevalence of CD in patients with epilepsy is 8.1% on the basis of a flat intestinal mucosa.[195] [D] Epilepsy is characterized by recurring seizures, with or without calcification, in the occipital area of the brain, that can develop without the more classic malabsorptive symptoms of CD. The majority of patients have complex partial attacks. There is also a subgroup of patients who develop the syndrome of CD, epilepsy, and cerebral calcifications which may be related to underlying folate deficiency.[181] Study conducted in a tertiary center investigating the occurrence CD in living patients with epilepsy of unknown etiology demonstrated the prevalence of CD was increased among patients with epilepsy of unknown etiology and of them 80% had supratentorial brain atrophy vs. 26% of controls. Screening of CD seems warranted in patients with epilepsy of unknown etiology, particularly when there is co-existent cerebral atrophy of unknown etiology.[191] Case report describes finding CD in a child with difficult to control seizures suggestive of Lennox-Gastaut syndrome. GFD led to progressive seizure control, allowing significant decrease in dosage of anti-epileptic drugs. Progressive seizure control corroborates the importance of serological screening tests for CD, at least in patients with difficult to control epilepsy.[196] Case report describes significant reduction in seizures on a GFD for 1 of 4 patients with CD. CD should be ruled out in all cases of epilepsy of unknown origin.[195] [M] Marked by recurrent seizures. [C] Results from gluten exposure and malabsorption in CD involving calcium, magnesium, and folate. The mechanism underlying these processes remains obscure but may be immunological or related to trace vitamin deficiency.[181] [R] CD-related epilepsy responds to GFD.	Calcium, Folic acid, Magnesium.
Nervous System	Brain: cerebrum	215	Fatigue, Chronic / Lassitude [1,5,103,104]	(S)	[P] Prevalence of CD is 3.3% in participants with fatigue.[104] Common complaint at diagnosis in 75% of patients.[103] [D] Chronic fatigue or lassitude is a state of weariness not relieved by rest. Study measuring IgG and IgA isotypes and IgG subclasses demonstrated significantly higher proportion of patients with positive IgA gliadin antibodies reported chronic fatigue.[5] [M] Marked by overwhelming sense of exhaustion and decreased capacity to do normal physical or mental work. [C] Results from nutritional deficiencies in CD involving vitamin C, protein, iron, and magnesium. [R] CD-related fatigue responds to GFD.	Iron, Magnesium, Protein, Vitamin C.

+ (S) = Classic sign/symptom; (AT) = Atypical sign/symptom; (AD) Associated Disorder; (C) = Complication.

++ [P] = Prevalance; [D] = Description; [M] = Sign/symptom; [C] = CD related cause; [R] = Response to gluten Free diet (GFD).

Health Manifestations of Celiac Disease (CD)
Section B: Signs, Symptoms, Associated Disorders and Complications

Affected System	Affected Organ	ID No.	Manifestation	Type[+]	Current Medical Information [++]	Deficient Nutrient
Nervous System	Brain: cerebrum	216	Fatigue, Chronic Syndrome [1,197,198]	(AD)	[P] New association with CD.[197] High prevalence of serum markers of CD in patients with chronic fatigue syndrome.[198] [D] Chronic fatigue syndrome (CFS) is a debilitating illness characterized by persistent or relapsing overwhelming and incapacitating fatigue not relieved by rest, having a definite onset and often accompanied by numerous symptoms involving various body systems.[197] The etiology of CFS remains unclear; however, a number of recent studies have shown oxidative stress may be involved in its pathogenesis. CD may be involved in CFS symptom presentation and oxidation via cytokine induction. CD should be included in the differential diagnosis of CFS.[197] [M] Marked by at least four symptoms present over 6 months: impaired short-term memory or decreased concentration severe enough to substantially reduce occupational, educational, social, or personal activities, recurrent sore throats, tender cervical or axillary lymph nodes, muscle pain, multijoint pain without joint swelling or tenderness, headaches, unrefreshing sleep, postexertional malaise lasting more than 24 hours. [C] Results from unclear etiology; malabsorption of antioxidants in CD may be involved.[197] [R] Responds to GFD with dietary supplementation.[197]	Carboydrate Omega-3 fatty acids, Omega-6 fatty acids, Protein, Vitamins, especially Vitamin C, and Minerals.
Nervous System	Brain: cerebrum	217	Migraine Headaches [180,199,200]	(AT)	[P] A significant proportion of patients with migraine (4.4%) have CD.[199] [D] Migraine headache is a neurologic disorder characterized by reduced cerebral blood flow. Single photon emission CT study investigating cerebral perfusion demonstrated a regional baseline reduction in brain tracer uptake in all patients with CD which completely resolved at 6 month follow-up for patients on a GFD.[199] Study screening neurologic disorders in children and young adults demonstrated that 35.5% migraine patients had classical early infantile enteropathic CD and 64.5% presented with late-onset symptoms, showing malabsorption did not play a significant role in the pathogenesis.[180] Case report describes a patient with untreated CD who presented with a state of acute migraine accompanied by multiple neurologic deficits including transient cortical blindness with CT and MRI alterations, and hypocoagulation due to factor VII deficiency. She was receiving estroprogestin therapy. There was a prompt response to cortisone therapy followed by a state of complete well-being, which also led to the disappearance of migraine attacks after 5 years of dietary treatment alone.[200] [M] Marked by periodic, usually one-sided pulsing headache with or without aura and light and noise sensitivity, nausea. [C] Results from unclear etiology involving gluten exposure in CD and malabsorption of folic acid. [R] GFD leads to normalization of blood flow and resolution or improvement in frequency, duration, and intensity of migraine within 6 months.[199]	Folic acid.

+ (S) = Classic sign/symptom; (AT) = Atypical sign/symptom; (AD) Associated Disorder; (C) = Complication.

++ [P] = Prevalance; [D] = Description; [M] = Sign/symptom; [C] = CD related cause; [R] = Response to gluten Free diet (GFD).

Health Manifestations of Celiac Disease (CD)
Section B: Signs, Symptoms, Associated Disorders and Complications

Affected System	Affected Organ	ID No.	Manifestation	Type+	Current Medical Information ++	Deficient Nutrient ++
Nervous System	Brain: cerebrum	218	Multiple Sclerosis [34,201,202]	(AD)	[P] Reports conflict regarding association of multiple sclerosis (MS) with CD. Screening for CD using IgA anti-endomysial antibodies found prevalence of 2%, and a 12% rate using IgG anti-gliadin antibodies.[201] Study using anti-tranglutaminase antibodies in a group of 95 patients with MS found none.[202] [D] Multiple sclerosis is an immune-mediated, chronic, slowly progressive, demyelinating disease of the central nervous system characterized by multiple and varied neurologic symptoms and signs, usually with exacerbations and remissions. [M] Marked by varied muscular weakness, numbness, visual disturbances. [C] Results from unclear etiology, but an immune mechanism is suspected based on certain HLA allotypes. Omega-3 fatty acid deficiency is suspected.[34] [R] Response to GFD varies.	Omega-3 fatty acids suspected.[34]
Nervous System	Brain: cerebrum	219	Occipital Lobe Epilepsy with Cerebral Calcifications [1,203,204]	(AD)	[P] New association with CD.[203,204] [D] Occipital lobe epilepsy with cerebral calcifications is characterized by repetitive abnormal electrical discharges within the brain that may manifest as paroxysmal visual disturbances. Case report of three school age boys who presented with partial seizures with visual symptoms describes subsequent diagnosis of CD based on positive serology and small intestinal biopsy showing grade 3 severe enteropathy. A tomography scan of the head revealed bilateral occipital calcifications in all cases. All 3 patients, following a GFD and taking anti-convulsants, were free of seizures in the follow-up (1,2, and 8 years). Investigators concluded that it is of vital importance to investigate CD in any patient with epilepsy and occipital calcifications, even in the absence of GI symptoms, since early diagnosis and treatment with exclusion of gluten affect how the syndrome courses later on.[203] Case report of three Australian patients with seizure types including simple partial, complex-partial, and secondarily generalized seizures illustrates the association between seizures of occipital origin, cerebral calcifications, and CD even in patients not of Mediterranean origin. The seizure semiology consisted of visual disturbances such as blurred vision, loss of focus, seeing colored dots, and brief stereotyped complex visual hallucinations like seeing unfamiliar faces or scenes. Symptoms of malabsorption were not always present. Routine EEG was unremarkable. In all cases, CT demonstrated cortical calcification of the occipital-parietal regions. Magnetic imaging showed no additional lesion. All patients had biopsy confirmed CD. Seizure control improved after treatment with GFD and anticonvulsants.[204] [M] Marked by paroxysmal visual disturbances representing seizures and alteration in consciousness. [C] Results from unclear etiology involving gluten exposure. [R] Occipital lobe epilepsy responds to GFD.	Not applicable.

+ (S) = Classic sign/symptom; (AT) = Atypical sign/symptom; (AD) Associated Disorder; (C) = Complication.

++ [P] = Prevalance; [D] = Description; [M] = Sign/symptom; [C] = CD related cause; [R] = Response to gluten Free diet (GFD).

Health Manifestations of Celiac Disease (CD)
Section B: Signs, Symptoms, Associated Disorders and Complications

Affected System	Affected Organ	ID No.	Manifestation	Type[+]	Current Medical Information [++]	Deficient Nutrient
Nervous System	Brain: cerebrum	220	Progressive Multifocal Leukoencephalopathy [1,205]	(AD)	[P] New association with CD.[205] [D] Progressive multifocal leukoencephalopathy, a progressive demyelinating disorder of the central nervous system, is characterized by tissue loss of subcortical white matter and active perivascular inflammatory foci with numerous eosinophilic granulocytes. It usually occurs as an opportunistic infection in patients with underlying depression of cell-mediated immunity. Case report describes a patient with history of anemia and hypoproteinemia for several years. Within a year after diagnosis of CD, progressive multifocal leukoencephalopathy developed with an unusual course of 10 years until death. GFD altered the morbidity dramatically in this case. It is postulated that this patient's immune deficiency was related to his malabsorption syndrome and hypoglobulinemia, and the course became unusually protracted (longest reported course in the American literature) because of restoration of plasma protein levels. Autopsy showed classic findings. Electron microscopy found oligodendrocyte nuclei and cytoplasm were crowded with virions, but many myelin sheaths invested by severely infected oligodendritic processes were remarkably well preserved. This fact would argue against a direct cause-and-effect relationship between infection of oligodendrocytes and myelin breakdown. The likelihood of an autoimmune mechanism at work in this disease is suggested, and the role of eosinophils and other cells in such processes is considered.[205] [M] Marked by rapid deterioration, usually 9 months to death. [C] Results from underlying depression of cell-mediated immunity; an autoimmimmune mechanism is likely.[205] [R] Responds to GFD.	Not applicable.

+ (S) = Classic sign/symptom; (AT) = Atypical sign/symptom; (AD) Associated Disorder; (C) = Complication.

++ [P] = Prevalance; [D] = Description; [M] = Sign/symptom; [C] = CD related cause; [R] = Response to gluten Free diet (GFD).

Health Manifestations of Celiac Disease (CD)
Section B: Signs, Symptoms, Associated Disorders and Complications

Affected System	Affected Organ	ID No.	Manifestation	Type[+]	Current Medical Information [++]	Deficient Nutrient
Nervous System	Brain: cerebrum	221	Vasculitis of the Central Nervous System [206]	(C)	[P] New association with CD.[206] [D] Vasculitis of the central nervous system is characterized by inflammation of large, medium, or small blood vessels which is often segmental with scattered foci of intense inflammation, and results in necrosis with scarring. Case report describes a patient with CD who developed vasculitis of the CNS. She presented with recurrent transient ischemic attacks (TIA) with right hemihypoesthesia and right hemiparesia, severe pre-tibial edema, decreased muscle tonus of extremities and decreased deep tendon reflexes. While hospitalized she suffered a reversible stroke. CT scan revealed multiple lacunar infarcts predominantly in frontotemporal regions. MR imaging (MRI) revealed cerebellar, corticosubcortical chronic atrophy, left frontoparietal corticosubcortical chronic atrophy, a variety of small edematous lesions in cortical areas on T2 weighted images. Digital subtraction angiography revealed indefinite segmental narrowing of the left middle cerebral artery. The histological examination of temporal superficial arteries revealed patchy inflammatory cell infiltrates of both lymphocytes and macrophages. Serum C3-C4 and albumin levels were decreased.[206] [M] Marked by fever, pain, malaise, and neurologic deficits depending in part on the size of the affected vessel(s) which may include seizure, TIA and/or stroke. [C] Results from immune-mediated processes. [R] Studies are inadequate to determine response to GFD.	Not applicable.

+ (S) = Classic sign/symptom; (AT) = Atypical sign/symptom; (AD) Associated Disorder; (C) = Complication.
++ [P] = Prevalance; [D] = Description; [M] = Sign/symptom; [C] = CD related cause; [R] = Response to gluten Free diet (GFD).

Section B   *Signs, Symptoms, Associated Disorders & Complications*   203

Health Manifestations of Celiac Disease (CD)
Section B: Signs, Symptoms, Associated Disorders and Complications

Affected System	Affected Organ	ID No.	Manifestation	Type[+]	Current Medical Information[++]	Deficient Nutrient
Nervous System	Brain: mind	222	Anxiety, Chronic Maladaptive [1,207,208,209]	(AD)	[P] Common in people with untreated CD and can be the only manifestation.[207] CD patients showed high levels of state anxiety in a significantly higher percentage compared to controls (71.4% vs 23.7%)[208] [D] Anxiety, a distressing emotional state, is characterized by a vague uneasiness or unpleasant feeling of apprehension and dysfunction. Deficiency of amino acids and vitamins implicate reduction of synthesis of neurotransmitters in the central nervous system and could be linked to immunological disregulation in CD patients.[207] Anxiety itself causes depletion of vitamins and minerals. Study evaluating the real nature of anxiety in newly diagnosed CD patients (classic type) by means of the State and Trait Anxiety Inventory test demonstrated anxiety is present in a predominantly reactive form rather than as a personality trait. After one year on GFD, a significant decrease in the percentage of state anxiety was found while there was no significant changes in the percentage of trait anxiety.[208] Study evaluating cerebral perfusion in untreated CD patients with no neurologic or psychiatric disorder other than anxiety or depression demonstrated evidence of significant regional cerebral blood flow alteration. Cerebral single photon emission CT scan examination showed 73% of untreated CD patients had at least one hypoperfused brain region compared with only 7% of patients on a GFD and none of controls.[209] [M] Marked by anticipation of danger and interference with normal functioning, ranging from mild qualms and easy startling to occasional panic, often with headaches and fatigue. [C] Results from unclear etiology involving gluten exposure, regional cerebral blood flow alteration, and malabsorption of multiple nutrients in CD including calcium, magnesium, iron, potassium, B vitamins, tryptophan, and thiamin. [R] Withdrawal of gluten usually results in disappearance of symptoms.[207]	B vitamins, Calcium, Iron, Magnesium, Potassium, Tryptophan, Vitamin B$_1$.
Nervous System	Brain: mind	223	Apathy [210]	(AT)	[P] Common in untreated CD.[210] [D] Apathy is an abnormal emotional state characterized by indifference to things which others find interesting, moving or exciting. Long before the onset of other symptoms of CD, there may be disinterest in regular daily activities, passage of three soft stools per day and hard-to-flush bulky stools.[210] [M] Marked by lack of feeling or absence of care. [C] Results from multiple nutritional deficiencies in CD including omega-3 and omega-6 fatty acids, thiamin, vitamin B$_{12}$, niacin, folic acid, iron, and copper. [R] CD-related apathy responds to GFD.	Copper, Folic acid, Iron, Omega-3 fatty acids, Omega-6 fatty acids, Vitamin B$_1$, Vitamin B$_3$, Vitamin B$_{12}$.

[+] (S) = Classic sign/symptom; (AT) = Atypical sign/symptom; (AD) Associated Disorder; (C) = Complication.

[++] [P] = Prevalance; [D] = Description; [M] = Sign/symptom; [C] = CD related cause; [R] = Response to gluten Free diet (GFD).

Recognizing Celiac Disease Signs, Symptoms, Associated Disorders & Complications

Health Manifestations of Celiac Disease (CD)
Section B: Signs, Symptoms, Associated Disorders and Complications

Affected System	Affected Organ	ID No.	Manifestation	Type[+]	Current Medical Information [++]	Deficient Nutrient
Nervous System	Brain: mind	224	Depression [1,207,208, 209,211,212,213]	(AT)	[P] Depression is a feature of adult CD.[211] Depression is typical in adults at diagnosis of CD.[212] Depression is a mood disorder characterized by absence of cheerfulness, dejection, and loss of interest or pleasure in living. It appears in untreated and treated CD patients. Malabsorption and amino acids and vitamin deficiency implicate reduction of synthesis of central nervous system (CNS) neuro-transmitters.[207] Initially present as a consequence of CD symptoms and malabsorption/malnutrition, depression may be sustained by reduced quality of life related in part to decreased sense of well-being, and in part to dietary restrictions, leading to social difficulties, such as fear of eating at restaurants or parties.[208] Study evaluating personality using the Minnesota Multiphasic Personality Inventory (MMPI) demonstrated high score for depression. The score correlated with daily fat excretion but was unrelated to GI complaints.[211] Study evaluating cerebral perfusion in untreated CD patients demonstrated evidence of regional cerebral blood flow alteration. 73% had at least one hypoperfused brain area vs. 7% of patients on a GFD and none of controls.[209] Study evaluating the real nature of depression in classic CD patients at diagnosis and 1 year follow-up using the State and Trait Inventory test demonstrated treatment after 1 year on a GFD failed to reduce depression in a significant percentage of patients. Results could suggest patients need psychological support.[208] Study using the MMPI to evaluate response to GFD of newly diagnosed patients demonstrated no improvement after one year despite improved intestinal mucosa. After 3 years, following 6 months of 80mg/day of oral pyridoxine therapy, scores became normalized indicating causal relationship between adult CD and concomitant depression and implicating metabolic effects from deficient vitamin B$_6$.[212] Case report describes depression related to CD in a patient, age 41, with Down's syndrome who showed spectacular and lasting improvement of both psychotic and depressive symptoms after 12 months on a GFD.[213] [M] Marked by persistent feelings of guilt/ self-criticism, sense of worthlessness, irritability, poor concentration, insomnia or excessive sleep, and recurring thoughts of suicide/ death. [C] Results from unclear etiology involving malabsorption, immunological disregulation,[207] and cerebral blood flow alterations in CD.[209] [R] Improvement can be obtained on GFD.	EPA (impulse transmission), Protein, especially tryptophan (low serotonin) and tyrosine (low dopamine/ adrenaline), magnesium, zinc, thiamin, vitamin C, vitamin B complex, pyridixine, folic acid, vitamin B$_{12}$.

[+] (S) = Classic sign/symptom; (AT) = Atypical sign/symptom; (AD) Associated Disorder; (C) = Complication.

[++] [P] = Prevalance; [D] = Description; [M] = Sign/symptom; [C] = CD related cause; [R] = Response to gluten Free diet (GFD).

Health Manifestations of Celiac Disease (CD)
Section B: Signs, Symptoms, Associated Disorders and Complications

Affected System	Affected Organ	ID No.	Manifestation	Type+	Current Medical Information ++	Deficient Nutrient
Nervous System	Brain: mind	225	Inability to Concentrate [180]	(AD)	[P] New association with CD.[180] [D] Inability to concentrate is a mental dysfunction characterized by trouble fixing the mind on one subject to the exclusion of all other thoughts. Study screening for occurrence of "soft" neurologic manifestations in children and young adults demonstrated that patients with CD are more prone to develop inability to concentrate than controls. It is not clear whether accumulative effects of nutritional, immunologic, or inflammatory factors might play some role on attention span or that the effect is direct and relates to non-specific effects of chronic disease. Kieslich et al. reported on the presence of multiple white matter lesions detected by brain magnetic resonance imaging. One cannot rule out that these lesions might also interfere with high cognitive functions, such as in other white matter diseases.[180] [M] Marked by easy distraction and altered ability to complete tasks. [C] Results from unclear etiology.[180] Nutritional deficiencies include thiamin and omega-3 fatty acid, especially DHA. [R] Future longitudinal prospective studies might better define the clinical response of concentration to GFD.[180]	Omega-3 fatty acid, especially DHA, Vitamin B_1.
Nervous System	Brain: mind	226	Insomnia [1,34]	(AD)	[P] Increased frequency in untreated CD. [D] Insomnia in CD is characterized by sleeplessness due to reduction of synthesis of neurotransmitters in the central nervous system, especially melatonin. [M] Marked by inability to fall asleep or stay asleep. [C] Results from multiple micronutrient malabsorption in CD including vitamin B_6, B-complex, magnesium, thiamin, calcium, EPA, and especially tryptophan (for synthesis of melatonin).[34] [R] CD-related insomnia responds to GFD.	B-complex, Calcium, EPA, and Tryptophan (melatonin), Magnesium, Vitamin B_1, Vitamin B_6.
Nervous System	Brain: mind	227	Irritability [3,55]	(AD)	[P] Increased frequency in CD.[55] Common presenting symptom in children.[3] [D] Irritability is a mental state characterized by excessive response to annoyance. [M] Marked by impatience and excessive response to annoyance. [C] Results from multiple deficiencies in CD including tryptophan (low serotonin), thiamin, pyridoxine, vitamin C, calcium and magnesium. Other CD-related causes include enteritis, upset stomach, and GERD. [R] CD-related irritability responds to GFD.	Calcium, Magnesium, Tryptophan (low serotonin), Vitamin B_6, Vitamin B_1, Vitamin B_6, Vitamin C.

+ (S) = Classic sign/symptom; (AT) = Atypical sign/symptom; (AD) Associated Disorder; (C) = Complication.

++ [P] = Prevalance; [D] = Description; [M] = Sign/symptom; [C] = CD related cause; [R] = Response to gluten Free diet (GFD).

Health Manifestations of Celiac Disease (CD)
Section B: Signs, Symptoms, Associated Disorders and Complications

Affected System	Affected Organ	ID No.	Manifestation	Type+	Current Medical Information ++	Deficient Nutrient
Nervous System	Brain: mind	228	Schizophrenia Spectrum Disorders 1,207,213,214,216,217, 218,219,220	(AT)	[P] Gluten sensitivity is common in schizophrenia.[207] Psychotic symptoms often occur in adult CD.[214] [D] Schizophrenia is a thought disorder characterized by psychotic symptoms and inappropriate and bizarre behavior affecting cognitive function, interpersonal relationships, work or education, and self care. Both schizophrenia and CD involve a genetic component. It can be hypothesized that the meeting point for the gene-environment interaction may be an alteration in gut permeability, in which the gut may lose its capacity to block exogenous psychosis-causing substances, thus causing the development of schizophrenia. The conditional test looking at the combined effect of the CLDN5 gene, involved in forming permeability barriers, and the DQB1 gene, associated with CD, demonstrated these two genes possibly work together in conferring a susceptibility to schizophrenia.[214] Study demonstrated more schizophrenics than controls showed IgA antibody levels above the upper limit to gliadin, beta-lactoglobulin, and casein.[215] Study demonstrated that gluten exerts a primary schizophrenia-promoting effect evidenced by improvement with gluten withdrawal after a two week period and exacerbation with reinstatement.[216] Study demonstrated that gluten may be a primary trigger for schizophrenia.[217] Study testing the hypothesis that neuroactive peptides from gluten grains are major agents evoking schizophrenia in those with the genotypes demonstrated gluten is harmful to schizophrenics.[218] Study determining the origin of peptides that exhibit opioid activity demonstrated a high opioid-like activity in isolated peptides from wheat gluten hydrolysates. While some peptides showed no activity, 0.5mg of the most active peptides were equivalent to 1 nM of morphine in the binding assay and were derived from the gliadin fraction of gluten.[219] Case report of SPECT examination of a patient with "schizophrenic disorder" with undiagnosed and untreated CD demonstrated hypoperfusion of the left frontal brain area, without structural cerebral abnormalities. Dysfunction disappeared after GFD.[220] Case report of a patient with Down's syndrome with psychosis, describes subsequent diagnosis of CD with spectacular and lasting improvement after 12 months on a GFD.[213] [M] Marked by confusion, delusions, hallucinations, disorganized speech and behavior, lack of insight, and by flat affect, social withdrawal, and absence of volition. [C] Results from exposure to gluten through increased intestinal permeability; malnutrition in CD.[213,214,216,220] [R] Schizophrenia improves and may resolve on GFD.[213,214,216,220]	EPA, Magnesium, Vitamin C, Vitamin B_{12} (causing paranoia).

+ (S) = Classic sign/symptom; (AT) = Atypical sign/symptom; (AD) Associated Disorder; (C) = Complication.

++ [P] = Prevalance; [D] = Description; [M] = Sign/symptom; [C] = CD related cause; [R] = Response to gluten Free diet (GFD).

Health Manifestations of Celiac Disease (CD)
Section B: Signs, Symptoms, Associated Disorders and Complications

Affected System	Affected Organ	ID No.	Manifestation	Type+	Current Medical Information ++	Deficient Nutrient
Nervous System	Peripheral nerves	229	Peripheral Neuropathy [1,181,221, 222, 223]	(AD)	[P] CD is commonly associated with sensory neuropathy, occurring in 2.5% of all neuropathy patients.[221] Chronic axonal neuropathy occurs in 23.1% of patients with treated CD.[222] [D] CD-associated peripheral neuropathy may be of axonal or demyelinating type181 involving sensory loss, paresthesis, and muscle weakness, alone or in any combination.[221] Case report of patient and literature review reveals that patients with chronic gluten enteropathy and severe steatorrhea may develop a generalized peripheral neuropathy of the distal axonopathy type. Vitamin levels are usually normal and the neuropathy appears to respond to gluten restriction.[223] Study of patients with biopsy confirmed CD and neuropathy demonstrated all patients had burning, tingling, and numbness in their hands and feet, with distal sensory loss. 45% had diffuse paresthesias and 10% had weakness. Agglutination assay revealed 65% were positive for ganglioside antibodies. Results of electrophysiologic studies were normal or mildly abnormal in 90% of the patients. 23% of well treated study patients showed an increased axonal neuropathy. Sural nerve biopsies from 3 of the patients revealed mild to severe axonopathy. CD should be considered even in the absence of GI symptoms because 30% of patients had neuropathic symptoms alone, without GI involvement, and neuropathic symptoms preceded other CD symptoms in another 10.5% of patients.[221] Study of well-treated patients with CD demonstrated an increased occurrence of axonal neuropathy. There were no significant differences in warm, cold, or vibration thresholds between patients with CD from controls, but means of heat pain thresholds and tactile thresholds were significantly higher in CD patients. Study further indicates that neurological manifestations occur even in patients without overt malabsorption.[222] [M] Marked by burning, tingling, and numbness in hands and feet with distal sensory loss and weakness of extremities. [C] Results from unclear immune mechanism; vitamin B deficiencies in CD. [R] Peripheral neuropathies may benefit from a GFD.[223]	Folic acid, Omega-3 fatty acids, Vitamin B_1, Vitamin B_3, Vitamin B_6, Vitamin B_{12}.

+ (S) = Classic sign/symptom; (AT) = Atypical sign/symptom; (AD) Associated Disorder; (C) = Complication.

++ [P] = Prevalance; [D] = Description; [M] = Sign/symptom; [C] = CD related cause; [R] = Response to gluten Free diet (GFD).

Health Manifestations of Celiac Disease (CD)
Section B: Signs, Symptoms, Associated Disorders and Complications

Affected System	Affected Organ	ID No.	Manifestation	Type[+]	Current Medical Information [++]	Deficient Nutrient
Pulmonary System	Lungs	230	Bronchiectasis [1,224]	(AD)	[P] New association with CD.[224] [D] Bronchiectasis is a pulmonary disease characterized by chronic dilation of a bronchus or bronchioles. Case report describes the course of a 48 year old woman in whom widespread bronchiectasis was the presenting sign of CD. The temporal relationship of the brochiectasis and CD, and the subsequent stabilization of her clinical symptoms and improvement in pulmonary physiology following treatment with inhaled corticosteroids, suggests a relationship between the two conditions which may be due to immunological mechanisms.[224] [M] Marked by fatigue, regular sputum production, and wheeze. [C] May result from immunological mechanism.[224] [R] Improves on GFD.[224]	Not applicable.
Pulmonary System	Lungs	231	Bronchoalveolitis, Lymphocytic [225] (Bronchial Pneumonia)	(C)	[P] New association with CD.[225] [D] Lymphocytic bronchoalveolitis (bronchial pneumonia) is a pulmonary disorder characterized by lymphocytic airway inflammation of the bronchi and alveoli (airsacs) next to them. It commonly occurs in weakened persons. Case report describes the course of bronchoscopic evidence of lymphocytic airway inflammation in association with newly diagnosed CD in a patient presenting with chronic cough with unclear cause after investigations. All features improved markedly on a GFD, suggesting causal relationship between CD, cough, and lymphocytic bronchoalveolitis.[225] [M] Marked by cough, fever, shortness of breath and sputum production. [C] Probable causal relationship with CD.[225] [R] Bronchoalveolitis improves markedly on GFD.[225]	Not applicable.

[+] (S) = Classic sign/symptom; (AT) = Atypical sign/symptom; (AD) Associated Disorder; (C) = Complication.

[++] [P] = Prevalance; [D] = Description; [M] = Sign/symptom; [C] = CD related cause; [R] = Response to gluten Free diet (GFD).

Health Manifestations of Celiac Disease (CD)
Section B: Signs, Symptoms, Associated Disorders and Complications

Affected System	ID No.	Manifestation	Type[+]	Current Medical Information [++]	Deficient Nutrient
Pulmonary System	232	Lungs Cavities or Abscess [226]	(C)	[P] Study found 1.2% prevalence in patients with CD. [226] [D] Lungs cavities or abcess constitute respiratory disease characterized by localized suppuration of the lung resulting from necrosis of lung tissue with surrounding inflammation. Next to malignancy, pulmonary abcess was found to be the commonest cause of death in the celiac population. [226] Study evaluating the occurrence of lung abscesses or cavities in 7 out of 600 patients with CD seen over a 20 year span demonstrated that the development of respiratory symptoms should be regarded as a potentially serious and life-threatening event in middle-aged celiac patients. Six of the 7 patients died. Staphylococcal infection, Klebsiella pneumoniae, bronchial carcinoma and previous TB accounted for the cavities in 4 patients. In the 3 other patients a definite cause could not be identified. Lung abcesses should be added to the list of respiratory diseases associated with CD. [226] [M] Marked by dyspnea, cough, irregular fever, and purulent sputum. Hyposplenism and malnutrition commonly occur. [C] Results from encapsulated bacterial infection, dysfunctional immune response and malnutrition. [R] Studies are inadequate to determine effect of GFD.	Iron, Omega-3 fatty acids, Protein, Vitamin C.

Pulmonary System	233	Pneumococal Septicemia [1,173,227,228]	(C)	[P] New association of susceptibility to fatal pneumonia in hyposplenism. [227]
				[D] Pneumococcal septicemia is characterized by a systemic response to lung infection.
				    Case report described course of fatal Streptococcus pneumoniae that developed in an elderly patient with hyposplenism complicating CD which was diagnosed 4 years previous to current hospitalization. Blood cultures confirmed Streptococcus pneumoniae and she was treated appropriately with ampicillin. Despite this, she died shortly after admission. Hyposplenism complicating CD is the presumed reason for development of fatal pneumococcal septicemia in this patient. Prophylactic vaccination may be appropriate in hyposplenism secondary to CD. [227]
				    Study evaluating pre- and postvaccination antibody levels in CD patients demonstrated appropriate response. Hyposplenism, as a complication of CD, confers an increased risk of pneumococcal sepsis, but such patients do not routinely receive pneumococcal vaccine despite reports of overwhelming pneumococcal sepsis. Vaccination of all patients with CD seems appropriate. [228]
				[M] Marked by vomiting, pleuritic chest pain, pyrexia, and bronchospasm.
				[C] Results from lowered resistance to infection due to hyposplenism. [227]
				[R] Non-significant tendency to improve morphologic changes of the spleen on strict GFD. [173]
					Not applicable.

[+] (S) = Classic sign/symptom; (AT) = Atypical sign/symptom; (AD) Associated Disorder; (C) = Complication.

[++] [P] = Prevalance; [D] = Description; [M] = Sign/symptom; [C] = CD related cause; [R] = Response to gluten Free diet (GFD).

Health Manifestations of Celiac Disease (CD)
Section B: Signs, Symptoms, Associated Disorders and Complications

Affected System	Affected Organ	ID No.	Manifestation	Type+	Current Medical Information ++	Deficient Nutrient
Pulmonary System	Lungs	234	Pulmonary Hemosiderosis, Idiopathic [229]	(AD)	[P] Rare association with CD.[229] [D] Idiopathic pulmonary hemosiderosis (IPH) is characterized by a triad of recurrent episodes of alveolar hemorrhage, hemoptysis, and iron deficiency anemia. The combination of IPH and CD is extremely rare, although both diseases may have a common pathogenetic link. As illustrated by this case report, CD should be looked for in patients with IPH, especially in those in whom the severity of anemia is disproportionate to radiologic findings even in the absence of GI symptoms, since both diseases may benefit from a GFD.[229] [M] Marked by bloody sputum, pulmonary hemorrhage, and anemia. [C] Results from iron deficiency in CD. [R] CD-related IPH responds to GFD.	Iron.
Pulmonary System	Lungs	235	Pulmonary Permeability, Increased [230]	(S)	[P] Increased frequency in patients with CD.[230] [D] Increased pulmonary permeability is a recognized subclinical pulmonary abnormality of CD characterized by abnormal clearance. Study investigating lung function in 25 patients with inflammatory bowel disease (IBD) and 18 patients with CD on a GFD compared to 20 normal patients, all without respiratory symptoms, demonstrated that airflow in patients on a GFD is not significantly different from controls, but there is an increase in pulmonary permeability. By contrast patients with IBD had decreased airflow and no change in permeability. These findings suggest that the mechanisms of lung disease in CD differs from that in IBD and supports the hypothesis of a common mucosal defect in lung and small intestine in CD, allowing increased permeability.[230] [M] Marked by mucosal changes. [C] Results from mucosal defect in lung in CD.[230] [R] Inadequate studies to determine response to GFD.	Not applicable.

+ (S) = Classic sign/symptom; (AT) = Atypical sign/symptom; (AD) = Associated Disorder; (C) = Complication.
++ [P] = Prevalance; [D] = Description; [M] = Sign/symptom; [C] = CD related cause; [R] = Response to gluten Free diet (GFD).

Health Manifestations of Celiac Disease (CD)
Section B: Signs, Symptoms, Associated Disorders and Complications

Affected System	Affected Organ	ID No.	Manifestation	Type+	Current Medical Information ++	Deficient Nutrient
Pulmonary System	Lungs	236	Tuberculosis, Increased Susceptibility [231]	(C)	[P] An increased prevalence of past tuberculosis is reported in 17% of adult CD population. [231] [D] Tuberculosis (TB), an infectious disease caused by Mycobacterium tuberculosis, is characterized by chronic bacterial infection most commonly affecting lungs in stages. It may be dormant or active, producing inflammation and formation of tubercles, necrosis, abcess, fibrosis, and calcification. Study evaluating CD patients for a history of TB demonstrated radiological evidence of past TB in 17% compared to 5% in controls. It is postulated that the increased prevalence of past TB in adult CD patients is the result of depressed cell-mediated immunity and/or malnutrition. [231] [M] Marked by chronic cough, sputum production, fever, sweats, and weight loss. [C] Results from depressed cell-mediated immunity and/or malnutrition in CD. [231] [R] GFD improves nutrition and immunity defense. Studies are inadequate to determine response to GFD.	Iron, Omega-3 fatty acids.
Pulmonary System	Lungs	237	Tuberculosis, Non-Response to Treatment [232]	(C)	[P] New association in patients with untreated CD. [232] [D] Non-response to treatment for tuberculosis (TB) is reported regarding two patients with tuberculosis who did not respond to adequate therapy. Both these patients were later found to have CD, which led to malabsorption of the TB medications. On treating the CD with GFD, the patients responded to TB treatment. [232] [M] Marked by failure to respond to adequate therapy. [232] [C] Resulted from malabsorption of TB medications due to gluten sensitive enteropathy. [232] [R] GFD resulted in response to TB treatment. [232]	Not applicable.
Sensory System	Eyes	238	Bitot's Spots [233]	(AD)	[P] Increased occurrence in patients with untreated CD. [D] Bitot's spots is a painless eye disorder in advanced vitamin A deficiency characterized by alteration in the exposed bulbar conjunctiva that is reversible. Superficial foamy patches are composed of epithelial debris and secretions. [233] Study investigating alterations in the anterior segment of the eye demonstrated vitamin A deficiency can be the reason for bilateral conjunctival manifestations. [233] [M] Marked by triangular shiny gray spots on the exposed conjunctiva. [C] Results from vitamin A and protein deficiency. [R] CD-related Bitot's spots resolve on GFD with supplementation.	Protein, Vitamin A.

+ (S) = Classic sign/symptom; (AT) = Atypical sign/symptom; (AD) Associated Disorder; (C) = Complication.

++ [P] = Prevalance; [D] = Description; [M] = Sign/symptom; [C] = CD related cause; [R] = Response to gluten Free diet (GFD).

Health Manifestations of Celiac Disease (CD)
Section B: Signs, Symptoms, Associated Disorders and Complications

Affected System	Affected Organ	ID No.	Manifestation	Type[+]	Current Medical Information [++]	Deficient Nutrient
Sensory System	Eyes	239	Blepharitis, Unexplained	(AD)	[P] Increased frequency in untreated CD. [D] Blepharitis is a feature of vitamin A deficiency characterized by non-ulcerative inflammation of the hair follicles and glands along the eyelid edges. [M] Marked by redness and tenderness of the eyelids with exudate and scaling on the edges. [C] Results from vitamin A, EPA and protein malabsorption in CD. [R] Resolves on GFD.	EPA, Vitamin A.
Sensory System	Eyes	240	Bloodshot Eyes, Chronic [233]	(AD)	[P] Increased frequency in patients with untreated CD. [D] Chronic bloodshot eyes is a feature of vitamin A deficiency characterized by congestion of the smaller blood vessels of the conjunctiva. [M] Marked by visible dilation of the smaller blood vessels of the conjunctiva in CD.[233] [C] Results from vitamin A malabsorption in CD.[233] [R] Resolves on GFD.	Vitamin A.
Sensory System	Eyes	241	Blurred Vision, Unexplained	(AT)	[P] Increased frequency in untreated CD. [D] Blurred vision is a feature of multiple micronutrient deficiencies. [M] Marked by unclear vision. [C] Results from malabsorption in CD including vitamin A, riboflavin (vitamin B$_2$), and EPA. [R] Resolves on GFD.	EPA, Vitamin A, Vitamin B$_2$.
Sensory System	Eyes	242	Cataracts [34,233]	(C)	[P] Increased frequency in untreated CD.[233] [D] Cataract formation, a feature of vitamin A deficiency and long standing hypocalcemia, is characterized by clouding of the lens of the eye. [M] Marked by distortion of vision especially at night or in very bright light that progressively leads to blindness. [C] Results from malabsorption of vitamin A and calcium.[34] Vitamin B$_2$ may be involved. [R] GFD is preventive and limits further changes.	Calcium, Vitamin A, Vitamin B$_2$.

[+] (S) = Classic sign/symptom; (AT) = Atypical sign/symptom; (AD) Associated Disorder; (C) = Complication.

[++] [P] = Prevalance; [D] = Description; [M] = Sign/symptom; [C] = CD related cause; [R] = Response to gluten Free diet (GFD).

Health Manifestations of Celiac Disease (CD)
Section B: Signs, Symptoms, Associated Disorders and Complications

Affected System	Affected Organ	ID No.	Manifestation	Type[+]	Current Medical Information [++]	Deficient Nutrient
Sensory System	Eyes	243	Keratoconjunctivitis Sicca [234]	(AD)	[P] Rare association with CD.[234] [D] Keratoconjunctivitis sicca is a chronic bilateral dessication with hyperemia of the conjunctiva and cornea due to tear abnormality. Thickening of the cornea may result, impairing vision. Case report of patient describes rare association of CD, keratoconjunctivitis sicca, and autoimmune thrombocytopenia. The development of three different autoimmune disorders in this patient may be related to the presence of HLA-B8 and HLA-Dw3, the prevalence of which is known to be increased in CD and keratoconjunctivitis sicca, and that of HLA-B8 in autoimmune thrombocytopenic purpura. Despite the fact that thrombocytopenia is rarely encountered in CD, it is suggested that an autoimmune mechanism should be excluded in patients with this combination.[234] [M] Marked by redness, itching, burning, photophobia, gritty sensation. [C] Results from autoimmune-mediated decreased lacrimal function. [R] It is unknown whether CD-related keratoconjunctivitis sicca responds to GFD.	Not applicable.
Sensory System	Eyes	244	Keratomalacia [233]	(AD)	[P] Increased frequency in untreated CD. [D] Keratomalacia, a late feature of vitamin A deficiency, is characterized by hazy, dry cornea that becomes softened and denuded. It is irreversible. The conjunctiva and lacrimal glands are also affected, resulting in ulceration. Study investigating alterations in the anterior segment of the eye demonstrated vitamin A deficiency can be the reason for bilateral painless cornea manifestations. An interdisciplinary cooperation is essential for the elaboration of the diagnosis and the treatment.[233] [M] Marked by loss of vision. [C] Results from advanced vitamin A and protein malabsorption in CD. [R] CD-related keratomalacia does not resolve on GFD.	Protein, Vitamin A.
Sensory System	Eyes	245	Night blindness (Nyctalopia)	(S)	[P] Increased frequency in untreated CD. [D] Nyctalopia, caused by lack of rhodopsin in the rods of the retina, is characterized by decreased ability to see at night. It is an early feature of vitamin A deficiency and decreased content of oxygen in the blood. [M] Marked by impaired ability to see in dim light or darkness. [C] Results from vitamin A malabsorption in CD. [R] CD-related night blindness resolves quickly on GFD.	Protein, Vitamin A.

[+] (S) = Classic sign/symptom; (AT) = Atypical sign/symptom; (AD) = Associated Disorder; (C) = Complication.

[++] [P] = Prevalance; [D] = Description; [M] = Sign/symptom; [C] = CD related cause; [R] = Response to gluten Free diet (GFD).

Health Manifestations of Celiac Disease (CD)
Section B: Signs, Symptoms, Associated Disorders and Complications

Affected System	Affected Organ	ID No.	Manifestation	Type[+]	Current Medical Information [++]	Deficient Nutrient
Sensory System	Eyes	246	Ocular Myopathy [184,187,235]	(AD)	[P] New association with CD.[187,235] Ocular signs were observed in 84% of CD patients with gluten ataxia.[184] [D] Ocular myopathy is characterized by abnormalities of eye movement. Case report describes the course of 31 year old female in whom stiff gait, stimulus-induced myoclonus, and difficulty initiating and maintaining horizontal and vertical voluntary saccades and maintaining eye contact with the visual target were the presenting signs of CD. CD has to be considered in the differential diagnosis of patients with neurologic symptoms of unknown origin, even in the absence of pronounced GI symptoms. Myoclonus responded well, but abnormalities of eye movement did not respond to a GFD in this patient.[187] Case report describes the course of a 12 year old girl in whom ocular myopathy was the presenting feature of biopsy-proven CD. Ocular myopathy responded well in this child. The process was apparantly reversed by a GFD and vitamin supplementation.[235] [M] Marked by difficulty initiating and maintaining eye movement and eye contact. [C] Results from causal relationship with CD.[187] [R] CD-related ocular myopathy may respond to GFD.	Magnesium.
Sensory System	Eyes	247	Uveitis, Bilateral [1,236]	(AD)	[P] Increased frequency in untreated CD. [D] Bilateral uveitis, a feature of riboflavin deficiency, is an intraocular inflammatory disorder involving the iris, ciliary body, and choroid (uveal tract structures). Case report of patient with uveitis and CD cured by a GFD.[236] [M] Marked by changes to membrane that hinders ability to protect against infection. Preceded by itching, burning of eyes. [C] Results from malabsorption of riboflavin (vitamin B$_2$) in CD; possible immune mechanism. [R] CD-related uveitis resolves on GFD.[236]	Vitamin B$_2$.
Sensory System	Eyes	248	Xerophthalmia [1]	(C)	[P] Increased frequency in untreated CD. [D] Xerophthalmia is a feature of vitamin A and/or omega-3 deficiency characterized by dryness of the cornea and conjunctiva, follows chronic inflammation. [M] Marked by dry, sandy eyes with thick, white mucosa. Keratinization or hardening leads to ulceration of cornea. [C] Results from malabsorption in CD. [R] Resolves on GFD. Supplementaion may be needed.	EPA, Vitamin A.

[+] (S) = Classic sign/symptom; (AT) = Atypical sign/symptom; (AD) Associated Disorder; (C) = Complication.

[++] [P] = Prevalance; [D] = Description; [M] = Sign/symptom; [C] = CD related cause; [R] = Response to gluten Free diet (GFD).

Health Manifestations of Celiac Disease (CD)
Section B: Signs, Symptoms, Associated Disorders and Complications

Affected System	Affected Organ	ID No.	Manifestation	Type[+]	Current Medical Information [++]	Deficient Nutrient
Sensory System	Nose	249	Loss of Smell [34]	(S)	[P] Increased frequency in untreated CD. [D] Loss of smell is characterized by impaired olfactory sense. [M] Marked by inability to detect chemical odors. [C] Results from zinc deficiency due to malabsorption. [34] [R] Loss of smell related to CD resolves on GFD.	Zinc.
Sensory System	Taste buds	250	Dysgeusia [34]	(S)	[P] Increased frequency in untreated CD. [D] Dysgeusia is characterized by impaired or perverted gustatory sense. [M] Marked by inability to distinguish the true flavor of a substance when tasted. [C] Results from multiple deficiencies including vitamin B_{12}, niacin, and zinc. [34] Other causes include associated disorders of CD such as diabetes, hypothyroidism, adrenal cortical insufficiency, liver disease, Sjögren's syndrome, and hypertension. [R] CD-related dygeusia resolves on GFD.	Vitamin B_3, Vitamin B_{12}, Zinc.

+ (S) = Classic sign/symptom; (AT) = Atypical sign/symptom; (AD) Associated Disorder; (C) = Complication.
++ [P] = Prevalance; [D] = Description; [M] = Sign/symptom; [C] = CD related cause; [R] = Response to gluten Free diet (GFD).

Recognizing Celiac Disease Signs, Symptoms, Associated Disorders & Complications

Health Manifestations of Celiac Disease (CD)
Section B: Signs, Symptoms, Associated Disorders and Complications

Affected System	Affected Organ	ID No.	Manifestation	Type[+]	Current Medical Information[++]	Deficient Nutrient
Skeletal System	Bones	251	Bone Fractures [1,237,238,239]	(C)	[P] 80% of fractures were detected before the diagnosis of CD or in patients who were noncompliant with the GFD; 7% occurred after start of GFD.[237] Fractures in classically symptomatic CD patients had a 47% occurrence vs.15% in controls.[238] [D] Bone fractures in CD are characterized by breaks in demineralized bones. Study investigating the prevalence of bone fractures and vertebral deformities in celiacs revealed that patients with CD had a high prevalence of fractures in the peripheral skeleton. Most of these events occurred before diagnosis or while patients were noncompliant with GFD. Early diagnosis and treatment were the most relevant measures to protect patients from the risk of fractures.[237] Study investigating celiac osteopathy revealed a wide variation in fracture risk, with increasing risk in the peripheral skeleton in classically symptomatic patients. Fractures in subclinical/silent CD patients were no different than controls. Compared with controls, CD patients had significantly more fractures produced by mild trauma. Diagnostic and therapeutic strategies to prevent bone loss and fracture should be preferentially used in the subgroup of patients with classic clinical disease.[238] Case report describes a 67 year old woman with a 20 year history of recurrent abdominal pain, diarrhea and diffuse bone pain. Diagnoses of iron deficiency disorder, iron absorption disorder, osteoporosis and hyperthyroidism had been made. Despite treatment with vitamin D3, calcium, fluorides and iron, patient's condition deteriorated to the point where she needed constant care. Celiac disease with secondary intestinal osteopathy was identified. High-dose parenteral treatment with vitamin D3, oral calcium supplementation and a GFD resulted in improvement within 3 months, and the patient can largely look after herself again.[239] [M] Marked by pain and dysfunction of the broken bone. [C] Results from multiple deficiencies in CD including calcium, vitamin D, phosphorus, magnesium, copper, and vitamin K. [R] GFD improves bone density and strength in CD-related bone demineralization. Supplementation with calcium and vitamin D3 suggested.	Calcium, Copper, Magnesium, Phosphorus Vitamin D, Vitamin K.

+ (S) = Classic sign/symptom; (AT) = Atypical sign/symptom; (AD) Associated Disorder; (C) = Complication.
++ [P] = Prevalance; [D] = Description; [M] = Sign/symptom; [C] = CD related cause; [R] = Response to gluten Free diet (GFD).

Health Manifestations of Celiac Disease (CD)

Section B: Signs, Symptoms, Associated Disorders and Complications

Affected System	ID No.	Manifestation	Type[+]	Current Medical Information [++]	Deficient Nutrient
Skeletal System	252	Bone Pain [1,239,240]	(C)	[P] Increased prevalence in untreated CD.[240] [D] Bone pain associated with demineralization is due to severe hyperparathyroidism. Case report describes a 67 year old woman with a 20 year history of recurrent abdominal pain, diarrhea and diffuse bone pain. Diagnoses of iron deficiency disorder, iron absorption disorder, osteoporosis and hyperthyroidism had been made. Despite treatment with vitamin D3, calcium, fluorides and iron, patient's condition deteriorated to the point where she needed constant care. Celiac disease with secondary intestinal osteopathy was identified. High-dose parenteral treatment with vitamin D3, oral calcium supplementation and a GFD resulted in improvement within 3 months, and the patient can largely look after herself again.[239] Case report describes the course of a 35 year old woman with recent fracture of right arm a year after fracture of left shoulder, following complaints of pain in her right leg on walking and low back pain 5 years preceding. Radiographs showed generalized demineralization and severe subperiostal bone resorption with typical brown tumors. Subsequently, she was diagnosed with CD and hyperparathyroidism with severe bone involvement: osteitis fibrosa cystica, bone pains, and multiple fractures. A parathyroid adenoma was identified and removed. Untreated CD, vitamin D deficiency, and concomitant hyperparathyroidism resulted in severe osteomalacia. The normal calcium values observed were likely to be a consequence of reduction of total body calcium content and vitamin D deficiency. Hypophosphatemia was present 10 years preceding, suggesting that there was hyperparathyroidism at that time.[240] [M] Marked by diffuse bone pain and pain in spine, pelvis and lower extremities in osteomalacia. [C] Results from vitamin D deficiency; consequent hypocalcemia and concomitant hyperparathyroidism.[240] [R] Bone pain resolves with therapy on GFD.[239,240]	Calcium, Magnesium, Vitamin D.

+ (S) = Classic sign/symptom; (AT) = Atypical sign/symptom; (AD) Associated Disorder; (C) = Complication.

++ [P] = Prevalance; [D] = Description; [M] = Sign/symptom; [C] = CD related cause; [R] = Response to gluten Free diet (GFD).

Health Manifestations of Celiac Disease (CD)
Section B: Signs, Symptoms, Associated Disorders and Complications

Affected System	Affected Organ	ID No.	Manifestation	Type[+]	Current Medical Information [++]	Deficient Nutrient
Skeletal System	Bones	253	Osteitis Fibrosa Cystica [240,241]	(C)	[P] New associations with CD.[240,241] [D] Osteitis fibrosa cystica is a bone disease characterized by decalcification and softening of bones with bone cyst formation and tumors. Metabolic bone disease due to secondary hyperparathyroidism is common in CD.[241] Case report describes the course of a 54 year old female patient found to have huge bone cysts due to osteitis fibrosa cystica in the long bones. A parathyroid adenoma was identified and removed. CD and Turner's syndrome were diagnosed.[241] Case report describes a 35 year old female patient with fracture of her right arm a year after fracture of left shoulder, following complaints of pain in her right leg on walking and low back pain 5 years preceding. Radiographs showed generalized demineralization and severe subperiostal bone resorption with typical brown tumors. Subsequently, she was diagnosed with CD and hyperparathyroidism with severe bone involvement: osteitis fibrosa cystica, bone pains, and multiple fractures. A parathyroid adenoma was identified and removed. Untreated CD, vitamin D deficiency, and concomitant hyperparathyroidism resulted in severe osteomalacia. Normal calcium values were likely to be a consequence of reduction of total body calcium content and vitamin D deficiency. Hypophosphatemia was present 10 years preceding, suggesting that there was hyperparathyroidism at that time.[240] [M] Marked by bone pain.[241] [C] Results from vitamin D deficiency, consequent hypocalcemia, and concomitant hyperparathyroidism.[240] [R] Responds to GFD with supplementation.[240]	Calcium, Vitamin D.
Skeletal System	Bones	254	Osteomalacia [1,242]	(C)	[P] Common in patients with untreated CD.[242] [D] Osteomalacia is a metabolic bone disorder characterized by generalized reduction in bone density in adults and pseudofractures with muscular weakness and bone tenderness. Study investigating bone metabolism in celiac patients demonstrated that static and dynamic histomorphometry of iliac crest bone biopsy are useful tools to evaluate bone metabolism in CD, especially if hyperparathyroidism or mineralization defect are suspected. Hyperparathyroidism may be a problem in patients before introducing a GFD. Mineralization defect and osteomalacic changes are common later on, irrespective of whether the patients are in remission or not.[242] [M] Marked by weakness of upper arms/thighs, waddling gait, elevated serum alkaline phosphatase, bone pain, skeletal changes and greater risk of fractures, especially of wrist and pelvis. [C] Results from vitamin D malabsorption with hypophosphatemia and calcium deficiency. [R] Osteomalacic changes may not respond to a GFD.[242]	Calcium, Phosphorus, Vitamin D.

[+] (S) = Classic sign/symptom; (AT) = Atypical sign/symptom; (AD) Associated Disorder; (C) = Complication.

[++] [P] = Prevalance; [D] = Description; [M] = Sign/symptom; [C] = CD related cause; [R] = Response to gluten Free diet (GFD).

Health Manifestations of Celiac Disease (CD)
Section B: Signs, Symptoms, Associated Disorders and Complications

Affected System	Affected Organ	ID No.	Manifestation	Type+	Current Medical Information ++	Deficient Nutrient
Skeletal System	Bones	255	Osteonecrosis [243]	(C)	[P] New association with CD requires high index of suspicion.[243] [D] Osteonecrosis is a bone disorder resulting from insufficient blood flow to a part of the skeleton characterized by ensuing death of bone cells. Case report describes a 39 year old male patient with CD and multiple osteonecrosis, a previously unrecognized association. His symptoms were mild hypocalcemia, diarrhea, and arthralgias. Secondary hyperparathyroidism, CD and extensive osteonecrosis were detected by hematologic and radiologic studies. The hematologic variables normalized after institution of a GFD and calcium supplementation.[243] [M] Marked by bone pain of various degree and intensity. [C] Results from secondary hyperparathyroidism due to malabsorption in CD. [R] CD-related osteonecrosis responds to GFD.[243]	Calcium.

+ (S) = Classic sign/symptom; (AT) = Atypical sign/symptom; (AD) Associated Disorder; (C) = Complication.

++ [P] = Prevalance; [D] = Description; [M] = Sign/symptom; [C] = CD related cause; [R] = Response to gluten Free diet (GFD).

220   *Recognizing Celiac Disease* Signs, Symptoms, Associated Disorders & Complications

Health Manifestations of Celiac Disease (CD)

Section B: Signs, Symptoms, Associated Disorders and Complications

Affected System	Affected Organ	ID No.	Manifestation	Type[+]	Current Medical Information [++]	Deficient Nutrient

Skeletal System	Bones	256	Osteoporosis [1,9,244, 245,246,247]	(C)	[P] At diagnosis of CD: 40% with osteopenia, 26% with osteoporosis, and 34% with normal bone mineral density (BMD).[244]
					
					[D] Osteoporosis is a metabolic bone disorder characterized by diminished bone mass with retention of normal cell appearance and high bone turnover. Elevated prolactin and follicle-stimulating hormone (FSH) in males indicate an imbalance an imbalance of hypothalmus-pituitary level increasing their risk.
					
					    Study investigating pathogenesis of bone loss and weakening in CD patients demonstrated that bone weakening might result from 1) metabolic disturbances of bone remodeling affecting trabecular and cortical bone masses and the mechanical quality of the bone material, and 2) a reduction of muscle strength impairing the modeling dependent optimization of bone architectural design and mass of cortical bone. GFD seems to correct almost exclusively the metabolically induced disturbances.[245]
					
					    Study evaluating the impact of a 1-year GFD on bone metabolism and nutritional status in newly diagnosed CD patients demonstrated that CD patients are at high risk for developing a low BMD and bone turnover impairment. A one year GFD improved this situation in the 57% which showed mucosal recovery. Between postmenopausal and fertile women there were significant differences in BMD and several bone markers.[244]
					
					    Study investigating calcium absorption and BMD over 4 years treatment with a GFD demonstrated that increased calcium intake could potentially compensate for the reduced fractional calcium absorption in treated adult CD patients, but may not normalize the BMD. Inverse correlation between parathyroid hormone (PTH) and time following treatment suggests continuing long-term benefit of gluten withdrawal on bone metabolism.[9]
					
					    Study evaluating 266 patients with and 574 without osteoporosis demonstrated the prevalence of CD in osteoporosis is high enough to justify a recommendation for serologic screening of all patients with osteoporosis for CD.[246]
					
					    Case report describes a 60 year old woman presenting with refractory osteoporosis. Osteoporosis was confirmed, osteomalacia was ruled out based on transiliac bone biopsy, and CD was revealed. Serum levels of calcium and phosphorus were normal; vitamin D, folic acid, and vitamin B$_{12}$ were low; AGA and EMA antibodies were significantly elevated. Careful diagnostic evaluation of osteoporosis is necessary due to consequences.[247]
					
					[M] Marked by back pain and skeletal changes, especially in height and form of spine and increased risk for fractures.
					
					[C] Results from deficiency of calcium, vitamin D in particular, and other micronutrients in CD.
					
					[R] GFD significantly improves BMD, bone metabolism and nutrition even in post-menopausal women and in patients with incomplete mucosal recovery.[244]
						Boron, Calcium, Copper, Iron, Magnesium, Manganese, Vitamin D, Vitamin K, Zinc.

+ (S) = Classic sign/symptom; (AT) = Atypical sign/symptom; (AD) Associated Disorder; (C) = Complication.

++ [P] = Prevalance; [D] = Description; [M] = Sign/symptom; [C] = CD related cause; [R] = Response to gluten Free diet (GFD).

Health Manifestations of Celiac Disease (CD)
Section B: Signs, Symptoms, Associated Disorders and Complications

Affected System	ID No.	Manifestation	Type[+]	Current Medical Information [++]	Deficient Nutrient
Skeletal System	257	Enteropathic Arthritis [1,11,248,249]	(AT) (AD)	[P] Increased frequency in CD.[248] [D] Enteropathic arthritis is a form of arthritis associated with chronic inflammatory bowel diseases characterized by peripheral joint disease. Abnormal bowel permeability and immunologic and genetic influences are probably involved in the pathogenesis of the joint disease in CD, although the exact mechanisms remain uncertain.[248] CD exemplifies the interplay between antigen entrance through the gastrointestinal (GI) canal and genetic host factors such as HLA B27. In most cases such an interplay results in formation of circulating immune complexes causing the development of peripheral joint disease.[249] [M] Marked by joint pain, chronic inflammation and swelling. [C] Results from uncertain autoimmune mechanism involving formation of circulating immune complexes and abnormal bowel permeability.[248] [R] CD-related enteropathic arthritis responds to GFD.	Not applicable.
Skeletal System	258	Psoriatic Arthritis [1,250,251]	(AT) (AD)	[P] 4.4% of patients with psoriatic arthritis (PsoA) had CD.[250] [D] Psoriatic arthritis is a joint manifestation of psoriasis, a systemic autoimmune disease, characterized by asymmetric involvement in one or more joints, especially affecting the distal phalangeal joints of fingers and toes. Joint symptoms may coincide with exacerbations and remissions of skin symptoms. Study investigating whether patients with PsoA have an increased prevalence of antigliadin antibodies (AGA) and of CD demonstrated that patients with PsoA have an increased prevalence of raised IgA and of CD. Patients with raised AGA have a more pronounced inflammation with a longer duration of morning stiffness than those with a low AGA concentration. None of the patients had IgA antibodies to endomysium.[250] Case report of a girl followed for 18 years describes psoriasis and CD presenting at age two. At age 12 she presented arthritis of the left knee while not following a GFD. Continuation of the GFD with non steroidal antiphlogistic drugs therapy afforded complete remission of articular symptoms and good pubertal and intellectual growth.[251] [M] Marked by inflammation of large and small joints including the sacroiliacs and spine. [C] Results from autoimmune mechanism not clearly understood. Omega-3 fatty acid deficiency may exacerbate. [R] Insufficient studies to determine response to GFD. Arthritis responded in case report patient.[251]	Omega-3 fatty acids.

[+] (S) = Classic sign/symptom; (AT) = Atypical sign/symptom; (AD) Associated Disorder; (C) = Complication.

[++] [P] = Prevalence; [D] = Description; [M] = Sign/symptom; [C] = CD related cause; [R] = Response to gluten Free diet (GFD).

Health Manifestations of Celiac Disease (CD)
Section B: Signs, Symptoms, Associated Disorders and Complications

Affected System	Affected Organ	ID No.	Manifestation	Type+	Current Medical Information ++	Deficient Nutrient
Skeletal System	Joints	259	Recurrent Monoarthritis [1,252]	(AT)	[P] Report of new association in childhood.[252] [D] Recurrent monoarthritis is a joint disorder characterized by peripheral arthritis involving one joint with a usual interval of up to 15 years to diagnosis of CD in adults. Case report describes the course of an 11 year old boy with a 2 year interval between the appearance of arthritis and the diagnosis of CD. The boy was asymptomatic for bowel disease and his nutritional status was normal. Diagnosis of CD was established using AGA and anti-EMA antibody tests and was confirmed by small bowel biopsy. A GFD resulted in the persistent remission of arthritis. As the treatment of CD-associated arthritis is based on dietary therapy, physicians should be alert to the possibility of occult CD in any child with arthritis of unclear origin.[252] [M] Marked by pain and swelling of one joint. [C] Results from exposure to gluten. [R] GFD resulted in the persistent remission of arthritis.[252]	Not applicable.
Urinary System	Kidneys	260	Hypocalciuria [1,20,22]	(S)	[P] Common lab result at diagnosis of CD.[20] [D] Hypocalciuria, or decreased calcium in the urine, indicates low urinary calcium excretion, an early renal compensatory mechanism in hypocalcemia (low blood calcium level). Study investigating the effect of a GFD on mineral and bone metabolism in women with CD and, using the strontium test, assessing intestinal calcium absorption demonstrated significantly abnormal urinary calcium and plasma calcium at diagnosis of CD.[20] Case report describes a 36 year old woman presenting with hypocalcemia and hypocalciuria with serum 25-hydroxyvitamin D and 1,25-hydroxyvitamin D that were normal and elevated, respectively, as the initial manifestations of CD. Hypocalciuria and secondary hyperparathyroidism were refractory to pharmacologic calcium and cholecalciferol supplementation. Discussion: the diagnosis of calcium malabsorption was considered despite the absence of GI symptoms because the serum 25-hydroxyvitamin D level seemed inappropriate for the degree of hypocalcemia, and the PTH and l alphahydroxylase responses to hypocalcemia appeared intact. Conclusion: primary intestinal malabsorption of calcium without concomitant vitamin D deficiency is possible in celiac disease because of the preferential involvement of the proximal small intestine early in the disease process. Our patient had hypocalcemia caused by celiac disease and values for serum 25-hydroxyvitamin D and 1,25- dihydroxyvitamin D that were normal and elevated, respectively. Correction was demonstrated after dietary gluten withdrawal.[22] [M] Marked by abnormal plasma calcium. [C] Results from calcium malabsorption in CD.[20] [R] Normalizes on a GFD.[20,22]	Calcium.

+ (S) = Classic sign/symptom; (AT) = Atypical sign/symptom; (AD) Associated Disorder; (C) = Complication.

++ [P] = Prevalance; [D] = Description; [M] = Sign/symptom; [C] = CD related cause; [R] = Response to gluten Free diet (GFD).

Health Manifestations of Celiac Disease (CD)
Section B: Signs, Symptoms, Associated Disorders and Complications

Affected System	Affected Organ	ID No.	Manifestation	Type+	Current Medical Information ++	Deficient Nutrient
Urinary System	Kidneys	261	IgA Nephropathy [1,253,254]	(AD)	[P] CD occurs in 3.6% of patients with IgA nephropathy (IgA NP), and 14% of HLA DQ2 positive patients with IgA nephropathy had CD.[253] [D] IgA nephropathy is a primary renal disease in which circulating IgA antigliadin antibodies (IgA-AGA) are often found and is characterized by recurrent hematuria, mild proteinuria, and glomerular changes.[254] Study examining the relationship between IgA-AGA and clinical data concludes that IgA-AGA are associated with the progression of IgA NP. Antireticulin and antiendomysium antibody tests were negative in all patients and control sera. Findings support the current concept about the pathogenesis of IgA NP, where the defective IgA production itself may be the primary and intestinal lesions as well as the production of IgA-AGA, the secondary phenomenon.[254] Study seeking to establish how common CD is in patients with IgA nephropathy, and whether the possible association can be explained by similar HLA DQ status demonstrates that although there is no increase in celiac-type HLA DQ, patients with IgA nephropathy carry a risk of developing CD. It can be hypothesized that the increased intestinal permeability in IgA nephropathy may predispose genetically susceptible patients to CD.[253] [M] Marked by protein in the urine. [C] Results from unclear autoimmune mechanism.[254] Increased intestinal permeability in IgA nephropathy may predispose genetically susceptible patients to CD.[253] [R] GFD had no apparent influence on the course of nephropathy.[253]	Not applicable.

+ (S) = Classic sign/symptom; (AT) = Atypical sign/symptom; (AD) Associated Disorder; (C) = Complication.

++ [P] = Prevalance; [D] = Description; [M] = Sign/symptom; [C] = CD related cause; [R] = Response to gluten Free diet (GFD).

Health Manifestations of Celiac Disease (CD)

Section B: Signs, Symptoms, Associated Disorders and Complications

Affected System	Affected Organ	ID No.	Manifestation	Type[+]	Current Medical Information [++]	Deficient Nutrient
Urinary System	Kidneys	262	Renal Calculus [1,255,256]	(AT) (AD)	[P] New association with CD.[255] [D] Renal calculi are hard formations in the kidneys composed of calcium oxalate, uric acid and cystine. They vary in size from microscopic crystalline foci to several centimeters in diameter. Case report of a 49 year old man with renal colic and left renal calculus describes CD presenting with a urinary calculus in the absence of gastrointestinal (GI) symptoms. Investigations showed hyperoxaluria for which there was no dietary or drug cause. The presence of hyperoxaluria with hypercalciuria prompted malabsorption studies. CD was diagnosed, and 3 months on a GFD led to normalization of urinary oxalate excretion, resolution of small bowel pathology and disappearance of endomysial antibodies. Enteric hyperoxaluria (EHO) is a common cause of hyperoxaluria and calcium urolithiasis.[255] In health, dietary calcium is complexed with luminal oxalate, limiting its absorption. In EHO, the excess free fatty acids, from fat malabsorption, compete with oxalate for calcium binding, leading to an increased availability of oxalate for absorption (solubility theory). This oxalate is absorbed in the colon, which is made more permeable to unabsorbed bile salt and fatty acids (permeability theory). The identification and correction of hyperoxaluria is important to prevent recurrent calculi and oxalate nephrosis, especially as patients with urolithiasis are often empirically advised to eat a low-calcium diet. Paradoxically, this promotes oxaluria, increasing the risk of further kidney stones in hyperoxaluric patients.[255] Case report describes a 10 year old girl with steatorrhea, hyperoxaluria, and a renal calculus in a single functioning kidney presenting with CD. Successful management of the steatorrhea corrected both the chronic diarrhea and hyperoxaluria. Pediatricians caring for children with malabsorptive conditions should be aware of the risk of urinary calculus formation as a result of increased dietary oxalate absorption.[256] [M] Marked by various pain - excruciating when passing stones or with obstruction, bleeding, chills, fever, genital pain, nausea, vomiting, and abdominal distention, although many calculi are asymptomatic. [C] Results from malabsorption of fats in CD.[255] [R] CD-related calculi formation improves on a GFD.[255]	Not applicable.

[+] (S) = Classic sign/symptom; (AT) = Atypical sign/symptom; (AD) Associated Disorder; (C) = Complication.

[++] [P] = Prevalance; [D] = Description; [M] = Sign/symptom; [C] = CD related cause; [R] = Response to gluten Free diet (GFD).

Health Manifestations of Celiac Disease (CD)
Section B: Signs, Symptoms, Associated Disorders and Complications

Affected System	Affected Organ	ID No.	Manifestation	Type+	Current Medical Information ++	Deficient Nutrient
Urinary System	Bladder	263	Urinary Tract Infection (UTI) [1,257]	(AT) (AD)	[P] Significantly higher risk of first time urinary tract infection (UTI) in children with CD than in controls.[257] [D] Urinary tract infection is a urinary disorder characterized by pyuria and dysuria. Study investigating the occurrence of UTI in children with CD demonstrated in the majority of cases UTI was associated with untreated, active CD.[257] [M] Marked by pain and burning on urination, urgency and frequency. [C] Results from lowered tissue integrity and resistance to infection, nutritional deficiencies in CD including vitamin A, vitamin C, omega-3 fatty acids, iron. [R] Insufficient studies to show if GFD may be preventive of CD-related UTI.	Iron, Omega-3 fatty acids, Vitamin A, Vitamin C.
Reproductive System: Female	Ovaries	264	Amenorrhea, Secondary [1,258,259,260]	(S)	[P] 38.8 % of patients with CD complained of amenorrhea compared with 9.2% of controls.[258] [D] Secondary amenorrhea is an adolescent menstrual disorder characterized by failure to menstruate due to lack of menarche or absence for more than 3 months in females who had previously menstruated. CD may impair the reproductive life of affected women, eliciting amenorrhea.[259] Study investigating the gynecological history of newly diagnosed patients with CD demonstrated that amenorrhea is frequently associated with celiac disease.[258] Study analyzing gynecological disturbances in patients with CD in relation to their nutritional status and adherence to a GFD demonstrated adolescents who were not adherent to a GFD presented delayed menarche and secondary amenorrhea. Gluten could explain the disturbances and malnutrition would worsen the disease in a consequent vicious cycle. CD should be included in screening of reproductive disorders.[260] [M] Marked by abnormal absence of menstruation. [C] Results from endocrine dysfunction involving gluten exposure and nutritional deficiencies in CD. Pathogenesis still awaits clarification.[259] [R] The possible prevention or treatment of amenorrhea in CD can only be achieved through a life-long maintenance of a GFD.[259]	Calcium, Magnesium, Omega-6 fatty acids, Vitamin D.

+ (S) = Classic sign/symptom; (AT) = Atypical sign/symptom; (AD) Associated Disorder; (C) = Complication.
++ [P] = Prevalance; [D] = Description; [M] = Sign/symptom; [C] = CD related cause; [R] = Response to gluten Free diet (GFD).

Health Manifestations of Celiac Disease (CD)
Section B: Signs, Symptoms, Associated Disorders and Complications

Affected System	Affected Organ	ID No.	Manifestation	Type[+]	Current Medical Information[++]	Deficient Nutrient
Reproductive System: Female	Ovaries	265	Infertility, Female 1,18,38,259,261, 262,263,264,265,266,267, 268,269	(S) (AD) (C)	[P] High incidence of CD found in women with impaired fertility.[261] 2.7% rate in Finnish women.[262] 1.13% rate in Czech women.[263] 3.03% rate in Northern Sardinian women.[264] Rate is 2.65% in Arab women.[266] 3.6% of French women with CD experienced infertility or low birth weight.[265] [D] Infertility is characterized by failure to conceive after one year of intercourse. Infertility is not related to the severity of CD.[267] Unexplained subfertility is often undiagnosed in CD. Consideration of CD can increase the probability of conception and uncomplicated pregnancy.[268] Infertility may be a consequence of the endocrine derangements caused by selective nutrient deficiencies.[269] An interaction among specific nutritional deficiencies, endocrine imbalances, and immune disturbances is suspected.[259] Zinc proteins have been shown to be involved in the transcription and translation of genetic material. Zinc deficiency has been incriminated in infertility.[38] Study investigating the incidence of infertility demonstrated that patients with CD are subfertile. Overall difference in fertility is due to relative infertility prior to diagnosis, and is corrected by a GFD.[261] Study investigating the incidence of subclinical forms of CD in women with decreased fertility demonstrated higher incidence in silent CD.[262] Study investigating prevalence of infertility in healthy blood donors and in high-risk groups of adults demonstrated that 1.13% of 365 women with infertility considered as immunologically mediated were found to be positive in screening IgA and IgG-AGA and IgA-tTG as step 1 and IgA-AGA and/or IgA-tTG and EMA as step 2.[263] Study investigating the prevalence of CD in couples being evaluated for infertility compared with the known prevalence of silent CD demonstrated higher prevalence.[264] Study investigating the proportion of adult patients with CD who had had undiagnosed symptoms during childhood and the consequences of such diagnostic delay demonstrated low fertility and short stature correlated with duration of symptoms before diagnosis.[265] [M] Marked by the inability to become pregnant. [C] Results from unknown pathogenesis.[265] Malnutrition, iron, folate, and zinc deficiencies have all been implicated.[18] [R] GFD and correction of deficient dietary elements can lead to a return of fertility.[18]	Calcium, Folic acid, Iron, Magnesium, Omega-6 fatty acids, Vitamin D, Zinc.

[+] (S) = Classic sign/symptom; (AT) = Atypical sign/symptom; (AD) Associated Disorder; (C) = Complication.

[++] [P] = Prevalence; [D] = Description; [M] = Sign/symptom; [C] = CD related cause; [R] = Response to gluten Free diet (GFD).

Health Manifestations of Celiac Disease (CD)
Section B: Signs, Symptoms, Associated Disorders and Complications

Affected System	Affected Organ	ID No.	Manifestation	Type[+]	Current Medical Information [++]	Deficient Nutrient
Reproductive System: Female	Ovaries	266	Menarche, Late [1,258,259,260,270]	(S)	[P] Significantly retarded in patients with untreated CD.[270] [D] Late menarche is a menstrual disorder characterized by abnormal delay of menstruation. CD may impair the reproductive life of affected women, eliciting delayed menarche.[259] In CD there is a high level of autoantibodies directed against self-antigens, so there could be antibodies against hormones or organs critical for pubertal development. Moreover, in CD there could be a selective malabsorption of micronutrients essential for the metabolism of carrier or receptor proteins for sex hormones.[270] Hyperprolactinemia results in delayed menarche.[18] Study investigating the gynecological history of newly diagnosed patients with CD demonstrated that delayed menarche is frequently associated with celiac disease. Mean age of menarche at 13.5 years vs.12.1 years in controls.[258] Study analyzing gynecological disturbances in patients with CD in relation to their nutritional status and adherence to a GFD demonstrated adolescents who were not adherent to a GFD presented delayed menarche and secondary amenorrhea. Gluten could explain the disturbances and malnutrition would worsen the disease in a consequent vicious cycle. CD should be included in screening of reproductive disorders.[260] [M] Marked by abnormal delay of initial menstrual period. [C] Results from endocrine dysfunction involving gluten exposure and nutritional deficiencies in CD.[260] Pathogenesis still awaits clarification.[259] [R] CD-related late menarche responds to GFD, and GFD is preventive of delay.[259,260,270]	Omega-6 fatty acids, cholesterol.

+ (S) = Classic sign/symptom; (AT) = Atypical sign/symptom; (AD) Associated Disorder; (C) = Complication.

++ [P] = Prevalance; [D] = Description; [M] = Sign/symptom; [C] = CD related cause; [R] = Response to gluten Free diet (GFD).

Health Manifestations of Celiac Disease (CD)
Section B: Signs, Symptoms, Associated Disorders and Complications

Affected System	Affected Organ	ID No.	Manifestation	Type+	Current Medical Information++	Deficient Nutrient

Reproductive System: Female	Ovaries	267	Menopause, Early [1,259,261,271]	(S)	[P] Increased frequency in CD.[259]
					[D] Early menopause is the permanent cessation of menstruation beginning 2 to 4 years earlier in celiac women characterized by vasomotor instability, psychologic and emotional symptoms and profound changes in the lower genital tract. CD may impair the reproductive life of affected women, eliciting precocious menopause.[259]
					    Study investigating the incidence of menopause in CD demonstated a difference of 2.5 years between CD patients and controls. Mean age at menopause in patients with CD is 47.6 years in CD patients and 50.1 years in controls.[261]
					    Case report describes course of a 23 year old woman with a diagnosis of hypothyroidism due to Hashimoto's thyroiditis, autoimmune Addison's disease, and kariotypically normal spontaneous premature ovarian failure. Search for CD revealed positive EMA antibodies and total villous atrophy at jejunal biopsy. Marked clinical improvement and a progressive decrease in the need for thyroid and adrenal replacement therapies occurred over a 3-month period. After 6 months serum EMA became negative and after 12 months a new jejunal biopsy showed complete mucosal recovery. After 18 months the anti-thyroid antibodies titre decreased significantly and thyroid substitution therapy was discontinued. The precocious identification of CD in polyglandular disease is clinically relevant not only for the high risk of complications inherent to untreated CD, but also because CD is a cause of substitute hormonal therapy failure in patients with autoimmune thyroid disease.[271]
					[M] Marked by variable symptoms including hot flashes, nervousness, fatigue, apathy, excitability, depression, headache, and myalgia.
					[C] Results from unclear etiology involving nutritional deficiencies in CD.
					[R] The possible prevention or treatment of early menopause in CD can only be achieved through a life-long maintenance of GFD.[259]
						Cholesterol, Omega-6 fatty acids.

Reproductive System: Female	Ovaries	268	Premenstrual Syndrome, (PMS) [34]	(AT)	[P] Increased frequency in CD. [D] Premenstrual syndrome (PMS) is a menstrual disorder that occurs regularly during the last week of the luteal phase and starts to subside a few days before menstruation begins. [M] Marked by greatly depressed mood, marked anxiety, marked emotional lability, persistent irritability, and increased interpersonal conflicts. [C] Results from nutritional deficiencies in CD including calcium, magnesium, vitamin D, and EPA. [R] CD-related PMS responds to a GFD.	Calcium, EPA, Magnesium, Vitamin D.

+ (S) = Classic sign/symptom; (AT) = Atypical sign/symptom; (AD) Associated Disorder; (C) = Complication.

++ [P] = Prevalance; [D] = Description; [M] = Sign/symptom; [C] = CD related cause; [R] = Response to gluten Free diet (GFD).

Health Manifestations of Celiac Disease (CD)
Section B: Signs, Symptoms, Associated Disorders and Complications

Affected System	Affected Organ	ID No.	Manifestation	Type[+]	Current Medical Information [++]	Deficient Nutrient
Reproductive System: Female	Uterus	269	Dysmenorrhea [272,273]	(AT)	[P] New association with CD. [272] [D] Dysmenorrhea is a menstrual disorder characterized by cramping, spasmodic pain that occurs regularly just before or during menstruation. Case report of a 43 year old woman with chronic abdominal pain and pelvic pain, deep dyspareunia, dysmenorrhea, diarrhea, and a 5 kg weight loss during the last 6 months, describes failure of surgical intervention followed by complete success with GFD therapy. At laparoscopy, numerous small leiomyomata were seen and a few filmy adhesions between the small bowel and the abdominal wall were lysed. Except for the deep dyspareunia, all symptoms remitted after surgery, only to recur at 6 months of follow-up. Subsequently, CD was diagnosed and a GFD prescribed on which the patient became free of symptoms. [272] Study investigating the effects of vitamin E in the treatment of dysmenorrhea demonstrated that vitamin E relieves the pain of primary dysmenorrhea and reduces blood loss. Vitamin E 200 units was given twice a day, beginning 2 days before the expected start of menstruation and continued through the first 3 days of bleeding. Treatment was continued over 4 months. In the vitamin E group, pain severity was lower at 2 months and 4 months, pain duration was shorter at 2 months and at 4 months, and blood loss assessed by PBLAC score was lower at 2 months and at 4 months than controls. [273] [M] Marked by pain located in the lower abdomen that may radiate to the back or thighs during menstruation. [C] Results from unclear etiology, thought to involve uterine ischemia mediated by increased production of prostaglandins with increased contractibility of the myometrium, involving deficiencies in CD of vitamin E and omega-3 fatty acids. [R] CD-related dysmenorrhea completely responds to GFD. [272,273]	Omega-3 fatty acids, Vitamin E.

[+] (S) = Classic sign/symptom; (AT) = Atypical sign/symptom; (AD) Associated Disorder; (C) = Complication.

[++] [P] = Prevalance; [D] = Description; [M] = Sign/symptom; [C] = CD related cause; [R] = Response to gluten Free diet (GFD).

Health Manifestations of Celiac Disease (CD)
Section B: Signs, Symptoms, Associated Disorders and Complications

Affected System	Affected Organ	ID No.	Manifestation	Type[+]	Current Medical Information [++]	Deficient Nutrient
Reproductive System: Female	Vagina	270	Dyspareunia [272]	(AT)	[P] New association with CD.[272] [D] Dyspareunia is a disorder characterized by pain during or after coitus involving the labia, vagina or pelvis. Case report of a 43 year old woman with chronic abdominal pain and pelvic pain, deep dyspareunia, dysmenorrhea, diarrhea, and a 5 kg weight loss during the last 6 months describes failure of surgical intervention followed by complete success with GFD therapy. At laparoscopy, numerous small leiomyomata were seen and a few filmy adhesions between the small bowel and the abdominal wall were lysed. Except for the deep dyspareunia, all symptoms remitted after surgery, only to recur at 6 months of follow-up. Subsequently, CD was diagnosed and a GFD prescribed on which the patient became free of symptoms.[272] [M] Marked by painful coitus. [C] Results from inadequate vaginal lubrication, vaginal atrophy, and uterine myomata due to gluten exposure and nutritional deficiencies in CD. [R] CD-related dyspareunia completely responds to GFD.[272]	Vitamin E.
Reproductive System: Female	Vagina	271	Vaginitis [1]	(S)	[P] Frequently associated with CD in females. [D] Vaginitis is a genital disorder characterized by non-infectious tissue inflammation. [M] Marked by itching and redness. [C] Results from nutritional deficiencies causing lack of tissue integrity which include folic acid, niacin (vitamin B_3), and vitamin A. [R] CD-related vaginitis responds to GFD and is preventive.	Folic acid, Vitamin A, Vitamin B_3.

+ (S) = Classic sign/symptom; (AT) = Atypical sign/symptom; (AD) Associated Disorder; (C) = Complication.

++ [P] = Prevalance; [D] = Description; [M] = Sign/symptom; [C] = CD related cause; [R] = Response to gluten Free diet (GFD).

Affected System	Affected Organ	ID No.	Manifestation	Type+	Current Medical Information ++	Deficient Nutrient
Reproductive System: Male	Testes	272	Hypogonadism, Unexplained in Adults [18,274,275,276]	(AD)	[P] Increased frequency in males with untreated CD.[274] [D] Hypogonadism is characterized by inadequate production of male hormones and/or spermatozoa. Gonadal dysfunction is believed to be due to reduced conversion of testosterone to dihydrotestosterone caused by low levels of 5 alpha-reductase in CD. This leads to derangement of the hypothalmic-pituitary axis.[18] Affected males show a picture of tissue resistance to androgens. Hormone alterations are reversible upon the start of a GFD, emphasizing the importance of early diagnosis. As regards the nutritional aspects, the folic acid deficiency of CD can affect rapidly proliferating tissues such as the seminiferous epithelium. More attention should be paid to deficiencies of fat-soluble vitamins, such as A and D, observed in CD. Vitamin A is important for Sertoli cell function as well as for early spermatogenetic phases. Vitamin E supports the correct differentiation and function of epididymal epithelium, spermatid maturation and secretion of proteins by the prostate. The detection of early biomarkers of andrological or endocrinological dysfunctions should trigger timely strategies for prevention and treatment.[274] Study investigating pituitary regulation of gonadal function in treated and untreated male patients with CD demonstrated a derangement of pituitary regulation of gonadal function. Exaggerated responses of follicle-stimulating hormone (FSH) (89%) and luteinizing hormone LH (49%) to luteinizing hormone-releasing hormone LHRH were found in celiacs with subtotal villous atrophy and were commonly found when basal gonadotropin concentrations were normal. LH response was closely linked to jejunal morphology.[275] Study investigating levels of plasma testosterone, dihydrotestosterone, sex-hormone binding globulin, estradiol, and luteinising hormone in men with CD and relating these findings to jejunal morphology; fertility; semen quality, and sexual function demonstrated androgen resistance and hypothalmic-pituitary dysfunction that appear to be relatively specific to CD and cannot be explained merely in terms of malnutrition or chronic ill-health. Endocrine disturbance may be related to sexual dysfunction in CD, but its relationship to disordered spermatogenesis in CD has not been clearly established.[276] [M] Marked by immature secondary sex characteristics and reduced semen quality.[18] [C] Results from unclear etiology involving gluten exposure and deficiencies including zinc and vitamins A, E, and D.[274,276] [R] CD-related hypogonadism in males responds to GFD.[274]	Omega-6 fatty acids, Vitamin A, Vitamin E, Vitamin D, Zinc.

+ (S) = Classic sign/symptom; (AT) = Atypical sign/symptom; (AD) Associated Disorder; (C) = Complication.

++ [P] = Prevalance; [D] = Description; [M] = Sign/symptom; [C] = CD related cause; [R] = Response to gluten Free diet (GFD).

Health Manifestations of Celiac Disease (CD)
Section B: Signs, Symptoms, Associated Disorders and Complications

Affected System	Affected Organ	ID No.	Manifestation	Type+	Current Medical Information ++	Deficient Nutrient
Reproductive System: Male	Testes	273	Impotence [18,274,276]	(AD)	[P] Increased incidence in celiac males. [18,274,276] [D] Impotence is erectile dysfunction characterized by the inability to achieve or maintain an erection satisfactory for coitus. Increases of follicle-stimulating hormone (FSH) and prolactin are not related to impotence, but they may indicate an imbalance at the hypothalmus-pituitary level. [274] Study investigating levels of plasma testosterone, dihydrotestosterone, sex-hormone binding globulin, estradiol, and luteinising hormone in men with CD and relating these findings to jejunal morphology, fertility, semen quality, and sexual function demonstrated androgen resistance and hypothalmic-pituitary dysfunction that appear to be relatively specific to CD and cannot be explained merely in terms of malnutrition or chronic ill-health. Findings suggest endocrine disturbance may be related to sexual dysfunction in CD. [276] [M] Marked by inability to achieve or maintain an erection. [C] Results from unclear etiology involving endocrine dysfunction, gluten exposure and nutritional deficiencies in CD. [274] [R] Hormone alterations are reversible upon start of the GFD, emphasizing the importance of early diagnosis. [274] Gluten withdrawal and correction of deficient dietary elements can lead to a return of fertility. [18]	Calcium, Magnesium, Vitamin D.

+ (S) = Classic sign/symptom; (AT) = Atypical sign/symptom; (AD) Associated Disorder; (C) = Complication.

++ [P] = Prevalance; [D] = Description; [M] = Sign/symptom; [C] = CD related cause; [R] = Response to gluten Free diet (GFD).

Health Manifestations of Celiac Disease (CD)
Section B: Signs, Symptoms, Associated Disorders and Complications

Affected System	Affected Organ	ID No.	Manifestation	Type[+]	Current Medical Information[++]	Deficient Nutrient
Reproductive System: Male	Testes	274	Infertility, Male [1,18,49,274,275,276]	(S)	[P] Celiac male has greater risk of infertility than celiac female.[274] [D] Infertility in males is characterized by inability to either produce sperm or to produce viable sperm or mobile sperm resulting in prohibiting fertilization of the female ovum. Gonadal dysfunction is believed due to reduced conversion of testosterone to dihydrotestosterone caused by low levels of 5 alpha-reductase in CD, leading to derangement of the hypothalmic-pituitary axis. Hyperprolactinemia seen in 25% of CD patients causes androgen deficiency and infertility.[18] The detection of early biomarkers of andrological or endocrinological dysfunctions should trigger timely strategies for prevention and treatment. Hormone alterations are reversible upon the start of the GFD, emphasizing the importance of early diagnosis; this should be performed in the case of clinical suspicion, e.g. unexplained hypoandrogenism. Nutritionally, the folic acid deficiency of CD can affect rapidly proliferating tissues such as the seminiferous epithelium. More attention should be paid to deficiencies of fat-soluble vitamins, such as A and D, observed in CD. Vitamin A is important for Sertoli cell function as well as for early spermatogenetic phases. Vitamin E supports the correct differentiation and function of epididymal epithelium, spermatid maturation and secretion of proteins by the prostate.[274] Study investigating the role of oxidative stress in CD demonstrated the level of markers for vitamin E were significantly lower in CD than in contols.[49] Study investigating pituitary regulation of gonadal function in treated and untreated male CD patients demonstrated derangement of pituitary regulation of gonadal function. Exaggerated responses of folliclestimulating hormone (89%) and luteinizing hormone (49%) to luteinizing hormone-release hormone were found in celiacs with sub-total villous atrophy and were commonly found when basal gonadotropin concentrations were normal. LH response was closely linked to jejunal morphology.[275] Study investigating increased plasma testosterone and free testosterone index, reduced dihydrotestosterone, and raised serum luteinising hormone related to jejunal morphology, fertility, semen quality, and sexual function in 41 celiac males demonstrated a pattern indicative of androgen resistance specific to CD. As jejunal morphology improved hormone levels appeared to return to normal. This specific combination of abnormalities was not present in any of the disease control groups and, to our knowledge androgen resisance has not been described previously in another non-endocrine disorder.[276] [M] Marked by low, unhealthy sperm count. [C] Results from endocrine disorders and deficiencies of micronutrients.[274] [R] Hormone alterations are reversible upon start of GFD.[274] GFD and correction of deficient dietary elements can lead to a return of fertility.[18]	Folic acid, Omega-6 fatty acids, Vitamin A, Vitamin E, Vitamin D, Zinc.

[+] (S) = Classic sign/symptom; (AT) = Atypical sign/symptom; (AD) Associated Disorder; (C) = Complication.

[++] [P] = Prevalance; [D] = Description; [M] = Sign/symptom; [C] = CD related cause; [R] = Response to gluten Free diet (GFD).

Health Manifestations of Celiac Disease (CD)
Section B: Signs, Symptoms, Associated Disorders and Complications

Affected System	Affected Organ	ID No.	Manifestation	Type+	Current Medical Information ++	Deficient Nutrient
Reproductive System: Male	Testes	275	Sperm abnormalities [49,274]	(S)	[P] Increased incidence in CD, affecting about 18%, requiring high index of suspicion.[274] [D] Sperm abnormalities are the result of gonadal dysfunction characterized by inability to either produce sperm or to produce viable sperm or mobile sperm resulting in prohibiting fertilization of the female ovum affecting about 18% of celiac males. Within the seminiferous tubules of the testes, Sertoli cells maintain and regulate maturation of sperm from germ cell and Leydig's cells produce testosterone required for sustaining spermatogenesis. Detection of early biomarkers of andrological or endrocrinological dysfunction should trigger timely strategies for prevention and treatment. Folic acid deficiency can affect the rapidly proliferating tissues such as the seminiferous epithelium. More attention should be paid to deficiencies of fat-soluble vitamins, such as A and D, observed in CD. Vitamin A is important for Sertoli cell function as well as for early spermatogenetic phases. Vitamin E supports the correct differentiation and function of epididymal epithelium, spermatid maturation and secretion of proteins by the prostate.[274] Study investigating the role of oxidative stress in CD demonstrated the level of markers for vitamin E were significantly lower in CD than in contols.[49] [M] Marked by impaired formation of spermatozoa, poorly mobile sperm, and reduced sperm count. [C] Results from andrological or endrocrinological dysfunction and deficiencies of micronutrients.[274] [R] Hormone alterations are reversible upon start of a gluten-free diet.[274]	Folic acid, Omega 6 fatty acids, Vitamin A, Vitamin E, Vitamin D, Zinc.
Reproduction: Pregnancy, Parturition, and Puerperium	Blood: plasma and cells	276	Severe Iron Deficiency Anemia in Pregnancy [1,277]	(S)	[P] Increased frequency in patients with CD.[277] [D] Severe iron deficiency anemia in pregnancy, characterized by abnormal formation of small, pale red blood cells and iron depletion refractory to oral iron supplementation, may present CD. Article "Not always a relapse ": All of the patients in their series had typical GI manifestations of CD in infancy that had resolved despite a normal diet, but subsequently relapsed in pregnancy or the puerperium. In most patients, a previous history of GI disease or anemia cannot be elucidated, and refractory sideropenic anemia during pregnancy may be the only sign of CD. Although the acute presentation of CD in pregnancy or the puerperium is concerning, potentially of more concern is the risk of spontaneous abortion and intrauterine growth retardation of undiagnosed CD.[277] [M] Marked by pallor, fatigue, dyspnea on exertion, susceptibility to infection, and risk to fetal organogenesis (formation and development of body organs). [C] Results from iron deficiency due to malabsorption in gluten sensitive enteropathy.[277] [R] Iron deficiency anemia responds to a GFD.	Iron.

+ (S) = Classic sign/symptom; (AT) = Atypical sign/symptom; (AD) Associated Disorder; (C) = Complication.

++ [P] = Prevalance; [D] = Description; [M] = Sign/symptom; [C] = CD related cause; [R] = Response to gluten Free diet (GFD).

Section B *Signs, Symptoms, Associated Disorders & Complications*

Health Manifestations of Celiac Disease (CD)
Section B: Signs, Symptoms, Associated Disorders and Complications

Affected System	Affected Organ	ID No.	Manifestation	Type+	Current Medical Information ++	Deficient Nutrient
Reproduction: Pregnancy, Parturition, and Puerperium	Breasts	277	Short Duration of Breast Feeding [1,259]	(C)	[P] Women with CD are at higher risk.[259] [D] Short duration of breast feeding is characterized by inadequate milk production. 96% of infants of celiac mothers are fed 2 months or less. [M] Marked by inability to produce sufficient milk to satisfy the infant's needs. [C] Results from nutritional deficiencies in CD including protein, calcium, phosphorus, and fat. [R] Milk production responds to a GFD. The possible prevention or treatment of reproductive effects can only be achieved through a life-long maintenance of a GFD.[259]	Fat, Calcium, Phosphorus, Protein.

+ (S) = Classic sign/symptom; (AT) = Atypical sign/symptom; (AD) Associated Disorder; (C) = Complication.

++ [P] = Prevalance; [D] = Description; [M] = Sign/symptom; [C] = CD related cause; [R] = Response to gluten Free diet (GFD).

Health Manifestations of Celiac Disease (CD)
Section B: Signs, Symptoms, Associated Disorders and Complications

Affected System	Affected Organ	ID No.	Manifestation	Type[+]	Current Medical Information[++]	Deficient Nutrient
Pregnancy, Parturition, and Puerperium	Uterus	278	Abortions, Spontaneous [1,38,129, 258, 259, 260,261,267,268]	(S) (C)	[P] 15% rate found in undiagnosed women with CD vs. 6% in controls.[261] After treatment 1.3% of patients presented spontaneous abortion.[260] [D] Spontaneous abortion is a reproductive failure characterized by loss of the products of conception before the 20th week of pregnancy. Zinc proteins have been shown to be involved in the transcription and translation of genetic material. Zinc deficiency has been incriminated in abortion.[38] A better knowledge of the relationship between CD and abortion may lead to correctly diagnosing and treating the cause of some cases of abortion, previously labeled as cases of unidentified origin.[267] 'Unexplained' is often undiagnosed. Considering CD, which is often subclinical, in the differential diagnosis increases the probability of conception and uncomplicated pregnancy.[268] Study investigating the obstetric and gynecological history of 54 women age 16-62 years showed significant rate of repeat abortions.[258] Study investigating obstetric and gynecological disturbances in untreated women with CD in relation to their nutritional status demonstrated a higher percentage of spontaneous abortions, anemia, and hypoalbuminemia vs. controls. After treatment, patients presented with normal pregnancies and one patient presented spontaneous abortion. CD should be included in the screening of spontaneous abortions.[260] Case control study investigating the incidence of abortions in CD women demonstrated significantly more conceptions ended in miscarriage prior to diagnosis than among controls. After diagnosis and treatment the rate of miscarriage was similiar.[261] [M] Marked by early loss of fetus. [C] Results from unclear etiology involving gluten.[260] The overall evidence suggest that CD patients can be a group particularly susceptible to reproductive toxicants; however, the pathogenesis still awaits clarification.[259] Antiphospholipid syndrome (an associated disorder) induces fetal loss.[129] [R] The possible prevention or treatment of the effect of spontaneous abortion in CD can only be achieved through a life-long maintenance of a GFD.[259]	Folic acid, Protein, Vitamin A, Zinc.

+ (S) = Classic sign/symptom; (AT) = Atypical sign/symptom; (AD) Associated Disorder; (C) = Complication.

++ [P] = Prevalance; [D] = Description; [M] = Sign/symptom; [C] = CD related cause; [R] = Response to gluten Free diet (GFD).

Health Manifestations of Celiac Disease (CD)
Section B: Signs, Symptoms, Associated Disorders and Complications

Affected System	ID No.	Manifestation	Type[+]	Current Medical Information [++]	Deficient Nutrient
Reproduction: Pregnancy, Parturition, and Puerperium	279	Obstetrical Complications [38,269]	(S) (C) (AD)	[P] Increased frequency in women with CD.[269] [D] Obstetrical complications are reproductive disorders that may be a consequence of the endocrine derangements caused by selective nutrient deficiencies.[269] Zinc proteins have been shown to be involved in the transcription and translation of genetic material. Zinc deficiency has been incriminated in fetal malformations, fetal death, and abnormal deliveries with dystocia and placental ablation. Zinc therapy in patients with low zinc has reduced the frequencies of premature birth, placental ablation, perinatal death, and postmaturity. It is suggested that these data are compatible with the presence of zinc–deficiency syndrome in pregnancy which includes increased maternal morbidity, abnormal taste sensations, abnormally short or prolonged gestations, inefficient labor, atonic bleeding, and increased risks to the fetus.[38] Because the early diagnosis and treatment of CD is possible and not very costly, CD must be seriously considered in the preconceptional screening and treatment of patients with reproductive disorders.[269] [M] Marked by abnormally short or prolonged gestations, inefficient labor with dystocia, atonic bleeding, increased maternal morbidity, and increased risks to the fetus such as prematurity, postmaturity, and perinatal death. [C] Results from endocrine derangements caused by selective nutrient deficiencies.[269] [R] CD-related obstetrical complications can be prevented on GFD.	Folic acid, Iron, Zinc.
Reproduction: Pregnancy, Parturition, and Puerperium	280	Puerperium Complicated by CD [1,278]	(C)	[P] New association with CD.[278] [D] CD complicating puerperium is the manifestation of CD during the 6 weeks after delivery of a baby(ies). Case report of CD manifesting after young female developed severe diarrhea resulting in malabsorption during both pregnancies. On the first presentation the gluten sensitive enteropathy was not diagnosed despite detailed gastrointestinal (GI) and endocrine workup. Following her first pregnancy she remained free of symptoms for years on a normal diet. After birth of her second child her symptoms flared up and she was admitted. Diagnosis was confirmed by small intesinal biopsy. Significant improvement was achieved with supportive therapy and a GFD. Despite the transient symptoms, the diagnosis of latent CD seems to be evident.[278] [M] Marked by diarrhea during the puerperium. [C] Results from gluten exposure. [R] Significant improvement on a GFD. Lifelong GFD is mandatory to prevent the late complications of the puerperium.[278]	Not applicable.

+ (S) = Classic sign/symptom; (AT) = Atypical sign/symptom; (AD) Associated Disorder; (C) = Complication.

++ [P] = Prevalance; [D] = Description; [M] = Sign/symptom; [C] = CD related cause; [R] = Response to gluten Free diet (GFD).

Health Manifestations of Celiac Disease (CD)
Section B: Signs, Symptoms, Associated Disorders and Complications

Affected System	Affected Organ	ID No.	Manifestation	Type[+]	Current Medical Information [++]	Deficient Nutrient
Zygote	Chromosome	281	Down Syndrome [1,279,280]	(AD)	[P] Prevalence rate ranges from 5 to 12% of Down syndrome (1 of 600 births). Rate in Malta is 8%.[279] Rate in Turkey is 12.77% EMA positive.[280] [D] Down syndrome is a genetic disorder characterized by consequence of having an extra chromosome 21 or 22. Study investigating the incidence of CD in children with Down syndrome, to assess the availability of IgA-AGA and EMA for serologic screening, and to highlight the importance of follow-up demonstrated children with Down syndrome should be carefully examined in their follow-up, and CD should be considered in cases with growth retardation (all study patients with abnormal biopsy were below the 10th percentile for weight and height). Positivity of both IgA-AGA and EMA serologic screening tests give the most reliable results. Hypothyroidism was detected in one of 11 cases where at least one serologic marker was positive.[280] Study investigating incidence of CD in children and adults demonstrated a much greater frequency than that in the general population. Screening in all cases of Down syndrome for CD is recommended.[279] [M] Marked by mental retardation, abnormal features including low set ears, slanted eyes, flattened faces, short stature, and microencephaly. [C] Results from chromosomal abnormality at conception. [R] GFD will improve their well-being.	Zinc.
Zygote	Chromosome	282	Turner's Syndrome [1,281]	(AD)	[P] Prevalence rate of 6.4% CD in Turner's Syndrome (TS) patients.[281] [D] Turner's syndrome (TS) is a sex chromosome abnormality characterized failure of the ovaries to respond to pituitary hormone stimulation, as a consequence of having complete or partial absence of the two sex chromosomes. Multicenter study of 389 TS patients investigating 1) the incidence of CD and 2) the clinical characteristics and laboratory data of affected patients demonstrated a high prevalence of CD in TS patients. Ten patients showed classic CD, 8 showed atypical symptoms, and 7 showed a silent CD. Other autoimmune disorders were observed in 40% of the patients. The subclinical picture in 60% of the cases, the diagnostic delay, and the incidence of the other autoimmune disorders suggest that routine screening of CD in TS is indicated.[281] [M] Marked by failure of sexual maturity with amenorrhea, loss of taste, usually short stature, and web neck in about one third. [C] Results from chromosomal abnormality at conception. [R] GFD will improve their well-being.	Zinc.

+ (S) = Classic sign/symptom; (AT) = Atypical sign/symptom; (AD) Associated Disorder; (C) = Complication.

++ [P] = Prevalance; [D] = Description; [M] = Sign/symptom; [C] = CD related cause; [R] = Response to gluten Free diet (GFD).

Health Manifestations of Celiac Disease (CD)
Section B: Signs, Symptoms, Associated Disorders and Complications

Affected System	Affected Organ	ID No.	Manifestation	Type+	Current Medical Information ++	Deficient Nutrient
Fetus	Any	283	Congenital Anomalies [38,259]	(AD)	[P] No adequate studies are available on the rate of birth defects in progeny.[259] [D] Congenital anomalies are malformations present at birth. CD induces malabsorption and deficiency of factors essential for organogenesis, eg: iron, folic acid and vitamin K. The overall evidence suggests that CD patients can be a group particularly susceptible to reproductive toxicants; however, the pathogenesis of CD-related reproductive disorders still awaits clarification.[259] Zinc deficiency syndrome in pregnancy includes fetal malformations.[38] [M] Marked by deformity and/or dysfunction, such as cleft lip and heart failure. [C] Results from nutritional deficiencies in CD including iron, zinc, folic acid and vitamin K. [R] The possible prevention or treatment of reproductive effects can only be achieved through a life-long maintenance of a GFD.[259]	Folic acid, Iron, Vitamin K, Zinc.
Fetus	Any	284	Intrauterine Growth Retardation [1,38,259,278]	(C)	[P] Women with untreated CD are at higher risk for low birth weight of the newborn.[259] Increased risk in progeny of women with untreated CD.[278] [D] Intrauterine growth retardation is a fetal development abnormality characterized by failure to grow normally for gestational period. Zinc deficiency has been incriminated in fetal intrauterine growth retardation.[38] Although the acute presentation of CD in pregnancy is concerning, potentially of more concern is the risk of intrauterine growth retardation of undiagnosed CD.[278] [M] Marked by a 30% reduction of baby's birth weight. [C] Results from untreated CD causing nutritional deficiencies in the mother. [R] GFD is preventive, and weight of fetus normalizes in response to mother's GFD.	Iron, Omega-6 fatty acids, Protein, Vitamin A, Zinc.

+ (S) = Classic sign/symptom; (AT) = Atypical sign/symptom; (AD) Associated Disorder; (C) = Complication.

++ [P] = Prevalance; [D] = Description; [M] = Sign/symptom; [C] = CD related cause; [R] = Response to gluten Free diet (GFD).

Health Manifestations of Celiac Disease (CD)
Section B: Signs, Symptoms, Associated Disorders and Complications

Affected System	Affected Organ	ID No.	Manifestation	Type[+]	Current Medical Information[++]	Deficient Nutrient
Fetus	Exocrine glands	285	Cystic Fibrosis [282,283]	(AD)	[P] Association with CD is classic.[282] [D] Cystic fibrosis is an inherited disease of the exocrine glands characterized by chronic obstructive pulmonary disease (COPD), exocrine pancreatic insufficiency, and abnormally high sweat electrolytes. Children manifest the neurologic syndrome of vitamin E deficiency including ataxia with loss of deep tendon reflexes, loss of vibration and position sense, ophthalmoplegia, muscle weakness, ptosis, and dysarthria. Case report describes the investigation and subsequent diagnosis of CD and cystic fibrosis in an 8 year old girl with a history of steatorrhea, abdominal distention, and abundant and fetid stools with frequent cough and respiratory infections, referred to cardiology for congestive cardiac insufficiency. Cystic fibrosis is a common cause of cardiopathy but this patient had idiopathic cardiomyopathy associated with CD, which is the reason why this situation must be investigated through anti-endomysium and anti-tranglutaminase antibodies and intestinal biopsy.[282] Case report describes the uncommon occurrence of CD and cystic fibrosis in an obese adult patient. Apart from its rarity, the case serves to highlight the elusive nature of these two diseases when presenting with atypical features in an adult.[283] [M] Marked by nasal polyps, bronchiectasis, bronchitis, pneumonia, respiratory failure, salt depletion, pancreatic exocrine deficiency with malabsorption of fats, proteins, and carbohydrates, nutritional deficiencies, arthritis, failure to thrive and delayed puberty. [C] Caused by gene mutation on chromosome 7. [R] CD-related cystic fibrosis improves on GFD.[282]	Not applicable.
Fetus	Vertebrae	286	Spina Bifida [259]	(S)	[P] No adequate studies are available on the rate of birth defects in the progeny of CD affected women.[259] [D] Spina bifida is a congenital defect in the walls of the spinal canal in the lumbar section caused by folate deficiency in the mother during the pregnancy. [M] Marked by urinary incontinence, loss of feeling in saddle or limb, gait disturbances, and structural changes in the pelvis. [C] Results from CD induced malabsorption and deficiency of folic acid essential for organogenesis.[259] [R] Studies are inadequate. GFD with folic acid supplementation in the mother may be preventive of spina bifida in the fetus.	Folic acid, Iron.

[+] (S) = Classic sign/symptom; (AT) = Atypical sign/symptom; (AD) Associated Disorder; (C) = Complication.

[++] [P] = Prevalance; [D] = Description; [M] = Sign/symptom; [C] = CD related cause; [R] = Response to gluten Free diet (GFD).

Health Manifestations of Celiac Disease (CD)
Section B: Signs, Symptoms, Associated Disorders and Complications

Affected System	Affected Organ	ID No.	Manifestation	Type+	Current Medical Information ++	Deficient Nutrient
Child	All	287	Failure to Thrive and Growth Retardation 1,2,39,49,265, 280, 284 ,285,286	(S)	[P] Most frequent presentation in CD in the pediatric age group, but severe growth delay is less commonly seen in developed countries.[284] Prevalence of CD is 16.6% of children with failure to thrive, diarrhea, and anemia, while failure to thrive was found in 90% of children with CD.[285] [D] Failure to thrive (FTT) and growth retardation are conditions affecting children characterized by weight consistently below the 3rd percentile for age or a decrease in the expected rate of growth based on the child's previously defined growth curve, irrespective of whether below the 3rd percentile.[39] FTT is related to zinc deficiency.[49] High incidence in Down's syndrome.[280] Recent epidemiologic studies suggest that CD associated growth retardation is becoming a tangible health problem in developing countries where the problem has been historically overlooked.[284] Study investigating the possible change in spontaneous growth hormone (GH) secretion during a standardized gluten challenge demonstrated there is no impaired growth hormone secretion. Decreased growth rate in CD may not be primarily caused by changes in GH secretion. Instead it may be caused by changed peripheral sensitivity to GH.[286] Study to determine the prevalence, clinical, anthropometric and histological profiles of CD in 246 children with FTT, chronic diarrhea, and anemia attending a tertiary referral center in India demonstrated CD in 16.6% of the children. 90% of the children with CD had a history of FTT, 88% had a history of chronic diarrhea, and 14.2% had a history of anemia. Examination showed 100% with short stature. The ages at onset of symptoms were 0.5 to 10 years. Onset of FTT was earlier in children with subtotal villous atrophy than in those with partial villous atrophy. CD should be considered in the differential diagnosis, particularly in children without any symptoms of diarrhea.[285] Study investigating the proportions of adult patients with CD who had undiagnosed symptoms during childhood and the consequences of such diagnostic delay demonstrated missing the diagnosis of CD in a symptomatic child may lead to short stature and low female fertility which correlated with duration of symptoms before diagnosis.[265] [M] Marked by failure to gain weight and/or weight loss and short stature. May include edema of the feet, anemia, rickets, and clubbing of the fingers, features of vitamin A deficiency and B-vitamin deficiency.[285] [C] Results from inadequate nutrition due to malabsorption; decreased growth rate may be due to changed peripheral sensitivity to GH.[286] [R] Growth responds to GFD.[284]	B complex vitamins, Iron, Omega-6 fatty acid, Protein, Vitamin A, Zinc.

+ (S) = Classic sign/symptom; (AT) = Atypical sign/symptom; (AD) Associated Disorder; (C) = Complication.

++ [P] = Prevalance; [D] = Description; [M] = Sign/symptom; [C] = CD related cause; [R] = Response to gluten Free diet (GFD).

Health Manifestations of Celiac Disease (CD)
Section B: Signs, Symptoms, Associated Disorders and Complications

Affected System	Affected Organ	ID No.	Manifestation	Type[+]	Current Medical Information [++]	Deficient Nutrient
Child	Blood: plasma and cells	288	Hematologic, Abnormal Values in Childhood [287]	(S)	[P] Common presentation in children with untreated CD.[287] [D] Abnormal hematologic values in childhood were investigated in a study of children at diagnosis of CD. Study demonstrated anemia alone (86.3%), leukopenia coexisting with anemia (9%), thrombocytopenia alone (4.5%), iron deficiency anemia alone (54.5%), iron deficiency coexisted with zinc and vitamin B_{12} deficiency (13.6%), copper and vitamin B_{12} deficiency (8%), vitamin B_{12} deficiency alone (8%), zinc deficiency alone (8%), and combined iron, zinc, and copper deficiency (4.5%). Males had significantly lower values of hemoglobin and mean corpuscular volume (MCV) compared to females. CD should be included in the differential diagnosis in children who present with anemia, leukopenia, thrombocytopenia or prolonged prothrombin time and APTT, especially in geographical areas where the prevalence of CD is high.[287] [M] Marked by blood abnormalities. [C] Results from malabsorption in CD. [R] All abnormalities respond to a GFD.[287]	Copper, Iron, Vitamin B_{12}, Vitamin K, Zinc.
Child	Blood: plasma and cells	289	Latent Anemia in Intestinal Enzymopathies of Small Intestine [41,288]	(S)	[P] Common in children with CD and intestinal enzymopathies and those with intestinal enzymopathies and disaccharide deficiency.[288] [D] Latent anemia is characterized by unrecognized abnormal formation and dysfunction of erythrocytes. Intestinal enzymopathies are characterized by insufficient production of the enzymes necessary to split small peptide chains of proteins into absorbable amino acids and the disaccharides, lactose, maltose, and sucrose, into absorbable sugars. Study investigating 154 children with intestinal enzymopathies, which included 57 with CD, 52 with intestinal enzymopathies and disaccharide deficiency, and 45 with disaccharide deficiency syndrome, demonstrated that the typical changes in blood of children with intestinal enzymopathies were presented in decreasing of mean corpuscular volume (MCV), mean corpuscular hemoglobin (MCH), mean corpusculare hemogobin concentration (MCHC) and increasing of red cell distribution width (RDW). Study of ferrokinetics has shown that an anemia was caused by deficiency in many elements with preponderence of iron-deficiency erythropoiesis. The most sensitive and reliable indicators of early detection of latent anemia without decrease in hemoglobin level were ferritin content, the coefficient of saturation of transferrin and transferrin's receptors.[288] [M] Marked by weakness, fatigue, pallor, and susceptibility to infection. [C] Results from iron malabsorption in CD. [R] CD-related anemia responds slowly to GFD.[41]	Iron.

[+] (S) = Classic sign/symptom; (AT) = Atypical sign/symptom; (AD) Associated Disorder; (C) = Complication.

[++] [P] = Prevalance; [D] = Description; [M] = Sign/symptom; [C] = CD related cause; [R] = Response to gluten Free diet (GFD).

Health Manifestations of Celiac Disease (CD)
Section B: Signs, Symptoms, Associated Disorders and Complications

Affected System	Affected Organ	ID No.	Manifestation	Type[+]	Current Medical Information [++]	Deficient Nutrient
Child	Blood: plasma and cells	290	Refractory Iron Deficiency Anemia in Childhood [40,41,289]	(S)	[P] Common in children with untreated CD.[40] Refractory anemia may be the sole presentation in children with subclinical CD.[289] [D] Refractory iron deficiency anemia in childhood is a microcytic anemia characterized by abnormal formation of small, pale red blood cells and iron depletion refractory to oral iron supplementation. Study evaluating the effect of iron supplementation, in addition to a GFD, on hematological profile of children with CD demonstrated that iron deficiency anemia is commonly associated with CD and iron deficiency state continues a long time even after excluding gluten from the diet and iron supplementation. In the follow-up evaluation of these cases on a GFD, mean hemoglobin levels were comparable with controls but the cases continued to have lower mean mean corpuscular volume (MCV), MCV serum ferritin levels and higher mean total iron binding capacity (TIBC). Seven children had mild anemia. Serum ferritin levels showed a negative correlation with the grade of villous atrophy and lamina propria infiltrate. Apart from offering children a GFD rich in iron, early detection and treatment of IDA and prophylactic iron folic acid supplementation will go a long way to optimize mental and psychomotor functions.[41] [M] Marked by pallor, fatigue, dyspnea on exertion, and susceptibility to infection. [C] Results from iron malabsorption in gluten sensitive enteropathy. [R] Iron deficiency anemia responds slowly to GFD.[41]	Iron.

[+] (S) = Classic sign/symptom; (AT) = Atypical sign/symptom; (AD) Associated Disorder; (C) = Complication.

[++] [P] = Prevalance; [D] = Description; [M] = Sign/symptom; [C] = CD related cause; [R] = Response to gluten Free diet (GFD).

Health Manifestations of Celiac Disease (CD)
Section B: Signs, Symptoms, Associated Disorders and Complications

Affected System	Affected Organ	ID No.	Manifestation	Type+	Current Medical Information++	Deficient Nutrient
Child	Bones	291	Osteopenia in Childhood [290,291,292, 293]	(C)	[P] 50% prevalence found at diagnosis of CD in children.[290] [D] Osteopenia in childhood is a metabolic bone disorder characterized by diminished bone mass with the retention of normal cell appearance and high bone turnover. Osteopenia is defined as a bone mineral test (BMD) expressed with a z score lower than -1.0. Study to investigate the prevalence of osteopenia, to identify the relationship between bone mineral density (BMD), serum calcium, and parathyroid hormone levels, and to determine the effect of a GFD on BMD in children with CD, demonstrated BMD and bone mineral content values in newly diagnosed patients were significantly lower than controls. The BMD values were significantly increased after a year on GFD. At one year, osteopenia was not resolved with the GFD, and this was especially true in patients without gastrointestinal (GI) manifestation. At least 4 years of GFD are required for a complete recovery of bone mineralization in some patients. The mean calcium level was lower in the patients who did not follow their diet strictly. There was a positive correlation between calcium level and BMD and bone mineral content. BMD evaluation recommended.[290] Study comparing the BMD of children and adolescents with CD on a GFD to BMD of controls and to evaluate lab analysis of calcium malabsorption of CD patients, demonstrated the BMD of adolescents was lower than controls; whereas was no difference was found between the BMD of children with CD and controls.[291] Study investigating BMD in children with CD at diagnosis and in patients after one year demonstrated children with CD are at risk for reduced BMD. Untreated patients had significantly lower serum calcium and significantly higher parathyroid hormone levels than did treated patients. A strict GFD improves bone mineralization, even at 1 year. Early diagnosis and treatment will protect the patient from osteoporosis.[292] Study investigating the changes in bone metabolism of children during consumption of a GFD demonstrated that the rate of bone metabolism is altered in children with untreated CD, and these alterations may be the cause of osteopathy. Serum bone-specific alkaline phosphatase concentrations of patients were significantly lower than controls at the time of diagnosis and increased gradually and significantly during the GFD. Remarkable changes occur after the start of a GFD, and they result in a more balanced equilibrium.[293] [M] Marked by increased risk of fractures. BMD z score below -1.0. [C] Results from defective calcium absorption sometimes associated with lactose intolerance, increased body use of calcium, loss in stool, and impaired vitamin D absorption.[290] [R] GFD results in rapid improvement of BMD.[290,292,293]	Calcium. Possibly Copper, Magnesium, Vitamin D, Vitamin K.

+ (S) = Classic sign/symptom; (AT) = Atypical sign/symptom; (AD) Associated Disorder; (C) = Complication.

++ [P] = Prevalance; [D] = Description; [M] = Sign/symptom; [C] = CD related cause; [R] = Response to gluten Free diet (GFD).

Affected System	Affected Organ	ID No.	Manifestation	Type⁺	Current Medical Information ⁺⁺	Deficient Nutrient
Child	Bones	292	Rickets [294]	(C)	[P] Increased frequency in CD. [D] Rickets is a disorder of cartilage cell growth and enlargement of epiphyseal growth plates in children characterized by inadequate mineralization of developing cartilage and newly formed bone. Case report of an 11 year old girl with undiagnosed CD who had rickets masquerading as proximal muscle weakness and bone pain describes the importance of identifying the etiology of metabolic bone disease that leads to myopathy. This type of muscle weakness often responds fully to treatment. [294] [M] Marked by abnormalities in the shape, structure and strength of the skeleton, lethargy and flaccid muscles. [C] Results from deficiency of vitamin D in CD. [R] CD-related rickets respond to GFD.	Vitamin D.

⁺ (S) = Classic sign/symptom; (AT) = Atypical sign/symptom; (AD) Associated Disorder; (C) = Complication.

⁺⁺ [P] = Prevalance; [D] = Description; [M] = Sign/symptom; [C] = CD related cause; [R] = Response to gluten Free diet (GFD).

246   *Recognizing Celiac Disease* Signs, Symptoms, Associated Disorders & Complications

Affected System	Affected Organ	ID No.	Manifestation	Type[+]	Current Medical Information [++]	Deficient Nutrient
Child (S)	Bones	293	Short Stature [1,180,265, 284,285,286]	(AT)	[P] Common presentation at diagnosis in patients with untreated CD (13.5%).[180] Prevalence of 26% in patients who had undiagnosed symptomatic CD in childhood compared to a matched control group and a cohort of patients who had been diagnosed with CD during childhood.[265] Prevalence of 100% in newly diagnosed children with failure to thrive (FTT), diarrhea, and anemia.[285] [D] Short stature is a result of failure to thrive and severe growth delay[284] characterized by normal physiology with normal growth hormone level.[286] Study to determine the prevalence, clinical, anthropometric and histological profiles of CD in 246 children with FTT, chronic diarrhea, and anemia attending a tertiary referral center in India demonstrated CD in 16.6% of the children. Examination showed 100% with short stature.[285] Study investigating the proportion of adult patients with CD who had had undiagnosed symptoms during childhood and the consequences of such diagnostic delay demonstrated that short stature and low fertility correlated with duration of symptoms before diagnosis and concluded that missing the diagnosis of CD in a symptomatic child may lead to short stature and low female fertility. Compared with the control group, patients with CD were shorter (men 171.4 +/- 9.0cm vs. 176.4 +/- 6.9 cm, P<0.01; women 159.7 +/- 7.3 cm vs 162.7 +/- 6.2 cm, P<0.01 and had a higher prevalence of symptomatic osteoporosis (5%), cancer (10%), and autoimmune disease (25%). Compared with matched controls, and with patients whose CD had been diagnosed during childhood (n=36), or who had remained symptom-free (n=95), patients who had undiagnosed symptomatic CD during childhood exhibited higher prevalence of short stature (26%), low female fertility or low birth weight (36%). Multivariate analysis showed that short stature and low fertility correlated with duration of symptoms before diagnosis; osteoporosis and cancer correlated with age. The prevalence of autoimmune disease was unrelated to early onset of symptoms or delay in diagnosis.[265] [M] Marked by failure to achieve normal height. May include edema of the feet, anemia, rickets, clubbing of the fingers, and features of vitamin A and B-vitamin deficiency.[285] [C] Results from malabsorption in CD. [R] Stature responds to a GFD while child is still growing.	B Vitamins, Calcium, Iron, Omega-6 fatty acids, Protein, Vitamin A, Zinc.

[+] (S) = Classic sign/symptom; (AT) = Atypical sign/symptom; (AD) Associated Disorder; (C) = Complication.

[++] [P] = Prevalance; [D] = Description; [M] = Sign/symptom; [C] = CD related cause; [R] = Response to gluten Free diet (GFD).

Health Manifestations of Celiac Disease (CD)
Section B: Signs, Symptoms, Associated Disorders and Complications

Affected System	Affected Organ	ID No.	Manifestation	Type⁺	Current Medical Information ⁺⁺	Deficient Nutrient
Child	Brain: mind	294	Autism and Learning Disabilities [295]	(AD)	[P] Associated with CD.[295] [D] Autism and learning disabilities constitute a non-progressive psychiatric syndrome appearing in childhood characterized by withdrawal from communication with others often accompanied by repetitive or primitive behaviors. Autistic children often manifest complex biochemical and immunological abnormalities. Primary gastrointestinal (GI) pathology may play an important role in the inception and clinical expression of autism. The route to the fetus is through the mother's intestine...could exogenous neurotoxic opioid peptides of gluten in the mother's bloodstream damage the developing central nervous system and cause autism in the offspring?[295] 1) Common clinical characteristics of hepatic encephalopathy and a form of autism associated with developmental regression in an apparently healthy child, accompanied by immune-mediated GI pathology, have led to the proposal that there may be analogous mechanisms of toxic encephalopathy. Aberrations in opioid biochemistry are common. 2) Increased intestinal permeability, including 50% of children without GI symptoms, leads to systemic opioid excess second to gliadin absorption and its direct effect on the central nervous system (CNS), permanently perturbing the developing brain. Same mechanism can be in utero. 3) Many autistic children with gut symptoms have a characteristic intestinal pathology - ileocolonic lymphoid nodular hyperplasia and enterocolitis. The colonic lesion consisting of a mucosal infiltrate of γδ T cells and CD8+ T cells and crypt cell proliferation is enhanced significantly, and the basement membrane is thicker than in normal or disease groups. Neutrophil and eosinophil mucosal infiltration and absence on colonic epithelium of HLA-DR antigen suggests a T-helper -2 dominated immune response. The corresponding small intestinal lesion also shows a distinct cell-mediated epithelial immunopatholgy in which immune-mediated epithelial damage is predominant, serum IgG colonizes with complement. (C1q) at the epithelial basolateral membrane and epithelial proliferation is increased. 4) Secondary colonic anaerobic dysbiosis produces neurotoxic encephalopathy. 5) Elimination of gluten and/or casein improves behavior and general well-being.[295] [M] Marked by self-absorption, inaccessibility, aloneness, inability to relate, repetitive play, rage reactions if interrupted, rhythmical movements, and many language disturbances. GI symptoms include pain, esophageal reflux, diarrhea, chronic constipation.[295] [C] Results from unclear mechanism; gluten exposure with toxicity from the gut and autoimmunity are the forerunners; lactic acidosis from acid tolerant bacterial overgrowth. [R] Mainly post-natal development of autism improves on GFD and casein-free diet.[295]	B vitamins, EPA, Iron.

⁰⁺ (S) = Classic sign/symptom; (AT) = Atypical sign/symptom; (AD) Associated Disorder; (C) = Complication.

⁺⁺ [P] = Prevalance; [D] = Description; [M] = Sign/symptom; [C] = CD related cause; [R] = Response to gluten Free diet (GFD).

Health Manifestations of Celiac Disease (CD)
Section B: Signs, Symptoms, Associated Disorders and Complications

Affected System	Affected Organ	ID No.	Manifestation	Type+	Current Medical Information ++	Deficient Nutrient
Child	Brain: mind	295	Attention Deficit Hyperactive Disorder (ADHD) and Learning Disabilities [180]	(AD)	[P] First prevalence study shows rate of 20.3% for female patients with untreated CD and 21.2% for male patients with untreated CD vs.10.5% in controls.[180] [D] Attention Deficit Hyperactive Disorder (ADHD) is a maladaptive disorder characterized by a persistent pattern of inattention and impulsivity, or both, that are developmentally inappropriate. Study screening for a wide spectrum of both hard and soft neurologic disorders, including ADHD in children and young adults who have CD, demonstrated that patients with CD are more prone to develop ADHD than controls.[180] [M] Marked by low frustration levels, intolerance for changes in immediate environment, and failure to respond to discipline, especially in a group setting. Temper tantrums and negativity appear in young children and restlessness and carelessness in older children. [C] Etiology is unclear whether accumulative effects of nutritional, immunologic, or inflammatory factors might play some role on learning disorders or attention span or that the effect is indirect.[180] Probably neurotransmitter abnormalities are due to malabsorption in CD. [R] Improves on GFD.[180]	EPA, Iron, Protein, Vitamin B₃.
Child	Brain: mind	296	Developmental Delay [1,180]	(AD)	[P] New association with CD with a 15.5% rate in patients with CD vs. 3.3% in controls.[180] [D] Developmental delay is a psychiatric condition characterized by abnormal social relations and is more characteristic of the classical infantile-onset CD, probably caused by nutritional deficits and toxic effects of severe malabsorption.[180] Study investigating 17 children and young adults (mean age 9 years) with CD and developmental delay demonstrated significant incidence of infantile symptoms of CD (70.6%) whereas chronic abdominal pain or late-onset gastrointestinal (GI) symptoms, anemia, and short stature were the presenting symptoms in the remainder. All the patients in this group had additional neurologic disorders. Ten had learning disabilities and/or ADHD and 2 were ataxic, five were hypotonic during infancy, one had cerebellar ataxia, and another epilepsy.[180] [M] Marked by inappropriate affect, aloofness, difficulty making friendships, and by strange mannerisms. [C] Results from gluten exposure and nutrient deficiencies in CD including essential fatty acids, protein, iron, and B vitamins. [R] Developmental delay responds to a GFD, except for coexisting epilepsy and ataxia.[180]	B vitamins, Iron, Omega-3 fatty acids, Omega-6 fatty acids, Protein.

+ (S) = Classic sign/symptom; (AT) = Atypical sign/symptom; (AD) Associated Disorder; (C) = Complication.

++ [P] = Prevalance; [D] = Description; [M] = Sign/symptom; [C] = CD related cause; [R] = Response to gluten Free diet (GFD).

Health Manifestations of Celiac Disease (CD)
Section B: Signs, Symptoms, Associated Disorders and Complications

Affected System	ID No.	Manifestation	Type[+]	Current Medical Information [++]	Deficient Nutrient
Child Brain	297	Stroke in Childhood [296]	(AD)	[P] New association with CD.[296] [D] Stroke in childhood is characterized by sudden loss of neurologic function caused by infarction. Case report of a child presenting with a recurrent transient hemiplegia describes investigation for CD. Magnetic resonance imaging of the brain confirmed infarction; transcranial Doppler studies and magnetic resonance angiography were abnormal. Although there were virtually no gastrointestinal (GI) symptoms and the child was thriving, CD serology was strongly positive and a duodenal biopsy confirmed the disease. Tissue transglutaminase is the major autoantigen in CD and is thought to maintain vascular endothelial integrity. Anti-endomysial immunoglobulin A antibodies, demonstrated to be the same autoantibody as anti-transglutaminase, react with cerebral vasculature, suggesting an autoimmune mechanism for CD associated vasculopathy. Because CD is a potentially treatable cause of cerebral vasculopathy, serology - specifically antitissue transglutaminase antibodies - should be included in the evaluation of cryptogenic stroke in childhood, even in the absence of gut symptoms.[296] [M] Marked by hemiplegia. [C] Results from suggested autoimmune reaction. [R] GFD is preventive.	Not applicable.
Child Esophagus	298	Glycogenic Acanthosis [297]	(AD)	[P] New association with CD.[297] [D] Glycogenic acanthosis is an esophageal disease characterized by presence of numerous, uniformly grey-white plaques, which are usually 2-10 mm in diameter and may be confluent, round elevations involving the entire esophageal surface. It is characterized microscopically by epithelial cell hypertrophy and hyperplasia with accumulation of glycogen in the cell cytoplasm.[297] Case report of 6 year old boy and 8 year old girl with iron deficient anemia, failure to thrive, and positive antigliadin antibodies (AGA) with confirmed intestinal biopsy for CD describes finding grey-white plaques on esophageal mucosa during endoscopic investigation for CD. Multicentric studies in larger pediatric population suggested to determine if there is a significant association.[297] [M] Marked by dysphagia. [C] Results from unclear etiology involving gluten exposure in CD. [R] Studies are inadequate to determine effect of GFD.	Not applicable.

[+] (S) = Classic sign/symptom; (AT) = Atypical sign/symptom; (AD) Associated Disorder; (C) = Complication.

[++] [P] = Prevalance; [D] = Description; [M] = Sign/symptom; [C] = CD related cause; [R] = Response to gluten Free diet (GFD).

Health Manifestations of Celiac Disease (CD)
Section B: Signs, Symptoms, Associated Disorders and Complications

Affected System	Affected Organ	ID No.	Manifestation	Type[+]	Current Medical Information [++]	Deficient Nutrient
Child	Joints	299	Juvenile Idiopathic Arthritis [1,298]	(AT)	[P] 6.6% occurrence of CD in juvenile idiopathic arthritis (JIA).[298] [D] Juvenile Idiopathic Arthritis (JIA) is a rheumatic disorder characterized by chronic, inflammatory disease of large and small synovial joints and other organs in children under age 16. Growth and development may be impaired. 　　Study investigating the thyroid function and the prevalence of antithyroid antibodies, autoimmune thyroiditis and CD in 151 children with JIA vs 158 matched controls demonstrated high prevalence of biopsy confirmed CD in patients with JIA. These data seem to suggest careful monitoring of CD in JIA children.[298] [M] Marked by fatigue, joint pain, stiffness, and swelling in the morning rather than after activities. [C] Results from autoimmune mechanism. [R] CD-related JIA response to GFD varies.	Not applicable.
Child	Lymphocytes	300	Cancer Predisposition in Children [299]	(C)	[P] New association with CD.[299] [D] Cancer predisposition in children with CD is characterized by an increased number of chromosome aberations in peripheral blood lymphocytes. Whether genetically determined or a secondary phenomenon in CD, chromosome abnormalities may be involved in the predisposition to cancer in CD patients.[299] 　　Study investigating a group of children with CD in whom the initial frequency of chromosome aberations at diagnosis was known and to measure the same variable after a minimum of 2 years on a GFD demonstrated that the frequency of chromosome aberations in peripheral blood lymphocytes decreased significantly on a GFD. Investigators concluded that genomic instability is a secondary phenomenon, possibly caused by intestinal inflammation. Frequency of chromosome aberations at followup remained unchanged in children who were not diet adherant.[299] [M] Asymptomatic. [C] Results from unclear etiology involving gluten exposure, possibly intestinal inflammation. [R] Chromosome aberations respond to a GFD.[299]	Not applicable.

+ (S) = Classic sign/symptom; (AT) = Atypical sign/symptom; (AD) Associated Disorder; (C) = Complication.
++ [P] = Prevalance; [D] = Description; [M] = Sign/symptom; [C] = CD related cause; [R] = Response to gluten Free diet (GFD).

Section B   *Signs, Symptoms, Associated Disorders & Complications*   251

Affected System	Affected Organ	ID No.	Manifestation	Type⁺	Current Medical Information ⁺⁺	Deficient Nutrient
Child	Peripheral nerves	301	Hypotonia [180,300]	(S)	[P] Occurrence of hypotonia in study of infantile CD was 21.6% vs. 3.8% in controls.[180] [D] Hypotonia is characterized by abnormally low muscle tension characterized by the term "floppy child". Rapid diagnosis of CD and initiation of GFD are essential to achieving catch-up growth in affected children.[300] Study investigating the medical files of 16 patients with a history of infantile CD and hypotonia revealed that with the exception of 3 patients, one of whom had Down syndrome, the hypotonia completely resolved on a GFD. Four patients presented with short stature, and 4 patients had chronic abdominal pains, chronic fatigue, or anemia. Two patients who were found hypotonic on a GFD had low serum carnitine levels, and with dietary supplements and reinforcement of the GFD, their symptoms improved.[180] Case report of a 13 month old child presenting with flaccid paraparesis after an upper respiratory infection describes subsequent diagnosis of CD based on positive IgA antibody serology against gliadin, reticulin, and endomysium and duodenal biopsy showing villous atrophy. Full blood count, serum electrolytes, creatine kinase, Lyme serlogy, and vitamin E were all within normal limits. Lumbar puncture was unremarkable, chest radiographs, and brain and spinal MRI showed no abnormalities. Review of her growth chart showed her height had shifted from the 25th percentile to the 5th percentile in the past 5 months, prompting the possibility of malabsorption. Within 2 weeks of starting a GFD, the child was sitting independently and pulling herself up. After 7 months her weight was at the 50th percentile. Her strength, tone, and reflexes returned to normal.[300] [M] Marked by flaccid muscles. [C] Results from nutritional deficits and toxic effects of severe malabsorption in CD.[180] Autoimmune mechanisms might also be responsible for the neuronal damage.[300] [R] Clear resolution with improved nutritional status on GFD.[180,300]	Protein.

⁺ (S) = Classic sign/symptom; (AT) = Atypical sign/symptom; (AD) Associated Disorder; (C) = Complication.

⁺⁺ [P] = Prevalance; [D] = Description; [M] = Sign/symptom; [C] = CD related cause; [R] = Response to gluten Free diet (GFD).

Health Manifestations of Celiac Disease (CD)
Section B: Signs, Symptoms, Associated Disorders and Complications

Affected System	Affected Organ	ID No.	Manifestation	Type[+]	Current Medical Information [++]	Deficient Nutrient
Child	Ovaries	302	Delayed Puberty in Girls [258,259,260,270]	(S)	[P] Puberty significantly retarded in girls with untreated CD compared with girls following a GFD.[270] [D] Delayed puberty in girls is characterized by decreased functional activity of the ovaries resulting in late onset of ovulation and secondary sex characteristics. CD may impair the reproductive life of affected women, eliciting delayed menarche.[259] Hyperprolactinemia results in delayed menarche.[18] Study investigating the gynecological history of newly diagnosed patients with CD demonstrated that delayed menarche is frequently associated with celiac disease. Mean age of menarche at 13.5 years vs.12.1 years in controls.[258] Study analyzing gynecological disturbances in patients with CD in relation to their nutritional status and adherence to a GFD demonstrated adolescents who were not adherent to a GFD presented delayed menarche and secondary amenorrhea. Gluten could explain the disturbances and malnutrition would worsen the disease in a consequent vicious cycle. CD should be included in screening of reproductive disorders.[260] [M] Marked by abnormal delay of breast and hair development and initial onset of menstrual period. [C] Results from endocrine dysfunction involving gluten exposure and nutritional deficiencies in CD.[260] Pathogenesis still awaits clarification.[259] In CD there is a high level of autoantibodies directed against self-antigens, so there could be antibodies against hormones or organs critical for pubertal development. Moreover, in CD there could be a selective malabsorption of micronutrients essential for the metabolism of carrier or receptor proteins for sex hormones.[270] [R] CD-related delayed puberty responds to GFD and is preventive of delay.[259,260,270]	B vitamins, Folic acid, Iron, Omega-6 fatty acids, Vitamin A, Vitamin D, Zinc.

[+] (S) = Classic sign/symptom; (AT) = Atypical sign/symptom; (AD) Associated Disorder; (C) = Complication.

[++] [P] = Prevalance; [D] = Description; [M] = Sign/symptom; [C] = CD related cause; [R] = Response to gluten Free diet (GFD).

Affected System	Affected Organ	ID No.	Manifestation	Type+	Current Medical Information ++	Deficient Nutrient
Child	Pancreas	303	Diabetes Mellitus, Juvenile Type 1 [115, 116,301,302,303,304,305]	(AD)	[P] Prevalence of CD in children with Type 1 diabetes mellitus in Wisconsin is at least 4.6%.[115] A nationwide German study found 6.7%.[301] A French study found 3.9%, and 82% of those were already positive for anti-tTG antibodies at Type 1 DM onset.[302] A Danish study found 12.3%.[304] [D] Juvenile DM Type 1 is characterized by lack of insulin production by the pancreas. Study investigating the influence of CD on growth and metabolic control in a nationwide cohort of German children and adolescents with type 1 DM demonstrated females were significantly more predisposed to have Type 1 DM and CD. CD patients were characterized by earlier onset of diabetes and decreased growth and weight than diabetic patients without CD. Evidence for thyroid disease was more common in the Type 1 DM with CD group (6.3% vs 2.3%) and HbA1c values were lower.[301] Study investigating the prevalence of CD in a diabetic population of children by measuring IgA anti-transglutaminase antibodies in parallel with classical markers (IgA and IgG antigliadin and IgA anti-endomysium) and measuring the temporal relationship between Type 1 diabetes onset and CD, demonstrated an excellent correlation between IgA-anti-EMA and IgA-anti-tTG antibodies and that CD is most often present before the onset of diabetes. Anti-tTG antibodies should alert pediatricians to the atypical forms of CD which are the most common forms in type 1 DM. CD-positive patients had earlier onset of diabetes and decreased growth and weight gain.[302] Study investigating the association of Type 1 diabetes, CD and some other diseases in children and adolescents with positive family history demonstrated risk of Type 1 diabetes was significantly associated with a positive family history for Type 1 DM, CD, allergic diseases, and Crohn's disease.[303] Study investigating 1) the prevalence of biopsy proven CD in 269 Danish children with Type 1 DM and 2) the clinical effects of a GFD in patients with diabetes and CD demonstrated the highest reported prevalence of CD in Type 1 DM in Europe. Patients were followed over a two year period while consuming a GFD, showing increase in weight, hemoglobin and ferritin, whereas HbA1c remained unchanged. Children less than 14 showed increased height. Screening for CD recommended in all children with Type 1 DM.[304] Study investigating breastfeeding, food supplementation, or age at introduction of gluten-containing foods in newborns of parents with Type 1 DM demonstrated that reduced total or exclusive breastfeeding did not significantly increase the risk of developing islet autoantibodies. Giving gluten-containing foods before age 3 months, however, was associated with significantly increased islet autoantibody risk.[305] [M] Marked by earlier onset of diabetes, decreased growth and weight gain, and poor diabetic control. [C] Results from a linked autoimmune mechanism. [R] GFD improves management of DM and reduces or eliminates risk of associated diseases.[116]	Not applicable.

+ (S) = Classic sign/symptom; (AT) = Atypical sign/symptom; (AD) Associated Disorder; (C) = Complication.

++ [P] = Prevalance; [D] = Description; [M] = Sign/symptom; [C] = CD related cause; [R] = Response to gluten Free diet (GFD).

Health Manifestations of Celiac Disease (CD)
Section B: Signs, Symptoms, Associated Disorders and Complications

Affected System	Affected Organ	ID No.	Manifestation	Type[+]	Current Medical Information [++]	Deficient Nutrient
Child	Skin	304	Chronic Bullous Dermatosis of Childhood [306]	(AD)	[P] New association with biopsy verified CD.[306] [D] Chronic bullous dermatosis (CBDC) of childhood is a bullous disease characterized by itchy, urticated papules and plaques as well as polycyclic lesions with blisters at the edge, located on the face and perineum. It exhibits linear deposits of IgA at the basement membrane zone. Patients with CBDC may have an atypical form of CD with an immunopathogenesis that differs from current concepts in CD and serological screening for CD may need to be repeated.[306] Case report of a 4 year old boy with CBDC contradicts the supposed non-association with gluten sensitive enteropathy. At 3.5 year of age the child was diagnosed with CBDC with fairly good response to Dapsone (an oral sulphone medication). Bouts of new lesions kept appearing due to a low dose (conceding to parents' fear of side effects) and topical steroids were added. At 4 years of age, subnormal levels of iron and zinc were found. S-anti-gliadin antibodies were normal but S-IgA anti-endomysium antibodies were positive at 1/20 (ref value >1/10). A peroral small bowel capsule biopsy from the distal duodenum showed a light microscopically normal mucosa without an increased number of intraepithelial lymphocytes. He was kept on a normal diet including gluten. At 6.1 years of age the AGA was still negative, but the EMA was higher at 1/640. Six months later the EMA was even higher at 1/1,280 without obvious GI symptoms. A re-biopsy of the small bowel showed hyperplastic villous atrophy of the crypts, severe inflammatory activity and increased numbers of intraepitheleal lymphocytes consistent with CD. A GFD was instituted and Dapsone dose decreased to half. At 4 month follow-up, the boy had only slight perioral changes. EMA and tTG antibodies were negative and Dapsone treatment was stopped. A small bowel biopsy after one year on a GFD showed a normal mucosa.[306] [M] Marked by long-standing or relapsing itchy wheals and blisters. [C] Results from unclear autoimmune mechanism involving gluten exposure. [R] Resolves on a GFD.[306]	Not applicable.

[+] (S) = Classic sign/symptom; (AT) = Atypical sign/symptom; (AD) Associated Disorder; (C) = Complication.

[++] [P] = Prevalance; [D] = Description; [M] = Sign/symptom; [C] = CD related cause; [R] = Response to gluten Free diet (GFD).

Health Manifestations of Celiac Disease (CD)
Section B: Signs, Symptoms, Associated Disorders and Complications

Affected System	Affected Organ	ID No.	Manifestation	Type[+]	Current Medical Information [++]	Deficient Nutrient
Child	Skin	305	Dermatitis Herpetiformis in Childhood [153,154,307]	(S)	[P] New association with CD.[307] [D] Dermatitis herpetiformis (DH) in childhood is a chronic inflammatory disease characterized by intensely itchy, red skin eruptions appearing on the extensor surfaces of the elbows, knees, back, buttocks, or scalp associated with sensitivity of the small intestine to gluten in the diet. Case report of DH in a 30 month old child is one of the youngest cases so far. After clinical investigations, an asymptomatic gluten-sensitive enteropathy was diagnosed. Skin lesions resolved on a GFD. DH should be considered in the differential diagnosis of chronic dermatitis in early childhood. Monitoring for complications is the greatest problem at this age.[307] [M] Marked by an extremely itchy, bullous skin rash affecting the extensor surfaces of the limbs, trunk, and scalp. All patients with DH have at least some degree of mucosal inflammation consistent with CD.[153] [C] Results from etiology not fully understood involving exposure to gluten; immune complex basis is most likely.[154] [R] Skin lesions resolve on a strict GFD.[153,307]	Not applicable.
Child	Small intestine	306	Fecal Occult Blood in Children [1,308]	(S)	[P] Occurs in 26.7% newly diagnosed children. None on a GFD.[308] [D] Fecal occult blood in children is characterized by bleeding in the gastrointestinal tract and may play a role in iron deficiency anemia.[308] Study prospectively evaluating 45 newly diagnosed children with CD for the presence of gluten in their diet, iron deficiency anemia, and fecal occult blood demonstrated occult blood testing may not be warranted in the absence of iron deficiency anemia or in children with iron deficiency anemia who are on GFD. Fecal occult blood was found in 4 iron deficient children, of whom 3 were newly diagnosed. Occult blood loss disappeared in 3 of the 4 children when gluten was removed from their diet. Fecal occult blood was found in 26.7% of children on a gluten-containing diet but not in children on a GFD or in control children.[308] [M] Marked by positivity to fecal occult stool test. [C] Results from GI inflammation, vitamin K and/or vitamin C deficiency, and small bowel ulceration in CD. Omega-3 fatty acid deficiency may contribute.[308] [R] Occult blood loss completely resolves on a GFD.[308]	Omega-3 fatty acids may contribute. Vitamin K, Vitamin C.

+ (S) = Classic sign/symptom; (AT) = Atypical sign/symptom; (AD) Associated Disorder; (C) = Complication.

++ [P] = Prevalence; [D] = Description; [M] = Sign/symptom; [C] = CD related cause; [R] = Response to gluten Free diet (GFD).

Health Manifestations of Celiac Disease (CD)
Section B: Signs, Symptoms, Associated Disorders and Complications

Affected System	Affected Organ	ID No.	Manifestation	Type+	Current Medical Information ++	Deficient Nutrient
Child	Small intestine	307	Penicillin V Impaired Absorption in Children [309]	(C)	[P] New association with CD. [309] [D] Penicillin V impairment of absorption in children is characterized by lack of ability to absorb penicillin V. Study investigating the gastrointestinal absorption of penicillin V (pc-V) in 6 children 6-12 months old with suspected CD demonstrated the absorption of calcium pc-V in oil suspension was impaired in the patients with suspected CD compared to that of the controls. The diagnosis of CD was set after small bowel biopsy and absorption tests of vitamin A and d-xylose. Control groups were 7 children with diarrhea but with normal small bowel biopsy and/or absorption tests and a group of 9 children with upper respiratory tract infection of the same age as the test group. After 6-8 months, the absorptive ability of oral calcium pc-V in suspension form in the children with suspected CD on a GFD was equal with that of a control group. [309] [M] Marked by poor response to antibiotic therapy. [C] Results from poor absorption of penicillin V in gluten sensitive enteropathy. [R] Impaired absorption of penicillin V resolved on GFD. [309]	Not applicable.

+ (S) = Classic sign/symptom; (AT) = Atypical sign/symptom; (AD) Associated Disorder; (C) = Complication.

++ [P] = Prevalance; [D] = Description; [M] = Sign/symptom; [C] = CD related cause; [R] = Response to gluten Free diet (GFD).

Health Manifestations of Celiac Disease (CD)
Section B: Signs, Symptoms, Associated Disorders and Complications

Affected System	Affected Organ	ID No.	Manifestation	Type[+]	Current Medical Information[++]	Deficient Nutrient
Child	Testes	308	Delayed Puberty in Boys [270,271,274,275]	(S)	[P] Increased frequency in boys with untreated CD.[271] [D] Delayed puberty in boys is characterized by decreased functional activity of the testes. Studies have found an abnormality pattern suggesting androgen resistance specific for CD. Gonadal dysfunction is believed to be due to reduced conversion of testosterone to dihydrotestosterone caused by low levels of 5 alpha-reductase in CD. This leads to derangement of the hypothalmic-pituitary axis.[270] Hormone alterations are reversible upon the start of a GFD, emphasizing the importance of early diagnosis. As regards the nutritional aspects, the folic acid deficiency of CD can affect rapidly proliferating tissues such as the seminiferous epithelium. More attention should be paid to deficiencies of fat-soluble vitamins, such as A and D, observed in CD. Vitamin A is important for Sertoli cell function as well as for early spermatogenetic phases. Vitamin E supports the correct differentiation and function of epididymal epithelium, spermatid maturation and secretion of proteins by the prostate. CD male patients should be regarded as vulnerable subjects, thus the detection of early biomarkers of andrological or endocrinological dysfunctions should trigger timely strategies for prevention and treatment.[274] Study investigating pituitary regulation of gonadal function in treated and untreated male patients with CD demonstrated a derangement of pituitary regulation of gonadal function. Exaggerated responses of follicle-stimulating hormone(FSH) (89%) and luteinizing hormone (LH) (49%) to luteinizing hormonereleasing hormone (LHRH) were found in celiacs with sub-total villous atrophy and were commonly found when basal gonadotropin concentrations were normal. LH response was closely linked to jejunal morphology.[275] [M] Marked by immature secondary sex characteristics.[270] [C] Results from unclear etiology involving gluten exposure and deficiencies of vitamin A, E, D, zinc, iron, folic acid, and group B vitamins. In CD there is a high level of auto-antibodies directed against self-antigens, so there could be antibodies against hormones or organs critical for pubertal development. Moreover, in CD there could be a selective malabsorption of micronutrients essential for the metabolism of carrier or receptor proteins for sex hormones.[271] [R] CD-related delayed puberty responds to GFD.[274]	B vitamins, Folic acid, Iron, Vitamin E, Vitamin A, Vitamin D, Zinc.

[+] (S) = Classic sign/symptom; (AT) = Atypical sign/symptom; (AD) Associated Disorder; (C) = Complication.

[++] [P] = Prevalance; [D] = Description; [M] = Sign/symptom; [C] = CD related cause; [R] = Response to gluten Free diet (GFD).

Health Manifestations of Celiac Disease (CD)
Section B: Signs, Symptoms, Associated Disorders and Complications

Affected System	Affected Organ	ID No.	Manifestation	Type+	Current Medical Information ++	Deficient Nutrient
Child	Thyroid	309	Juvenile Autoimmune Thyroid Disease [271,310]	(AD)	[P] Prevalence of juvenile autoimmune thyroid disease is 26.2% in patients with CD vs.10% of controls. Hypothyroidism was observed in 8.1% of CD children vs. 3.5% of controls and hyperthyroidism in 1.1% of CD children vs. none of control subjects. 15.7% of CD children had euthyroidism vs. 6% of controls.[310] [D] Juvenile autoimmune thyroid disease is characterized by abnormal circulating thyroid hormone levels. The precocious identification of CD in polyglandular disease is clinically relevant not only for the high risk of complications inherent to untreated CD, but also because CD is one of the causes for the failure of substitute hormonal therapy in patients with autoimmune thyroid disease.[271] Study to establish the prevalence of autoimmune thyroid involvement in a large series of pediatric patients with CD (256 patients were following a GFD, 87 patients were untreated), demonstrated high frequency of autoimmune thyroid disease among patients with CD both treated and untreated, and concluded these findings may justify a thyroid status assessment at diagnosis and at follow-up evaluation of children with CD. Hypothyroidism was observed in 8.1% of CD children vs. 3.5% of controls and hyperthyroidism in 1.1% of CD children vs. none of controls. 15.7% of CD children had euthyroidism vs. 6% of controls.[310] [M] Marked by changes in metabolism. [C] Results from linked autoimmune mechanism. [R] Poor response of juvenile autoimmune thyroid disease to GFD.	Not applicable.

+ (S) = Classic sign/symptom; (AT) = Atypical sign/symptom; (AD) Associated Disorder; (C) = Complication.

++ [P] = Prevalance; [D] = Description; [M] = Sign/symptom; [C] = CD related cause; [R] = Response to gluten Free diet (GFD).

Recognizing Celiac Disease Signs, Symptoms, Associated Disorders & Complications

References

Part 1
Part 2, Section A
Part 2, Section B

PART 1 REFERENCES

1. "Celiac Disease." National Digestive Diseases Information Clearinghouse. (NIH Publication No. 98-4269), April 1998.
2. Hill I, Dirks M, Liptak G, et al. Guideline for the diagnosis and treatment of celiac disease in children: recommendations of the North American Society for Pediatric Gastroenterology, Hepatology and Nutrition. *Journal of Pediatric Gastroenterology and Nutrition.* Jan 2005; 40:1-19.
3. Fasano, A. Where have all the american celiacs gone? *Acta Paediatrica Supplement.* 1996; 412:20-24.
4. National Institutes of Health, "National Institutes of Health Consensus Development Conference Statement, Celiac Disease," August 9, 2004; 1-14.
5. Hollén E, Högberg L, Stenhammar L, Fälth-Magnusson K, Magnusson KE. Antibodies to oat prolamines (avenins) in children with coeliac disease. *Scandanavian Journal of Gastroenterology.* 2003; 7:742-6.
6. Rudert C. "Updates in Celiac Disease – Getting Your Questions Answered," Derby City Celiac Newsletter, Fall 2001.
7. Guest JE. Gluten-Free Diet Self Management Three Step Process. Celiac Sprue Association USA. PO Box 31700, Omaha, NE, 68131-0700. http://www.csaceliacs.org.
8. Fasano A. Celiac disease – how to handle a clinical chameleon. *The New England Journal of Medicine.* Jun 2003; 348:2568-2570.
9. Semrad C. "Is cross contamination an issue?" Speech by Carol Semrad, M.D., Associate Professor, University of Chicago given at Columbia University Topics in Gastroenterology, Nutrition, Celiac Disease and Beyond Seminar. Friday, Sep 9, 2005.
10. Murray J. The widening spectrum of celiac disease. *American Journal of Clinical Nutrition.* Mar 1999; 69(3):354-365.
11. Green P. The many faces of celiac disease: clinical presentation of celiac disease in the adult population. *Gastroenterology.* 2005; 128:s74-s78.
12. Matysiak-Budnik T, Candalh C, Cellier C, et al. Limited efficiency of prolyl-endopeptidase in the detoxification of gliadin peptides in celiac disease. *Gastroenterology.* Sep, 2005; 129(3):786-96.
13. Nelsen D. Gluten-sensitive enteropathy (celiac disease): more common that you think. *American Family Physician.* Dec 15, 2002; 66(12):2259.
14. Qiao S-W, Berseng E, Molberg Ø, Xia J, Fleckenstein B, Khosla C, Sollid L. Antigen presentation to celiac lesion-derived T cells of a 33-mer gliadin peptide naturally formed by gastrointestinal digestion. *The Journal of Immunology.* 2004; 173:1757-1762.
15. Shan L, Qiao S-W, Arentz-Hansen H, Molberg Ø, Gray GM, Sollid LM, Khosla C. Identification and analysis of multivalent proteolytically resistant peptides from gluten: implications for celiac sprue. *J Proteome Res.* Sep-Oct, 2005; 4(5):1732-41.
16. Thomas K, Sapone A, Fasano A, Vogel S. Gliadin stimulation of murine macrophage inflammatory gene expression and intestinal permeability are MyD88-dependent: role of the innate immune response in celiac disease. *The Journal of Immunology.* 2006; 176:2512-2521.
17. Farhadi A, Banan A, Fields J, Keshavarzian A. Intestinal barrier: an interface between health and disease. *Journal of Gastroenterology and Hepatology.* 2003; 18:479-497.
18. Liu Z, Li N, Neu J. Tight junctions, leaky intestines, and pediatric diseases. *Acta Paediatrica.* 2005; 94:386-393.
19. Taber Cyclopedic Medical Dictionary, 19th ed. F A Davis Company, Philadelphia, PA.
20. Clemente MG, De Virgiliis S, Kang JS, et al. Early effects of gliadin on enterocyte intracellular signalling involved in intestinal barrier function. *Gut.* Feb 2003; 52(2):218-23.
21. N. K. Harms und W. F. Caspary: Die Zöliakie und Sprue - Zöliakie des Erwachsenen. (Hrsg.: Deutsche Zöliakie-Gesellschaft, e.V. Filderhauptstraße 61, 70599 Stuttgart.)
22. Kamaeva OI, Reznikov IP, Pimenova NS, Dobritsyna LV. Antigliadin antibodies in the absence of celiac disease. *Klinicheskaia Meditsina.* 1998; 76(2):33-5.

23. Wakefield AJ, Puleston JM, Montgomery SM, Anthony A, O'Leary JJ, Murch SH. Review article: the concept of entero-colonic encephalopathy, autism and opioid receptor ligands. Blackwell Science Ltd, *Aliment Pharmacol Ther.* 2002; 16:663-674.

24. Cook M. "Common errors in diagnosing celiac disease in adults." *Physician Assistant.* March 2001; 4.

25. Hoffenberg EJ, MacKenzie T, Barriga KJ, et al. A prospective study of the incidence of childhood celiac disease. *Journal of Pediatrics.* Sep 2003; 143 (3),308-14.

26. Castaño L, Blarduni E, Ortiz L, et al. Prospective population screening for celiac disease: high prevalence in the first 3 years of life. *Journal of Pediatric Gastroenterology and Nutrition.* Jul 2004; 39:80-84.

27. Dubé C, Rostom A, Sy R, et al. The prevalence of celiac disease in average-risk and at-risk western european populations: a systematic review. *Gastroenterology.* Apr 2005; 128(4 Suppl 1):S57-67.

28. Luostarinen L, Himanen SL, Luostarinen M, Collin P, Pirttila T. Neuromuscular and sensory disturbances in patients with well treated coeliac disease. *Journal of Neurology, Neurosurgery, and Psychiatry.* Apr 2003; 74(4):490-4.

29. Green P. Speech by Peter Green, M.D. Clinical Professor of Medicine and Director of The Center for Celiac Disease Research given at Columbia University Topics in Gastroenterology, Nutrition, Celiac Disease and Beyond Seminar. Friday, Sep 9, 2005.

30. Lepers S, Couignoux S, Colombel JF, Dubucquol S. Celiac disease in adults: new aspects. *La Revue de Medecine Interne.* Jan 2004; 25(1):22-34.

31. Ventura A, Magazzu G, Greco L. Duration of exposure to gluten and risk for autoimmune disorders in patients with celiac disease. *Gastroenterology.* Aug 1999; 117(2):287-303.

32. La Villa G, Pantaleo P, Tarquini R, Cirami L, Perfetto F, Mancuso F, Laffi G. Multiple immune disorders in unrecognized celiac disease: a case report, ed. Xu XQ. *The World Journal of Gastroenterology.* Jun 15, 2003; 9(6):1377-1380.

33. Greco L, Errichiello S. "Carmela?? Where is this lady? Where to identify symptoms and diseases associated to coeliac disease." Department of Pediatrics, University of Naples Federico II, Via S. Pansini 5, 80131, Naples, Italy; received by email 2003.

34. Rousset H. A great imitator for the allergologist: intolerance to gluten. *Allergie Et Immunologie.* Mar 2004; 36(3):96-100.

35. Horvath K. "Comments on Celiac Screening Tests" given to Philadelphia Celiac-Sprue Support Group. Pediatric Gastroenterology and Nutrition Laboratory, UMAB/Bressler Research Building, Room 10-047, 655 West Baltimore Street, Baltimore, MD 21201.

36. Kumar V, Jarzabek-Chorzelska M, Sulej J, Karnewska K, Farrell T, Jablonska S. Celiac disease and immunoblobulin A deficiency: how effective are the serological methods of diagnosis? *Clin Diagn Lab Immunol.* Nov 2002; 9(6):1295-1300.

37. Harewood GC, Holub JL, Lieberman DA. Variation in small bowel biopsy performance among diverse endoscopy settings: results from a national endoscopic database. *American Journal of Gastroenterology.* Sep 2004; 99(9):1790-4.

38. Sbarbati A, Valletta E, Bertini M, Cipolli M, Morroni M, Pinelli L, Tato L. Gluten sensitivity and 'normal' histology: is the intestinal mucosa really normal? *Digestive and Liver Disease: Official Journal of the Italian Society of Gastroenterology and the Study of the Liver.* Nov 2003; 35(11):768-73.

39. Riccabona M, Rossipal E. Sonographic findings in celiac disease. *Journal of Pediatric Gastroenterology and Nutrition.* Aug 1993; 17(2):198-200.

40. Doolan A, Donaghue K, Fairchild J, Wong M, Williams AJ. Use of HLA typing in diagnosing celiac disease in patients with type 1 diabetes. *Diabetes Care.* Apr 2005; 28(4):806-09.

41. Cummins AG, Thompson FM, Butler RN, et al. Improvement in intestinal permeability precedes morphometric recovery of the small intestine in coeliac disease. *Clinical Science.* April 2001; 100(4);379-86.

42. Lee SK, Lo W, Memeo L, Rotterdam H, Green PH. Duodenal histology in patients with celiac disease after treatment with a gluten-free diet. *Gastrointestinal Endoscopy.* 2003; 57:187-91.

43. Freeman H. Celiac disease: a review by Hugh Freeman, M.D., FRCPC, FACP, FACG. *BC Medical Journal.* Sep 2001; 43(7):390-395.

44. Ciacci C, Cirillo M, Cavallaro R, Mazzacca G. Long-term follow-up of celiac adults on gluten-free diet: prevalence and correlates of intestinal damage. *Digestion.* 2002; 66(3):178-85.

45. Culliford AN, Green PH. Refractory sprue. *Current Gastroenterology Reports.* 2003 Oct; 5(5):373-8.

46. Catassi C, Bearzi I, Holmes GK. Association of celiac disease and intestinal lymphomas and other cancers. *Gastroenterology.* Apr 2005: 128(4 Suppl 1):S79-86.

47. "Talking Glossary of Genetic Terms." National Human Genome Research Institute. National Institutes of Health. http://www.genome.gov/glossary.cfm. Accessed Jan 21, 2006.

48. "Genetic Basics." National Institutes of Health. NIH Publication No. 01-662. May 2001. http://publications.nigms.nih.gov/genetics/genetics.pdf Accessed Jan 30, 2006.

49. "Developing a Haplotype Map of the Human Genome for Finding Genes Related to Health and Disease." National Human Genome Research Institute. National Institutes of Health. http://www.genome.gov/10001665. Accessed Jan 30, 2006.

PART 2, SECTION A REFERENCES

1. Murray JA, The widening spectrum of celiac disease. *American Journal of Clinical Nutrition.* Mar 1999; 69(3):354-365.
2. Kathleen Mahan and Sylvia Escott-Stump, ed. Krause's Food, Nutrition, & Diet Therapy, 10th Edition. Philadelphia, PA, USA: W.B. Saunders Company, 2000.
3. Krums LM, Parfenov AI, Ekisenina NI. Disorders of lipid metabolism in patients with chronic diseases of the small intestine. *Klinicheskaia Meditsina.* Nov 1990; 68(11):54-7.
4. Richardson AJ. The importance of omega-3 fatty acids for behaviour, cognition and mood. *Scandanavian Journal of Nutrition.* 2003; 47(2):92-8.
5. Das UN. Long-chain polyunsaturated fatty acids interact with nitric oxide, superoxide anion, and transforming growth factor-ß to prevent human essential hypertension. *European Journal of Clinical Nutrition.* 2004; 58:195-203.
6. Valagussa F, Franzosi MG, Geraci E, et al. Dietary supplementation with n-3 polyunsaturated fatty acids and vitamin E after myocardial infarction: results of the GISS Prevensione trial. *Lancet.* Aug 7, 1999; 354(9177):447,9p,1 diagram,6 graphs.
7. Molteni N, Bardella MT, Vezzoli G, Pozzoli E, Bianchi P. Intestinal calcium absorption as shown by stable strontium test in celiac disease before and after gluten-free diet. *American Journal of Gastroenterology.* Nov 1995; 90(11):2025-8.
8. Colston KW, Mackay AG, Finlayson C, Wu JC, Maxwell JD. Localisation of vitamin D receptor in normal human duodenum and in patients with coeliac disease. *Gut.* Sep 1994; 35(9):1219-25.
9. Jameson S, Hellsing K, Magnusson S. Copper malabsorption in coeliac disease. *Science of the Total Environment.* Mar 15, 1985; 42(1-2):29-36.
10. Mark Beers and Robert Berkow. The Merck Manual, 17th Edition. Whitehouse Station, NJ, USA: Merck Research Laboratories, 1999.
11. Stazi AV, Mantovani A. A risk factor for female fertility and pregnancy: celiac disease. *Gynecological Endocrinology: The Official Journal of the International Society of Gynecological Endocrinology.* Dec 2000; 14(6):454-63.
12. Sher KS, Jayanthi V, Probert CS, Stewart CR, Mayberry JF. Infertility, obstetric and gynaecological problems in celiac sprue. *Digestive Diseases.* May-Jun 1994; 12(3):186-90.
13. Arnason JA, Gudjonsson H, Freysdottir J, Jonsdottir I, Valdimarsson H. Do adults with high gliadin antibody concentrations have subclinical gluten intolerance? *Gut.* Feb 1992; 33(2):194-7.
14. Rujner J, Wojtasik A, Kunachowicz H, Iwanow K, Syczewska M, Piontek E. Magnesium status in children and adolescents with celiac disease. *Wiadomosci Lekarskie: Organ Polskiego Towarzystwa Lekarskiego.* 2001; 54(5-6):277-85.
15. Rude RK, Olerich M. Magnesium deficiency: possible role in osteoporosis associated with gluten sensitive enteropathy. *Osteoporosis International.* 1996; 6(6):453-61.
16. Hinks LJ, Inwards KD, Lloyd B, Clayton BE. Body content of selenium in coeliac disease. *British Medical Journal.* Jun 23, 1984; 288(6434):1862-3.
17. Yüce A, Demir H, Temizel IN, Kocak N. Serum carnitine and selenium levels in children with celiac disease. *Indian Journal of Gastroenterology: Official Journal of the Indian Society of Gastroenterology.* May-Jun 2004; 23(3):87-8.
18. Scholmerich J, Wietholtz H, Buchsel R, Kottgen E, Lohle E, Gerok W. Zinc and vitamin A deficiency in gastrointestinal diseases. *Leber, Magen, Darm.* Nov 1984; 14 (6):288-95.
19. Giorgi PL, Catassi C, Guerrieri A. Zinc and chronic enteropathies. *La Pediatria Medica E Chirurgica: Medical and Surgical Pediatrics.* Sep-Oct 1984; 6(5):625-36.
20. Solomons NW, Rosenberg IH, Sandstead HH. Zinc nutrition in celiac sprue. *The American Journal of Clinical Nutrition.* Apr 1976; 29(4):371-5.
21. Jameson S. Zinc status in pregnancy: the effect of zinc therapy on perinatal mortality, prematurity, and placental ablation. *Annals of the New York Academy of Sciences.* Mar 1993; 15(678): 178-92.

22. Rasmussen M, Michalsen H, Lie SO, Nilsson A, Petersen LB, Norum KR. Intestinal retinol esterification and serum retinol in children with cystic fibrosis. *Journal of Pediatric Gastroenterology and Nutrition.* May-Jun 1986; 5(3):397-403.

23. Odetti P, Valentini S, Aragno I, Garibaldi S, Pronzato MA, Rolandi E, Barreca T. Oxidative stress in subjects affected by celiac disease. *Free Radical Research.* Jul 1998; 29(1):17-24.

24. Hozyasz KK, Chelchowska M, Laskowska-Klita T. Vitamin E levels in patients with celiac disease. *Medycyna Wieku Rozwojowego.* Oct-Dec 2003; 7(4 Pt 2):593-604.

25. Ziaei S, Zakeri M, Kazemnejad A. A randomised controlled trial of vitamin E in the treatment of primary dysmenorrhea. *BJOG: An International Journal of Obstetrics and Gynaecology.* Apr 2005; 112(4):466-9.

26. Aslam A, Misba SA, Talbot K, Chapel H. Vitamin E deficiency induced neurological disease in common variable immunodeficiency: two cases and a review of the literature of vitamin E deficiency. *Clinical Immunology.* Jul 2004; 112(1):24-9.

27. Bottaro G, Fichera A, Ricca O, et al. Effect of the therapy with vitamin K on coagulation factors in celiac disease in children. *La Pediatria Medica E Chirurgica: Medical and Surgical Pediatrics.* Jul-Aug 1986; 8(4):551-4.

28. Schattner A. A 70-year-old man with isolated weight loss and a pellagra-like syndrome due to celiac disease. *The Yale Journal of Biology and Medicine.* Jan-Feb 1999; 72(1):15-8.

29. Thien KR, Blair JA, Leeming RJ, Cooke WT, Melikan V. Serum folates in man. *Journal of Clinical Pathology.* May 1977; 30(5):438-48.

30. Wills AJ. The neurology and neuropathology of celiac disease. *Neuropathology and Applied Neurobiology.* 2000; 26:493-496.

31. Bye AM, Andermann F, Robitaille Y, Oliver M, Bohane T, Andermann E. Cortical vascular abnormalities in the syndrome of celiac disease, epilepsy, bilateral occipital calcifications, and folate deficiency. *Annals of Neurology.* Sep 1993; 34(3):399-403.

32. Dahele A, Ghosh S. Vitamin B_{12} deficiency in untreated celiac disease. *American Journal of Gastroenterology.* Mar 2001; 96(3):745-50.

33. Dickey W. Low serum vitamin B_{12} is common in celiac disease and is not due to autoimmune gastritis. *European Journal of Gastroenterology and Hepatology.* Apr 2002; 14(4):425-427.

Other Sources:

"US Department of Agriculture Nutrient Database for Standard Reference." Available at http://www.nal.usda.gov/fnic/cgi-bin/nut. Accessed June 15, 2006.

PART 2, SECTION B REFERENCES

1. Greco L, Errichiello S. "Carmela?? Where is this lady? Where to identify symptoms and diseases associated to Coeliac Disease." Department of Pediatrics, University of Naples Federico II, Via S. Pansini 5, 80131, Naples, Italy; received by email 2003.

2. National Institutes of Health, "National Institutes of Health Consensus Development Conference Statement, Celiac Disease," August 9, 2004; 1-14.

3. Murray JA. The widening spectrum of celiac disease. *American Journal of Clinical Nutrition.* Mar 1999; 69(3):354-365.

4. Vogelsang H, Genser D, Wyatt J, et al. Screening for celiac disease: a prospective study on the value of noninvasive tests. *The American Journal of Gastroenterology.* Mar 1995; 90(3):394-8.

5. Arnason JA, Gudjonsson H, Freysdoyyir J, Valdimarsson H. Do adults with high gliadin antibody concentrations have subclinical gluten intolerance? *Gut.* Feb 1992; 33(2):194-7.

6. Rostom A, Dube C, Cranney A, et al. The diagnostic accuracy of serologic tests for celiac disease: a systematic review. *Gastroenterology.* Apr 2005; 128(4 Suppl 1):S38-46.

7. Ventura A, Magazzi G, Greco L. Duration of exposure to gluten and risk for autoimmune disorders in patients with celiac disease. SIGEP study group for autoimmune disorders in celiac disease. *Gastroenterology.* Aug 1999; 117(2):297-303.

8. Ambroszkiewicz J, Gajewska J, Laskowska-Klita T. Bone alkaline phosphatase: characteristics and its clinical applications. *Medycyna Wieku Rozwojowego.* Apr-Jun 2002; 6(2):99-110.

9. Pazianas M, Butcher GP, Subhani JM, et al. Calcium absorption and bone mineral density in celiacs after long term treatment with gluten-free diet and adequate calcium intake. *Osteoporosis International.* Jan 2005; 16(1):56-63.

10. Ciacci C, Cirillo M, Giorgetti G, et al. Low plasma cholesterol: a correlate of nondiagnosed celiac disease in adults with hypochromic anemia. *American Journal of Gastroenterology.* Jul 1999; 94(7):1888-91.

11. Vuoristo M, Kesäniemi YA, Gylling H, Miettinen TA. Metabolism of cholesterol and apolipoprotein B in celiac disease. *Metabolism: Clinical and Experimental.* Nov 1993; 42(11): 1386-91.

12. Cavallaro R, Iovino P, Castiglione F, et al. Prevalence and clinical associations of prolonged prothrombin time in adult untreated coeliac disease. *European Journal of Gastroenterology and Hepatology.* Feb 2004; 16(2):219-23.

13. Bottaro G, Fichera A, Ricca O, et al. Effect of the therapy with vitamin K on coagulation factors in celiac disease in children. *La Pediatria Medica E Chirurgica: Medical and Surgical Pediatrics.* Jul-Aug 1986; 8(4):551-4.

14. Hallert C, Grant C, Grehn S, et al. Evidence of poor vitamin status in coeliac patients on a gluten-free diet for 10 years. *Alimentary Pharmacology and Therapeutics.* Jul 2002; 16(7):1333-9.

15. Nowakowska E, Chodera A, Bobkiewicz-Kozlowska T, Hertmanowska H. Folic acid: new indications for an old well-known drug. *Polski Merkuriusz Lekarski: Organ Polskiego Towarzystwa Lekarskiego.* Nov 2003; 15(89):449-51.

16. Lim PO, Tzemos N, Farquharson CA, et al. Reversible hypertension following coeliac disease treatment: the role of moderate hyperhomocysteinaemia and vascular endothelial dysfunction. *Journal of Human Hypertension.* Jun 2002; 16(6):411-5.

17. Kapur G, Patwari AK, Narayan S, Anand VK. Serum prolactin in celiac disease. *Journal of Tropical Pediatrics.* Feb 2004; 50(1):37-40.

18. Sher KS, Jayanthi V, Probert CS, Stewart CR, Mayberry JF. Infertility, obstetric and gynaecological problems in coeliac sprue. *Digestive Diseases.* May-Jun 1994; 12(3):186-90.

19. Novacek G, Miehsler W, Wrba F, Ferenci P, Penner E, Vogelsang H. Prevalence and clinical importance of hypertransaminasaemia in coeliac disease. *European Journal of Gastroenterology and Hepatology.* Mar 1999; 11(3):283-8.

20. Molteni N, Bardella MT, Vezzoli G, Pozzoli E, Bianchi P. Intestinal calcium absorption as shown by stable strontium test in celiac disease before and after gluten-free diet. *American Journal of Gastroenterology.* Nov 1995; 90(11):2025-8.

21. Cohen O, River Y, Zelinger I. Convulsive disorder in celiac disease. *Harefuah.* Jun 15, 1994; 126(12):707-10,763.

22. Rickels MR, Mandel SJ. Celiac disease manifesting as isolated hypocalcemia. *Endocrine Practice: Official Journal of the American College of Endocrinology and the American Association of Clinical Endocrinologists.* May-Jun 2004; 10(3):203-7.

23. Waeber G, Pralong G, Breitenstein E, Nicod P. Laryngospasm: unusual manifestation of celiac disease. *Schweizerische Medizinische Wochenschrift.* Mar 13, 1993; 123(10):432-4.

24. Jameson S, Hellsing K, Magnusson S. Copper malabsorption in coeliac disease. *Science of the Total Environment.* Mar 15, 1985; 42(1-2):29-36.

25. Goyens P, Brasseur D, Cadranel S. Copper deficiency in infants with active celiac disease. *Journal of Pediatric Gastroenterology and Nutrition.* Aug 1985; 4(4):677-80.

26. Williams SG, Davison AG, Glynn MJ. Hypokalaemic rhabdomyolsis: an unusual presentation of coeliac disease. *European Journal of Gastroenterology and Hepatology.* Feb 1995; 7(2):183-4.

27. Rujner J, Socha A, Wojtasik A, Kunachowicz H, Iwanow K, Syczewska M, Piontek E. Magnesium status in children and adolescents with celiac disease. *Wiadomosci Lekarskie: Organ Polskiego Towarzystwa Lekarskiego.* 2001; 54(5-6):277-85.

28. Rude RK, Olerich M. Magnesium deficiency: possible role in osteoporosis associated with gluten-sensitive enteropathy. *Osteoporosis International: A Journal Established as Result of Cooperation Between the European Foundation for Osteoporosis and the National Osteoporosis Foundation of the USA.* 1996; 6(6):453-61.

29. Russell JA. Osteomalacic myopathy. *Muscle and Nerve.* Jun 1994; 17(6):578-80.

30. La Villa G, Pantaleo P, Tarquini R, Cirami L, Perfetto F, Mancuso F, Laffi G. Multiple immune disorders in unrecognized celiac disease: a case report. *World J Gastroenterology.* 2003; 9(6):1377-1380, Available at: http://www.wjgnet.com/1007-9327/9/1377.asp. Accessed Jan 3, 2005.

31. Bermejo JF, Carbone J, Rodriguez JJ, et al. Macroamylasaemia, IgA hypergammaglobulinaemia and autoimmunity in a patient with Down syndrome and coeliac disease. *Scandanavian Journal of Gastroenterology.* Apr 2003; 38(4):445-7.

32. Brigden ML. A systematic approach to macrocytosis. Sorting out the causes. *Postgraduate Medicine.* May 1995; 97(5):171-2,175-7,181-4 passim.

33. Oita T, Yamashiro A, Mizutani F, Tamura A, Sakizono K, Okada A. Simultaneous presence of macroamylase and macrolipase in a patient with celiac disease. Rinsho Byori. *The Japanese Journal of Clinical Pathology.* Oct 2003; 51(10):974-7.

34. Kathleen Mahan and Sylvia Escott-Stump, ed. Krause's Food, Nutrition, & Diet Therapy. 10th Edition. Philadelphia, USA: W.B. Saunders Company, 2000.

35. Ciacci C, Cirillo M, Cavallaro R, Mazzacca G. Long-term follow-up of celiac adults on gluten-free diet: prevalence and correlates of intestinal damage. *Digestion.* 2002; 66(3):178-85.

36. Rea F, Polito C, Marotta A, et al. Restoration of body composition in celiac children after one year of gluten-free diet. *Journal of Pediatric Gastroenterology and Nutrition.* Nov 1996; 23(4):408-12.

37. Roth EB, Sjoberg K, Stenberg P. Biochemical and immuno-pathological aspects of tissue transglutaminase in coeliac disease. *Autoimmunity.* Jun 2003; 36(4):221-6.

38. Jameson S. Zinc status in pregnancy: the effect of zinc therapy on perinatal mortality, prematurity, and placental ablation. *Annals of the New York Academy of Sciences.* Mar 15, 1993; 678:178-92.

39. Mark Beers and Robert Berkow. The Merck Manual, 17th Edition. Whitehouse Station, NJ, USA: Merck Research Laboratories, 1999.

40. Karnam US, Felder LR, Raskin JB. Prevalence of occult celiac disease in patients with iron-deficiency anemia: a prospective study. *Southern Medical Journal.* Jan 2004; 97(1):30-4.

41. Kapur G, Patwari AK, Narayan S, Anand VK. Iron supplementation in children with celiac disease. *Indian Journal of Pediatrics.* Dec 2003; 70(12):955-8.

42. Singhal A, Moreea S, Reynolds PD, Bzeizi KI. Coeliac disease and hereditary haemochromatosis: association and implications. *European Journal of Gastroentorology and Hepatology.* Feb 2004; 16(2):235-7.

43. Côté HC, Huntsman DG, Wu J, Wadsworth LD, MacGrillivray RT. A new method for characterization and epitope determination of a lupus anticoagulant-associated neutralizing antiprothrombin antibody. *American Journal of Clinical Pathology.* Feb 1997; 107(2):197-205.

44. Williams SF, Mincey BA, Calamia KT. Inclusion body myositis associated with celiac sprue and idiopathic thrombocytopenic purpura. *Southern Medical Journal.* Jul 2003; 96(7):721-3.

45. Kahn O, Fiel MI, Janowitz HD. Celiac sprue, idiopathic thrombocytopenic purpura, and hepatic granulomatous disease. An autoimmune linkage? *Journal of Clinical Gastroenterology.* Oct 1996; 23(3):214-6.

46. Pittschieler K, Neutropenia, granulocytic hypersegmentation and celiac disease. *Acta Paediatrica.* Jun 1995; 84(6):705-6.

47. La Placa G, Arlati S, Verdura C, Andreotti M. Report of a case of celiac disease associated with transient erythroblastopenia in pediatric age. *La Pedriatria Medica e Chirurgica : Medical and Surgical Pediatrics.* Mar-Apr 1998; 20(2):153-4.

48. Stadlmaier E, Spary A, Tillich M, Pilger E. Midaortic syndrome and celiac disease: a case of local vasculitis. *Clinical Rheumatology.* Jun 2005; 24 (3):301-4.

49. Odetti P, Valentini S, Aragno I, Garibaldi S, Pronzato MA, Rolandi E, Barreca T. Oxidative stress in subjects affected by celiac disease. *Free Radical Research.* Jul 1998; 29(1):17-24.

50. Heidinger K, Kemkes-Matthes B, Matthes KJ, Franke F, Voss R, Heckers H. Endemic sprue: its first diagnosis based on bleeding complications. *Deutsche Medizinische Wochenschrift.* Nov 10, 1995; 120(45):1543-6.

51. Bhattacharyya A, Patel MK, Tymms DJ. Coeliac disease in adults: variations on a theme. *Journal of the Royal Society of Medicine.* Jun 1999; 92(6):286-9.

52. Yasunobu Y, Hayashi K, Shingu T, Yamagata T, Kajiyama G, Kambe M. Coronary atherosclerosis and oxidative stress as reflected by autoantibodies against oxidized low-density lipoprotein and oxysterols. *Atherosclerosis.* Apr 2001; 155(2):445-53.

53. Curione M, Barbato M, De Biase L, Viola F, Lo Russo L, Cardi E. Prevalence of coeliac disease in idiopathic dilated cardiomyopathy. *Lancet.* Jul 17, 1999; 354(9174):222-3.

54. Curione M, Barbato M, Viola F, Francia P, De Biase L, Cucchiara S. Idiopathic dilated cardiomyopathy associated with coeliac disease: the effect of a gluten-free diet on cardiac performance. *Digestive and Liver Disease: Official Journal of the Italian Society of Gastroenterology and the Italian Association for the Study of the Liver.* Dec 2002; 34(12):866-9.

55. Delcò F, El-Serag HB, Sonnenberg A. Celiac sprue among US military veterans: associated disorders and clinical manifestations. *Digestive Diseases and Sciences.* May 1999; 44(5):966-72.

56. Lahteenoja H, Toivanen A, Viander M, Maki M, Irjala K, Raiha I, Syrjanen S. Oral mucosal changes in coeliac patients on a gluten-free diet. *European Journal of Oral Sciences.* Oct 1998; 106(5):899,8p.

57. Mariani P, Mazzilli MC, Margutti G, et al. Coeliac disease, enamel defects and HLA typing. *Acta Paediatrica.* Dec 1994; 83(12):1272-5.

58. Patinen P, Aine L, Collin P, et al. Oral findings in coeliac disease and Sjögren's syndrome. *Oral Diseases.* Nov 2004; 10(Issue 6):330,5p.

59. Wright DH. The major complications of coeliac disease. *Bailliere's Clinical Gastroenterology.* Jun 1995; 9(2):351-69.

60. Green PH, Fleischauer AT, Bhagat G, Goyal R, Jabri B, Neugut AI. Risk of malignancy in patients with celiac disease. *American Journal of Medicine.* Aug 15, 2003; 115(3):191-5.

61. Usai P, Usai Satta P, Lai M, et al. Autonomic dysfunction and upper digestive functional disorders in untreated adult coeliac disease. *European Journal of Clinical Investigation.* Dec 1997; 27(12):1009-15.

62. Cuomo A, Romano M, Rocco A, Budillon G, Del Vecchio Blanco C, Nardone G. Reflux oesophagitis in adult coeliac disease: beneficial effect of a gluten free diet. *Gut.* Apr 2003; 52(4):514-7.

63. Makharia GK, Nandi B, Garg PK, Tandon RK. Plummer Vinson syndrome: unusual features. *Indian Journal of Gastroenterology: Official Journal of the Indian Society of Gastroenterology.* Mar-Apr 2002; 21(2):74-5.

64. Cuoco L, Cammarota G, Jorizzo RA, et al. Link between helicobacter pylori infection and iron-deficiency anaemia in patients with coeliac disease. *Scandanavian Journal of Gastroenterology.* Dec 2001; 36(12):1284-8.

65. Domagk D, Avenhaus W, Ullerich H, Henschke F, Menzel J, Domschke W. Heliobacter pylori-negative gastric ulcerations associated with celiac disease at first presentation. *Zeitschrift Fur Gastroenterologie.* Jul 2001; 39(7):529-32.

66. Stancu M, De Petris G, Palumbo TP, Lev R. Collagenous gastritis associated with lymphocytic gastritis and celiac disease. *Archives of Pathology & Laboratory Medicine.* Dec 2001; 125(12):1579-84.

67. Drut R, Drut RM. Lymphocytic gastritis in pediatric celiac disease – immunohistochemical study of the intraepithelial lymphocytic component. *Medical Science Monitor: International Medical Journal of Experimental and Clinical Research.* Jan 2004; 10(1):CR38-42.

68. Sedlack RE, Smyrk TC, Czaja AJ, Talwalkar JA. Celiac disease-associated autoimmune cholangitis. *American Journal of Gastroenterology.* Dec 2002; 97(12):3196-8.

69. Fraquelli M, Pagliarulo M, Colucci A, Paggi S, Conte D. Gallbladder motility in obesity, diabetes mellitus and coeliac disease. *Digestive and Liver Disease: Official Journal of the Italian Society of Gastroenterology and the Italian Association for the Study of the Liver.* Jul 2003; 35(Suppl 3):S12-6.

70. Floreani A, Betterle C, Baragiotta A, et al. Prevalence of coeliac disease in primary biliary cirrhosis and of antimitochondrial antibodies in adult coeliac disease patients in Italy. *Digestive and Liver Disease: Official Journal of the Italian Society of Gastroenterology and the Italian Association for the Study of the Liver.* Apr 2002; 34(4):258-61.

71. Gillett HR, Cauch-Dudek K, Jenny E, Heathcote EJ, Freeman HJ. Prevalence of IgA antibodies to endomysium and tissue transglutaminase in primary biliary cirrhosis. *Canadian Journal of Gastroenterology = Journal Canadien de Gastroenterologie.* Sep 2000; 14(8);672-5.

72. Wurm P, Dixon AD, Rathbone BJ. Ulcerative colitis, primary sclerosing cholangitis and coeliac disease: two cases and review of the literature. *European Journal of Gastroenterology and Hepatology.* Jul 2003; 15(7):815-7.

73. Murray JA, Watson T, Clearman B, Mitros F. Effect of a gluten-free diet on gastrointestinal symptoms in celiac disease. *American Journal of Clinical Nutrition.* Apr 2004; 79(4):669-73.

74. Rampertab SD, Fleischauer A, Neugut AI, Green PH. Risk of duodenal adenoma in celiac disease. *Scandanavian Journal of Gastroenterology.* Aug 2003; 38(8):831-3.

75. Hinks LJ, Inwards KD, Lloyd B, Clayton BE. Body content of selenium in coeliac disease. *British Medical Journal.* Jun 23, 1984; 288(6434):1862-3.

76. Nieuwenhuizen WF, Pieters RH, Knippels LM, Jansen MC, Koppelman SJ. Is Candida albicans a trigger in the onset of coeliac disease? *Lancet.* Jun 21, 2003; 361(9375):2152-4.

77. Wolf I, Mouallem M, Farfel Z. Adult celiac disease presented with celiac crisis: severe diarrhea, hypokalemia, and acidosis. *Journal of Clinical Gastroenterology.* Apr 2000; 30(3):324-6.

78. Mennecier D, Rimlinger H, Rapp C, Bredin C, Corberand D, Vergeau B. Acute diarrhoea revealing a coeliac disease. *La Presse Medicale.* Apr 24, 2004; 33(8):530-2.

79. Fine KD, Meyer RL, Lee EL. The prevalence and causes of chronic diarrhea in patients with celiac sprue treated with a gluten-free diet. *Gastroenterology.* Jun 1997; 112(6);1830-8.

80. Giorgi PL, Catassi C, Guerrieri A. Zinc and chronic enteropathies. *La Pediatria Medica e Chirurgica: Medical and Surgical Pediatrics.* Sep-Oct 1984; 6(5):625-36.

81. Mehta DI, Lebenthal E, Blecker U. Chronic diarrhea: causes, presentation, and management. *Indian Journal of Pediatrics.* Jul-Aug 1996; 63(4):459-71.

82. Dickey W, Hughes D. Erosions in the second part of the duodenum in patients with villous atrophy. *Gastrointestinal Endoscopy.* Jan 2004; 59(1):116-8.

83. Riccabona M, Rossipal E. Sonographic findings in celiac disease. *Journal of Pediatric Gastroenterology and Nutrition.* Aug 1993; 17(2):198-200.

84. Farhadi A, Banan A, Fields J, Keshavarzian A. Intestinal barrier: an interface between health and disease. *Journal of Gastroenterology and Hepatology.* 2003; 18:479-91.

85. Sabra A, Bellanti JA, Rais JM, Castro HJ, de Inocencio JM, Sabra S. IgE and non-IgE food allergy. *Annals of Allergy, Asthma, & Immunology.* Jun 2003; 90(6 Suppl 3):71-6.

86. Johnston SD, Smye M, Watson RGP. Intestinal permeability and morphometric recovery in coeliac disease. *Lancet.* Jul 28, 2001; 358(9278):259, 2p.

87. Abazia C, Ferrara R, Corsaro MM, Barone G, Coccoli P, Parrilli G. Simultaneous gas-chromatographic measurement of rhamnose, lactulose and sucrose and their application in the testing gastrointestinal permeability. *Clinica Chimica Acta; International Journal of Clinical Chemistry.* Dec 2003; 338(1-2):25-32.

88. Cummins AG, Thompson FM, Butler RN, et al. Improvement in intestinal permeability precedes morphometric recovery of the small intestine in coeliac disease. *Clinical Science.* Apr 2001; 100(4):379-86.

89. Kuitunen P, Visakorpi JK, Savilahti E, Pelkonen P. Malabsorption syndrome with cow's milk intolerance. Clinical findings and course in 54 cases. *Archives of Disease in Childhood.* May 1975; 50(50:351-6.

90. Monetini L, Cavallo MG, Manfrini S. Antibodies to bovine beta-casein in diabetes and other autoimmune diseases. *Hormone and Metabolic Research.* Aug 2002; 34(8):455-9.

91. Schweiger GD, Murray JA. Postbulbar duodenal ulceration and stenosis associated with celiac disease. *Abdominal Imaging.* Jul-Aug 1998; 23(4):347-9.

92. Lastennet F, Piloquet H, Camby C, Moussally F, Siret D. Acute intestinal invagination revealing celiac disease in a 9-month-old infant. *Archives De Pediatrie: Organe Officiel De La Societe Francaise De Pediatrie.* Feb 2002; 9(2):151-4.

93. Bret P, Francoz JB, Bret P, Cuche C, Gérard C. Lacunar images and invagination in 25 patients with celiac disease. *Journal Da Radiologie.* Nov 1980; 61(11):723-7.

94. Martinez G, Israel NR, White JJ. Celiac disease presenting as entero-enteral intussusception. *Pediatric Surgery International.* 2001; 17(1):68-70.

95. Cox MA, Lewis KO, Cooper BT. Sucrosemia in untreated celiac disease: a potential screening test. *Digestive Diseases and Sciences.* May 1998; 43(5):1096-101.

96. Smecuol E, Vazquez H, Sugai E, et al. Sugar tests detect celiac disease among first-degree relatives. *The American Journal of Gastroenterology.* Dec 1999; 94(12):3547-52.

97. Riobó P, Turbí C, Banet R, et al. Colonic volvulus and ulcerative jejunoileitis due to occult celiac sprue. *American Journal of the Medical Sciences.* May 1998; 315(5):317-8.

98. Koskela RM, Niemelä SE, Karttunen TJ, Lehtola JK. Clinical characteristics of collagenous and lymphocytic colitis. *Scandanavian Journal of Gastroenterology.* Sep 2004; 39(9):837-45.

99. Freeman HJ. Collagenous colitis as the presenting feature of biopsy-defined celiac disease. *Journal of Clinical Gastroenterology.* Sep 2004; 38(8):664-8.

100. Abdo AA, Urbanski SJ, Beck PL. Lymphocytic and collagenous colitis: the emerging entity of microscopic colitis. An update on pathophysiology, diagnosis and management. *Canadian Journal of Gastroenterology = Journal Canadien de Gastroenterologie.* Jul 2003; 17(7):425-32.

101. Cottone M, Marrone C, Casà A, Oliva L, et al. Familial occurrence of inflammatory bowel disease in celiac disease. *Inflammatory Bowel Diseases.* Sep 2003; 9(5):321-3.

102. Barta Z, Csípö I, Szabó GG, Szegedi G. Seroreactivity against saccharomyces cerevisiae in patients with Crohn's disease and celiac disease. *World Journal of Gastroenterology.* Oct 2003; 9(10):2308-12.

103. Gregory C, Ashworth M, Eade OE, Holdstock G, Smith CL, Wright R. Delay in diagnosis of adult coeliac disease. *Digestion.* 1983; 28(3):201-4.

104. Sanders DS, Patel D, Stephenson TJ, et al. A primary care cross-sectional study of undiagnosed adult coeliac disease. *European Journal of Gastroenterology and Hepatology.* Apr 2003; 15(4)407-13.

105. Longstreth GF, Drossman DA. New developments in the diagnosis and treatment of irritable bowel syndrome. *Current Gastroenterology Reports.* Oct 2002; 4(5):427-34.

106. Mein SM, Ladabaum U. Serological testing for coeliac disease in patients with symptoms of irritable bowel syndrome: a cost-effectiveness analysis. *Alimentary Pharmacology and Therapeutics.* Jun 1, 2004; 19(11):1199-210.

107. Sanders DS, Carter MJ, Hurlstone DP, et al. Association of adult coeliac disease with irritable bowel syndrome: a case-control study in patients fulfilling ROME II criteria referred to secondary care. *Lancet.* Nov 3, 2001; 358:1504-8.

108. Treem WR. Emerging concepts in celiac disease. *Current Opinion in Pediatrics.* Oct 2004; 16(5):552-9.

109. Myhre AG, Aarsetøy H, Undlien DE, Hovdenak N, Aksnes L, Husebye ES. High frequency of coeliac disease among patients with autoimmune adrenocortical failure. *Scandanavian Journal of Gastroenterology.* May 2003; 38(5):511-5.

110. Volta U, De Franceschi L, Molinaro N, et al. Frequency and significance of anti-gliadin and anti-endomysial antibodies in autoimmune hepatitis. *Digestive Diseases and Sciences.* Oct 1998; 43(10):2190-5.

111. Abdo A, Meddings J, Swain M. Liver abnormalities in celiac disease. Clinical Gastroenterology and Hepatology. Feb 2004;2(2):107-12.

112. Bardella MT, Valenti L, Pagliari C, et al. Searching for coeliac disease in patients with non-alcoholic fatty liver disease. *Digestive and Liver Disease: Official Journal of the Italian Society of Gastroenterology and the Italian Association for the Study of the Liver.* May 2004; 36(5):333-6.

113. Husová L, Senkyrík M, Lata J, et al. Large-droplet liver steatosis in celiac disease. *Vnitrni Lekarstvi.* Mar 2004; 50(3):244-8.

114. Not T, Tommasini A, Tonini G, et al. Undiagnosed coeliac disease and risk of autoimmune disorders in subjects with Type 1 diabetes mellitus. *Diabetologia.* Feb 2001; 44(2):151-5.

115. Aktay AN, Lee PC, Kumar V, Parton E, Wyatt DT, Werlin SL. The prevalence and clinical characteristics of celiac disease in juvenile diabetes in Wisconsin. *Journal of Pediatric Gastroenterology and Nutrition.* Oct 2001; 33(4):462-5.

116. Book LS. Diagnosing celiac disease in 2002: who, why, and how? *Pediatrics.* May 2002; 109(5):952,3p.

117. Liu E, Eisenbarth GS. Type 1A diabetes mellitus-associated autoimmunity. *Endocrinology and Metabolism Clinics of North America.* Jun 2002; 31(2):391-410, vii-viii.

118. Bouguerra R, Salem B, Chaâbouni H, et al. Celiac disease in adult patients with type 1 diabetes mellitus in Tunisia. *Diabetes and Metabolism.* Feb 2005; 31(1):83-6.

119. Dretzke J, Cummins C, Sandercock J, Fry-Smith A, Barrett T, Burls A. Autoantibody testing in children with newly diagnosed type 1 diabetes mellitus. *Health Technology Assessment: HTA.* Jun 2004; 8(22):iii-xi,1-183.

120. Perusicová J. Gastrointestinal complications in diabetes mellitus. *Vnitri Lekarstvi.* May 2004; 50(5):338-43.

121. Gannage MH, Abikaram G, Nasr F, Awada H. Osteomalacia secondary to celiac disease, primary hyperparathyroidism, and Grave's disease. *American Journal of the Medical Sciences.* Feb 1998; 315(2):136-9.

122. Lemieux B, Bolvin M, Brossard JH, et al. Normal parathyroid function with decreased bone mineral density in treated celiac disease. *Canadian Journal of Gastroenterology.* May 2001; 15(5):302-7.

123. Matsueda K, Rosenberg IH. Malabsorption with idiopathic hypoparathyroidism responding to treatment for coincident celiac sprue. *Digestive Diseases and Sciences.* Mar 1982; 27(3):269-73.

124. Boyle NH, Ogg CD, Hartley RB, Owen WJ. Parathyroid carcinoma secondary to prolonged hyperplasia in chronic renal failure and in coeliac disease. *European Journal of Surgical Oncology: The Journal of the European Society of Surgical Oncology and the British Association of Surgical Oncology.* Feb 1999; 25(1):100-3.

125. Mainardi E, Montanelli A, Dotti M, Nano R, Moscato G. Thyroid-related autoantibodies and celiac disease: a role for a gluten-free diet? *Journal of Clinical Gastroenterology.* Sep 2002; 35(3):245-8.

126. Reunala T, Collin P. Diseases associated with dermatitis herpetiformis. *British Journal of Dermatology.* Mar 1997; 136(3):315-8.

127. Ch'ng CL, Biswas M, Jones MK, Kingham JG. Prospective screening for celiac disease in patients with Graves' hyperthyroidism using anti-gliadin and tissue transflutaminase antibodies. *Clinical Endocrinology.* Mar 2005; 62 (3):303-6.

128. Villarrubia N, León F, Bootello A. T gamma-delta lymphocytes and their role in hypersensitivity processes in the digestive and respiratory mucosa. *Allergologia et Immunopathologia.* Sep-Oct 2002; 30(5):273-82.

129. Shamir R, Shoenfeld Y, Blank M, et al. The prevalence of coeliac disease antibodies in patients with the antiphospholipid syndrome. *Lupus.* 2003; 32:394-9.

130. Kero J, Gissler M, Hemminki E, Isolauri E. Could TH1 and TH2 diseases coexist? Evaluation of asthma incidence in children with coeliac disease, type 1 diabetes, or rheumatoid arthritis: a register study. *The Journal of Allergy and Clinical Immunology.* Nov 2001; 108(5)781-3.

131. Volta U, De Franceschi L, Molinaro N, Tetta C, Bianchi FB. Organ-specific autoantibodies in coeliac disease: do they represent an epiphenomenon or the expression of associated autoimmune disorders? *Italian Journal of Gastroenterology and Hepatology.* Feb 1997; 29(1):18-21.

132. Cataldo F, Marino V. Increased prevalence of autoimmune diseases in first degree relatives of patients with celiac disease. *Journal of Pediatric Gastroenterology and Nutrition.* Apr 2003; 36(4):470-3.

133. Rousset H. A great imitator for the allergologist: intolerance to gluten. *Allergie Et Immunologie.* Mar 2004; 36(3):96-100.

134. Iughetti L, Bulgarelli S, Forese S, Lorini R, Balli F, Bernasconi S. Endocrine aspects of coeliac disease. *Journal of Pediatric Endocrinology & Metabolism : JPEM.* Jul-Aug 2003; 16(6):805-18.

135. Femiano P, Castaldo V, Iossa C. Complex family association in autoimmune polyendocrine syndrome. *Minerva Pediatrica.* Apr 2003; 55(2):163-70.

136. Fracchia M, Galatola G, Corradi F, et al. Coeliac disease associated with Sjogren's syndrome, renal tubular acidosis, primary biliary cirrhosis and autoimmune hyperthyroidism. *Digestive and Liver Disease: Official Journal of the Italian Society of Gastroenterology and the Italian Association for the Study of the Liver.* Jul 2004; 36(7):489-91.

137. Béchade D, Desramé J, De Fuentès G, Camparo P, Raynaud JJ, Algayres JP. Common variable immunodeficiency and celiac disease. *Gatroenterologie Clinique et Biologique.* Oct 2004; 28(10 Pt 1):909-12.

138. Aslam A, Misba SA, Talbot K, Chapel H. Vitamin E deficiency induced neurological disease in common variable immunodeficiency: two cases and a review of the literature of vitamin E deficiency. *Clinical Immunology.* Jul 2004; 112(1):24-9.

139. Cataldo F, Lio D, Marino V, Scola L, Crivello A, Corazza GR. Plasma cytokine profiles in patients with celiac disease and selective IgA deficiency. *Pediatric Allergy Immunology: Official Publication of the European Society of Pediatric Allergy and Immunology.* Aug 2003; 14(4):320-4.

140. Dahlbom I, Olsson M, Forooz NK, Sjöholm AG, Truedsson L, Hansson T. Immunoglobulin G (IgG) anti-tissue transglutaminase antibodies used as markers for IgA-deficient celiac disease patients. *Clinical and Diagnostic Laboratory Immunology.* Feb 2005; 12(2):254-8.

141. Rutherford RM, Brutsche MH, Kearns M, Bourke M, Stevens F, Gilmartin JJ. Prevalence of coeliac disease in patients with sarcoidosis. *European Journal of Gastroenterology and Hepatology.* Sep 2004; 16(9):911-5.

142. Loche F, Bazex J. Celiac disease associated with cutaneous sarcoidosic granuloma. *La Revue de Medicine Interne.* 1997; 18(2):975-8.

143. Luft LM, Barar SG, Martin LO, Chan EK, Fritzler MJ. Autoantibodies to tissue transglutaminase in Sjögren's syndrome and related rheumatic diseases. *Journal of Rheumatology.* Dec 2003; 30(12):2613-9.

144. Zitouni M, Daoud W, Kallel M, Makni S. Systemic lupus erythematosus with celiac disease: a report of five cases. *Joint, Bone, Spine: Revue Du Rhuatisme.* Jul 2004; 71(4):344-6.

145. Liutu M, Kalimo K, Uksila J, Kalimo H. Etiologic aspect of chronic urticaria. *International Journal of Dermatology.* Jul 1998; 37(7):515-9.

146. Scala E, Giani M, Pirrotta L, Guerra EC, DePità O, Puddu P. Urticaria and adult celiac disease. *Allergy.* 1999; 54:1008-9.

147. Poon E, Nixon R. Cutaneous spectrum of coeliac disease. *Australian Journal of Dermatology.* May 2001; 42(2):136-8.

148. Fessatou S, Kostaki M, Karpathios T. Coeliac disease and alopecia areata in childhood. *Journal of Paediatrics and Child Health.* Mar 2003; 39(2):152-4.

149. Naveh Y, Rosenthal E, Ben-Arieh Y, Etzioni A. Celiac disease-associated alopecia in childhood. *Journal of Pediatrics.* Mar 1999; 134(3):362-4.

150. Várkonyi A, Boda M, Endreffy E, Németh I, Timár E. Coeliac disease: always something to discover. *Scandanavian Journal of Gastroenterology.* 1998; 228:122-9.

151. Meyers S, Dikman S, Spiera H, Schultz N, Janowitz HD. Cutaneous vasculitis complicating coeliac disease. *Gut.* Jan 1981; 22(1):61-4.

152. García-Patos V, Pujol RM, Barnadas MA, et al. Generalized acquired cutis laxa associated with coeliac disease: evidence of immunoglobulin A deposits on the dermal elastic fibres. *The British Journal of Dermatology.* Jul 1996; 135(1):130-4.

153. Collin P, Reunala T. Recognition and management of the cutaneous manifestations of celiac disease: a guide for dermatologists. American Journal of Clinical Dermatology. 2003;4(1):13-20.

154. Kárpáti S. Dermatitis herpetiformis: close to unraveling a disease. *Journal of Dermatological Science.* Apr 2004; 34(2):83-90.

155. Hervonen K, Vornanen M, Kautiainen H, Collin P, Reunala T. Lymphoma in patients with dermatitis herpetiformis and their first-degree relatives. *British Journal of Dermatology.* Jan 2005; 152(Issue 1):82,5p.

156. Smecuol E, Sugai E, Niveloni S, et al. Permeability, zonulin production, and enteropathy in dermatitis herpetiformis. *Clinical Gastroenterology and Hepatology: The Official Clinical Practice Journal of the American Gastroenterological Association.* Apr 2005; 3(4):335-41.

157. Marie I, Lecomte F, Hachulla E, et al. An uncommon association: celiac disease and dermatomyositis in adults. *Clinical and Experimental Rheumatology.* Mar-Apr 2001; 19(2):201-3.

158. Tasanen K, Raudasoja R, Kallioinen M, Ranki A. Erythema elevatum diutinum in association with coeliac disease. *The British Journal of Dermatology.* Apr 1997; 136(4)624-7.

159. Bartyik K, Várkonyi A, Kirschner A, Endreffy E, Túri S, Karg E. Erythema nodosum in association with celiac disease. *Pediatric Dermatology.* May-Jun 2004; 21(3):227-30.

160. Menni S, Boccardi D, Brusasco A. Ichthyosis revealing coeliac disease. *European Journal of Dermatology : EJD.* Jul-Aug 2000; 10(5):398-9.

161. Randle HW, Winkelmann RK. Pityriasis rubra pilaris and celiac sprue with malabsorption. *Cutis: Cutaneous Medicine for the Practitioner.* Jun 1980; 25(6):626-7.

162. Francesco Stefanini G, Resta F, Marsigli L, et al. Prurigo nodularis (Hyde's prurigo) disclosing celiac disease. *Hepato-Gastroenterology.* Jul-Aug 1999; 46(28):2281-4.

163. Ojetti V, Aguilar Sanchez J, Guerriero C, et al. High prevalence of celiac disease in psoriasis. *American Journal of Gastroenterology.* Nov 2003; 98(11):2574-5.

164. Addolorato G, Parente A, de Lorenzi G, et al. Rapid regression of psoriasis in a coeliac patient after gluten-free diet. A case report and review of the literature. *Digestion.* 2003; 68(1):9-12.

165. Marguerie C, Kaye S, Vyse T, Mackworth-Young C, Walport MJ, Black C. Malabsorption caused by coeliac disease in patients who have scleroderma. *British Journal of Rheumatology.* Sep 1995; 34(9):858-61.

166. Smedby KE, Akerman N, Hildebrand H, Glimelius B, Ekbom A, Askling J. Malignant lymphomas in celiac disease: evidence of increased risks for lymphoma types other than enteropathy-type T cell lymphoma. *Gut.* Jan 2005; 54(1):54-59.

167. Catassi C, Bearzi I, Holmes GK. Association of celiac disease and intestinal lymphomas and other cancers. *Gastroenterology.* Apr 2005; 128(4 Suppl 1):S79-86.

168. Culliford AN, Green PH. Refractory sprue. *Current Gastroenterology Reports.* Oct 2003; 5(5):373-8.

169. Yang DH, Myung SJ, Chang HS, et al. A case of enteropathy-associated T-cell lymphoma presenting with recurrent hematochezia. *Korean Journal of Gastroenterology = Taehan Sohwagi Hakhoe Chi.* Dec 2003; 42(6):527-32.

170. Meijer JWR, Mulder CJJ, Goerres MG, Boot H, Schweizer JJ. Coeliac disease and (extra)intestinal T-cell lymphomas: definition, diagnosis and treatment. *Scandanavian Journal of Gastroenterology.* Dec 2004; 39(Suppl 241):78,7p.

171. Kakar S, Nehra V, Murray JA, Dayharsh GA, Burgart LJ. Significance of intraepithelial lymphocytosis in small bowel biopsy samples with normal mucosal architecture. *The American Journal of Gastroenterology.* Sep 2003; 98(9):2027-33.

172. Howat AJ, McPhie JL, Smith DA, Aqel NM, Taylor AK, Cairns SA, et al. Cavitation of mesenteric lymph nodes: a rare complication of celiac disease, associated with a poor outcome. *Histopathology.* Oct 1995; 27(4):349-54.

173. Vázquez H, Martinez C, Xavier L, Mazure R, Boerr L, Bai J. Hyposplenism in celiac disease. Role of a gluten-free diet. *Acta Gastroenterologica Latinoamericana.* 1991; 21(1):17-21.

174. Brigden ML. Detection, education, and management of the asplenic or hyposplenic patient. *American Family Physician.* Feb 1, 2001; 63(3):499, 8p, 1 diagram, 1bw.

175. Ertekin V, Selimoglu MA, Tan H, Kiliçaslan B. Rhabdomyolysis in celiac disease. *Yonsei Medical Journal.* Apr 2003; 44(2):328-30.

176. Barta Z, Miltenyi Z, Illes A. Hypokalemic myopathy in a patient with gluten-sensitive enteropathy and dermatitis herpetiformis Duhring: a case report. *World Journal of Gastroenterology.* Apr 2005; 11(13):2039-40.

177. Cano Ruiz A, Barbado Hernández FJ, Martín Scapa MA, Gómez-Cerezo J, Vazquez Rodríguez JJ. Adult celiac disease presenting as tetany. *Anales de Medicina Interna: Organo Oficial de la Sociedad Espanola de Medicina Interna.* Dec 1996; 13(12):592-4.

178. Rubinstein A, Liron M, Bodner G, Gefel A. Bilateral femoral neck fractures as a result of celiac disease. *Postgraduate Medical Journal.* Jan 1982; 58(675):61-2.

179. Moltu SJ, Bentsen BS. Tetany – a first symptom of celiac disease. Tidsskrift for den Norske Laegeforening. Mar 30, 2000; 120(9):1034-6.

180. Zelnick N, Pacht A, Obeid R, Lerner A. Range of neurologic disorders in patients with celiac disease. *Pediatrics.* Jun 2004; 113(6):1672-1676.

181. Wills AJ. The neurology and neuropathology of celiac disease. *Neuropathology and Applied Neurobiology.* 2000; 26:493-496.

182. Usai P, Serra A, Marini, et al. Frontal cortical perfusion abnormalities related to gluten intake and associated autoimmune disease in adult celiac disease: 99 mTc-ECD brain SPECT study. *Digestive Liver Disease.* Aug 2004; 36(8):513-8.

183. Hadjivassiliou M, Grunewald R, Sharrack B, et al. Gluten ataxia in perspective: epidemiology, genetic susceptibility and clinical characteristics. *Brain.* Mar 2003; 126(Pt 3):685-91.

184. Ghezzi A, Zaffaroni M. Neurological manifestations of gastrointestinal disorders, with particular reference to the different diagnosis of multiple sclerosis. *Neurological Sciences: Official Journal of the Italian Neurological Society and of the Italian Society of Clinical Neurophysiology.* Nov 2001; 22(2):S117-22.

185. Hadjivassiliou M, Grunewald RA, Chattopadhyay AK, et al. Clinical, radiological, neurophysiological, and neuropathological characteristics of gluten ataxia. *Lancet.* Nov 14, 1998; 352(9140):1582-5.

186. Hadjivassiliou M, Boscolo S, Davies-Jones, et al. The humoral response in the pathogenesis of gluten ataxia. *Neurology.* Apr 23, 2002; 58(8):1221-6.

187. Hanagasi HA, Gurol E, Sahin HA, Emre M. Atypical neurological involvement associated with celiac disease. *European Journal of Neurology.* 2001; 8:67-69

188. Bhatia KP, Brown P, Gregory R, et al. Progressive myoclonic ataxia associated with coeliac disease. The myoclonus is of cortical origin, but the pathology is in the cerebellum. *Brain.* Oct 1995; 118(Pt 5):1087-93.

189. Pereira AC, Edwards MJ, Buttery PC, et al. Choreic syndrome and coeliac disease: a hitherto unrecognized association. *Movement disorders: Official Journal of the Movement Disorder Society.* Apr 2004; 19(4):478-82.

190. Collin P, Pirttilä T, Nurmikko T, Somer H, Erilä T, Keyriläinen O. Celiac disease, brain, and dementia. *Neurology.* Mar 1991; 41(3):372-5.

191. Luostarinen, Dastidar, Collin, Peräajo, Mäki, Erilä, Pirttilä. Association between coeliac disease and brain atrophy. *European Neurology.* 2001; 46(4):187,5.

192. Bye AM, Andermann F, Robitaille Y, Oliver M, Bohane T, Andermann E. Cortical vascular abnormalities in the syndrome of celiac disease, epilepsy, bilateral occipital calcifications, and folate deficiency. *Annals of Neurology.* Sep 1993; 34(3):399-403.

193. La Mantia L, Pollo B, Svoiardo M, et al. Meningo-cortical calcifying angiomatosis and celiac disease. *Clinical Neurology and Neurosurgery.* Sep 1998; 100(3):209-15.

194. Cicarelli G, Della Rocca G, Amboni M. Clinical and neurological abnormalities in adult celiac disease. *Neurological Sciences: Official Journal of the Italian Neurological Society and of the Italian Society of Clinical Neurophysiology.* Dec 2003; 24(5):311-7.

195. Essid M, Trabelsi K, Jerbi E, et al. Villous atrophy and idiopathic epilepsy. *La Tunisie Medicale.* Apr 2003; 81(4):270-2.

196. Pratesi R, Modelli IC, Martins RC, Almeida PL, Gandolfi L. Celiac disease and epilepsy: favorable outcome in a child with difficult to control seizures. *Acta Neurologica Scandanavica.* Oct 2003; 108(4):290-3.

197. Logan AC, Wong C. Chronic fatigue syndrome: oxidative stress and dietary modifications. *Alternative Medicine Review : A Journal of Clinical Therapeutic.* Oct 2001; 6(5):450-9.

198. Skowera A, Peakman M, Cleare A, Davies E, Deale A, Wessely S. High prevalence of serum markers of coeliac disease in patients with chronic fatigue syndrome. *Journal of Clinical Pathology.* Apr 2001; 54(40:335-6.

199. Gabrielli M, Cremonini F, Fiore G, et al. Association between migraine and celiac disease: results from a preliminary case control and therapeutic study. *American Journal of Gastroenterology.* Mar 2003; 98(3):625-9.

200. Morello F, Ronzani G, Cappellari F. Migraine, cortical blindness, multiple cerebral infarctions and hypocoagulapathy in celiac disease. *Neurological Sciences: Official Journal of the Italian Neurological Society and of the Italian Society of Clinical Neurophysiology.* Jun 2003; 24(2):85-9.

201. Pengiran Tengah CD, Lock RJ, Unsworth DJ, Wills AJ. Multiple sclerosis and occult gluten sensitivity. *Neurology.* Jun 22, 2004; 62(12):2326-7.

202. Salvatore S, Finazzi S, Ghezzi, et.al. Multiple sclerosis and celiac disease: is there an increased risk? Multiple Sclerosis: *Clinical and Laboratory Research.* Dec 2004; 10(6):711-2.

203. Díaz RM, González-Rabelino G, Delfino A. Epilepsy, cerebral calcifications and coeliac disease. The importance of an early diagnosis. *Revista de Neurologia.* Apr 1-15, 2005; 40(7):417-20.

204. Pfaender M, D'Souza WJ, Trost N, Litewka L, Paine M, Cook M. Visual disturbances representing occipital lobe epilepsy in patients with cerebral calcifications and coeliac disease: a case series. *Journal of Neurology, Neurosurgery, and Psychiatry.* Nov 2004; 75(11):1623-5.

205. Kepes JJ, Chou SM, Price LW Jr. Progressive multifocal leukoencephalopathy with 10-year survival in a patient with nontropical sprue. Report of a case with unusual light and election microscopic features. *Neurology.* Nov 1975; 25(11):1006-12.

206. Ozge A, Karakelle and H Kaleagasi; Celiac disease associated with recurrent stroke: a coincidence or cerebral vesculitis? *European Journal of Neurology.* 2001; 8:373-374.

207. Potocki P, Hozyasz K. Psychiatric symptoms and coeliac disease. *Psychiatria Polska.* Jul-Aug 2002; 36(4):567-78.

208. Addolorato G, Capristo E, Ghittoni G, et al. Anxiety but not depression decreases in coeliac patients after one-year gluten-free diet: a longitudinal study. *Scandanavian Journal of Gastroenterology.* May 2001; 36(5):502-6.

209. Addolorato G, Di Giuda D, De Rossi G, et al. Regional cerebral hypoperfusion in patients with celiac disease. *American Journal of Medicine.* Mar 1, 2004; 116(5):312-7.

210. Bosseckert H. Clinical aspects and differential diagnosis of malabsorption. *Deutsche Zeitschrift fur Verdauungs-und Stoffwechselkrankheiten.* 1983; 43(1):27-32.

211. Hallert C, Aström J. Psychic disturbances in adult coeliac disease. II. Psychological findings. *Scandanavian Journal of Gastroenterology.* Jan 1982; 17(1):21-4.

212. Hallert C, Aström J, Walan A. Reversal of psychopathology in adult coeliac disease with the aid of pyridoxine (vitamin B6). *Scandanavian Journal of Gastroenterology.* Mar 1983; 18(2):299-304.

213. Serratrice J, Disdier P, Kaladjian A, et al. Psychosis revealing a silent celiac disease in a young woman with trisomy 21. *La Presse Medicale.* Oct 12, 2002; 31(33):1551-3.

214. Wei J, Hemmings GP. Gene, gut and schizophrenia: the meeting point for the gene-environment interaction in developing schizophrenia. *Medical Hypotheses.* 2005; 64(3):547-52.

215. Reichelt KL, Landmark J. Specific IgA antibody increases in schizophrenia. *Biological Psychiatry.* Mar 15, 1995; 37(6):410-3.

216. Singh MM, Kay SR. Wheat gluten as a pathogenic factor in schizophrenia. *Science.* Jan 30, 1976; 191(4225):401-2.

217. Rudin DO. The choroid plexus and system disease in mental illness. III. The exogenous peptide hypothesis of mental illness. *Biological Psychiatry.* May 1981; 16(5):489-512.

218. Dohan FC, Harper EH, Clark MH, Rodriguez RB, Zigas V. Is schizophrenia rare if grain is rare? *Biological Psychiatry.* Mar 1984; 19(3):385-99.

219. Huebner FR, Lieberman KW, Rubino RP, Wall JS. Demonstration of high opioid-like activity in isolated peptides from wheat gluten hydrolysates. *Peptides.* Nov-Dec 1984; 5(6):1139-47.

220. De Santis A, Addolarato G, Romito A, et al. Schizophrenic symptoms and SPECT abnormalities in a coeliac patient: regression after a gluten-free diet. *Journal of Internal Medicine.* Nov 1997; 242(5):421-3.

221. Chin RL, Sander HW, Brannigan TH, et al. Celiac neuropathy. *Neurology.* May 27, 2003; 60(10):1581-5.

222. Luostarinen L, Himanen SL, Luostarinen M, Collin P, Pirttilä T. Neuromuscular and sensory disturbances in patients with well treated coeliac disease. *Journal of Neurology, Neurosurgery, and Psychiatry.* Apr 2003; 74(4):490-4.

223. Kaplan JG, Pack D, Horoupian D, DeSouza T, Brin M, Schaumburg H. Distal axonopathy associated with chronic gluten enteropathy: a treatable disorder. *Neurology.* Apr 1988; 38(4)642-5.

224. Mahadeva R, Flower C, Shneerson J. Bronchiectasis in association with coeliac disease. *Thorax.* Jun 1998; 53(6):527-9.

225. Brightling CE, Symon FA, Birring SS, Wardlaw AJ, Robinson R, Pavrod ID. A case of cough, lymphocytic bronchoalveolitis and coeliac disease with improvement following a gluten free diet. *Thorax.* Jan 2002; 57(1):91-2.

226. Stevens FM, Connolly CE, Murray JP, McCarthy CF. Lung cavities in patients with celiac disease. *Digestion.* 1990; 46(2):72-80.

227. Johnston SD, Robinson J. Fatal pneumococcal septicaemia in a coeliac patient. European Journal of Gastroenterology and Hepatology. Apr 1998;10(4):353-4

228. McKinley M, Leibowitz S, Bronzo R, Zanzi I, Weissman G, Schiffman G. Appropriate response to pneumococcal vaccine in celiac sprue. *Journal of Clinical Gastroenterology.* Mar 1995; 20(2):113-6.

229. Malhotra P, Aggarawal R, Aggarwal AN, Jindal SK, Awasthi A, Radotra BD. Coeliac disease as a cause of unusually severe anaemia in a young man with idiopathic pulmonary haemosiderosis. *Respiratory Medicine.* Apr 2005; 99(4):451-3.

230. Robertson DA, Taylor N, Sidhu H, Britten A, Smith CL, Holdstock G. Pulmonary permeability in coeliac disease and inflammatory bowel disease. *Digestion.* 1989; 42(2):98-103.

231. Williams AJ, Asquith P, Stableforth DE. Susceptibility to tuberculosis in patients with coeliac disease. *Tubercle.* Dec 1998; 69(4):267-74.

232. Shetty A, Mckendrick M. TB and coeliac disease. *Journal of Infection.* Jan 2004; 48(1):109-11.

233. Sadowski B, Rohrback JM, Steuhl KP, Weidle EG, Castrillón-Obendorfer WL. Corneal manifestations in Vitamin A deficiency. *Klinische Monatsblatter fur Augenheilkunde.* Aug 1994; 205(2)76-85.

234. Eliakim R, Heyman S, Kornberg A. Celiac disease and keratoconjunctivitis. Occurrence with thrombocytopenic purpura. *Archives of Internal Medicine.* May 1982; 142(5):1037.

235. Sandyk R, Brennan MJ. Isolated ocular myopathy and celiac disease in childhood. *Neurology.* Jun 1983; 33(6):792.

236. Hyrailles V, Desprez D, Beaurere L, et.al. Uveitis complicating celiac disease and cured by gluten-free diet. *Gastroenterologie Clinique et Biologique.* May 1995; 19(5):543-4.

237. Vasquez H, Mazure R, Gonzalez D, et al. Risk of fractures in celiac disease patients: a cross-sectional, case control study. *The American Journal of Gastroenterology.* Jan 2000; 95(1):183-9.

238. Moreno ML, Vazquez H, Mazure R, et al. Stratification of bone fracture risk in patients with celiac disease. *Clinical Gastroenterology and Hepatology.* Feb 2004; 2(2):127-34.

239. Dorst AJ, Ringe JD. Severe osteomalacia in endemic sprue. An important differential diagnosis in osteoporosis. *Fortschritte der Medizin.* Mar 20, 1998; 116(8):42-5.

240. Bertoli A, De Daniele N. A woman with bone pain, fractures, and malabsorption. *Lancet.* Feb. 3, 1996; 347(8997):300, 3/4p,1 chart.

241. Sleiman I, Godi D, Villanacci V, Pelizzari G, Balestrieri GP. Osteitis fibrosa cystica, coeliac disease and Turner syndrome. A case report. *Digestive and Liver Disease: Official Journal of the Italian Society of Gastroenterology and the Italian Association for the Study of the Liver.* Jul 2004; 36(7):486-8.

242. Arnala I, Kemppainen T, Kröger H, Janatuinen E, Alhava EM. Bone histomorphology in celiac disease. *Annales Chirurgiae Et Gynaecologiae.* 2001; 90(2):100-4.

243. Agrawal MD, Face L. Polyostotic osteonecrosis in a patient with celiac disease. *Endocrine Practice: Official Journal of the American College of Endocrinology and the American Association of Clinical Endocrinologists.* 1996; 2(6):385-8.

244. Sategna-Guidetti C, Grosso SB, Grosso S, et al. The effects of 1-year gluten withdrawal on bone mass, bone metabolism and nutritional status in newly-diagnosed adult coeliac disease patients. *Alimentary Pharmacology and Therapeutics.* Jan 2000; 14(1):35-43.

245. Ferretti J, Mazure R, Tanoue P, et al. Analysis of the structure and strength of bones in celiac disease patients. *American Journal of Gastroenterology.* Feb 2003; 98(2):382-90.

246. Stenson WF, Newberry R, Lorenz R, Baldus C, Civitelli R. Increased prevalence of celiac disease and need for routine screening among patients with osteoporosis. *Archives of Internal Medicine.* Feb 28, 2005; 165(4):393-9.

247. Scharla S. Causes of osteoporosis: don't forget celiac disease. *Deutsche Medizinische Wochenschrift.* Apr 25, 2003; 128(17):916-9.

248. Holden W, Orchard T, Wordsworth P. Enteropathic arthritis. *Rheumatic Diseases Clinics of North America.* Aug 2003; 29(3):513-30,viii.

249. Gran JT, Husby G. Joint manifestations in gastrointestinal diseases. 2. Whipples's disease, enteric infections, intestinal bypass operations, gluten-sensitive enteropathy, pseudomembranous colitis and collagenous colitis. *Digestive Diseases.* 1992; 10(5):295-312.

250. Lindquist U, Rudsander A, Boström, Nilsson B, Michaëlsson G. IgA antibodies to gliadin and coeliac disease in psoriatic arthritis. *Rheumatology.* 2002 Jan; 41(1),31-7.

251. Cottafava F, Cosso D. Psoriatic arthritis and celiac disease in childhood. A case report. *Medical and Surgical Pediatrics.* 1991 Jul-Aug; 13 (4), 431-3.

252. Falcini F, Ferrari R, Simonini G, Calabri GB, Pazzaglia A, Lionetti P. Recurrent monoarthritis in an 11-year-old boy with occult celiac disease. *Clinical and Experimental Rheumatology.* 1999 Jul-Aug; 17 (4), 509-11.

253. Collin P, Syrjänen J, Partanen J, et al. Celiac disease and HLA DQ in patients with IgA nephropathy. *The American Journal of Gastroenterology.* Oct 2002; 97(10):2572-6.

254. Ots M, Uibo O, Metsküla K, Uibo R, Salupere V. IgA-antigliadin in patients with IgA nephropathy: the secondary phenomenon? *American Journal of Nephrology.* 1999; 19(4):453-8.

255. Gama R, Schweitzer FAW. Renal calculus: a unique presentation of coeliac disease. *BJU International.* 1999; 84:528-9.

256. Jones DP, Stapleton FB, Whitington G, Noe HN. Urolithiasis and enteric hyperoxaluria in a child with steatorrhea. *Clinical Pediatrics.* Jun 1987; 26(6):304-6.

257. Saalman R, Fällström SP. High incidence of urinary tract infection in patients with coeliac disease. *Archives of Disease in Childhood.* Feb 1996; 74(2):170-1.

258. Molteni N, Bardella MT, Bianchi PA. Obstetric and gynecological problems in women with untreated celiac sprue. *Journal of Clinical Gastroenterology.* Feb 1999; 12(1)37-9.

259. Stazi AV, Mantovani A. A risk factor for female fertility and pregnancy: celiac disease. *Gynecologica endocrinology: the Official Journal of the International Society of Gynecological Endocrinology.* Dec 2000; 14(6):454-63.

260. Kotze LM. Gynecologic and obstetric findings related to nutritional status and adherence to a gluten-free diet in Brazilian patients with celiac disease. *Journal of Clinical Gastroenterology.* Aug 2004; 38(7):567-74.

261. Sher KS, Mayberry JF. Female fertility, obstetric and gynaecological history in coeliac disease: a case control study. *Acta Paediatrica. Supplementum.* May 1996; 412:76-7.

262. Collin P, Vilska S, Heinonen PK, Hällström O, Pikkarainen P. Infertility and coeliac disease. *Gut.* Sep 1996; 39(3):382-4.

263. Vanciková Z, Chlumecký V, Sokol D, et al. The serologic screening for celiac disease in the general population (blood donors) and in some high-risk groups of adults (patients with autoimmune diseases, osteoporosis and infertility) in the Czech republic. *Folia Microbiologica.* 2002; 47(6):753-8.

264. Meloni GF, Dessole S, Vargiu N, Tomasi PA, Musumeci S. The prevalence of celiac disease in infertility. *Human Reproduction.* Nov 1999; 14(11):2759-61.

265. Cosnes J, Cosnes C, Cosnes A, et al. Undiagnosed celiac disease in childhood. *Gastroenterologie Clinique et Biologique.* Jun-Jul 2002; 26(6-7)616-23.

266. Shamaly H, Mahameed A, Sharony A, Shamir R. Infertility and celiac disease: do we need more than one serological marker? *Acta Obstetricia et Gynecologica Scandinavica.* Dec 2004; 83(12)1184-8.

267. Caramaschi P, Biasi D, Carletto A, Randon M, Pacor ML, Bambara LM. Celiac disease and abortion: focusing on a possible relationship. *Recenti Progressi in Medicina.* Feb 2000; 91(2):72-5.

268. Bradley RJ, Rosen MP. Subfertility and gastrointestinal disease: 'unexplained' is often undiagnosed. *Obstetrical and Gynecological Survey.* Feb 2004; 59(2):108-17.

269. Rostami K, Steegers EA, Wong WY, Braat DD, Steegers-Theunissen RP. Coeliac disease and reproductive disorders: a neglected association. *European Journal of Obstetrics, Gynecology, and Reproductive Biology.* Jun 2001; 96(2):156-9.

270. Bona G, Marinello D, Orderda G. Mechanisms of abnormal puberty in coeliac disease. *Hormone Research.* 2002; 57(Suppl 2):63,3p.

271. Valentino R, Savastano S, Tommaselli AP. Unusual association of thyroiditis, Addison's disease, ovarian failure and celiac disease in a young woman. *Journal of Endocrinological Investigation.* May 1999; 22(5):390-4.

272. Porpora MG, Picarelli A, Prosperi Porta R, Di Tola M, D'Elia C, Cosmi EV. Celiac disease as a cause of chronic pelvic pain, dysmenorrhea, and deep dyspareunia. *Obstetrics and Gynecology.* May 2002; 99(5pt2):937-9.

273. Ziaei S, Zakeri M, Kazemnejad A. A randomised controlled trial of vitamin E in the treatment of primary dysmenorrhea. *BJOG: An International Journal of Obstetrics and Gynaecology.* Apr 2005; 112(4):466-9.

274. Stazi AV, Mantovani A. Celiac disease and its endocrine and nutritional implications on male reproduction. *Minerva Medica.* Jun 2004; 95(3):243-54.

275. Farthing MJ, Rees LH, Edwards CR, Dawson AM. Male gonadal function in coeliac disease: III. Pituitary regulation. *Clinical Endocrinology.* Dec 1983; 19(6):661-71.

276. Farthing MJ, Rees LH, Edwards CR, Dawson AM. Male gonadal function in coeliac disease: 2. Sex hormones. *Gut.* Feb 1983; 24(2):127-35.

277. Mitchell RMS, Robinson TJ. Celiac disease in pregnancy – not always a relapse. *Acta Obstetricia Et Gynecologica Scandanavica.* Aug 2003; 82(8):777, 1p.

278. Bajor J, Lomb Z, Anga B, Beró T. Manifestation of adult celiac disease during the puerperium. *Orvosi Hetilap.* Dec 28, 2003; 144(52):2565-9.

279. Sciberras C, Vella C, Grech V. The prevalence of coeliac disease in Down's syndrome in Malta. *Annals of Tropical Paediatrics.* Mar 2004; 24(1):81-3.

280. Cogulu O, Ozkinay F, Gunduz C, et al. Celiac disease in children with Down syndrome: importance of follow-up and serological screening. *Pediatrics International: Official Journal of the Japan Pediatric Society.* Aug 2003; 45(4):395-9.

281. Bonamico M, Pasquino AM, Mariani P, et al. Prevalence and clinical picture of celiac disease in Turner syndrome. *Journal of Clinical Endocrinology and Metabolism.* Dec 2002; 87(12):5495-8.

282. Lima Rm, Rocha C, Alvares S, Rocha A, Senra V, Rocha H. Celiac disease, cystic fibrosis and dilated cardiomyopathy. *Anales de Pediatria : Publacacion Oficial de la Asociacion Espanola de Pediatria.* Aug 2004; 61(2)193-4.

283. Rabinowitz I. Diagnosis of cystic fibrosis and celiac disease in an adult: one patient, two diseases, and three reminders. *Respiratory Care.* May 2005; 50(5):644-5.

284. Catassi C, Fasano A. Celiac disease as a cause of growth retardation in childhood. *Current Opinion in Pediatrics.* Aug 2004; 16(4):445-9.

285. Mohindra S, Yachha SK, Srivastava A, Krishnani N, Aggarwal R, Ghoshal UC. Coeliac disease in Indian children: assessment of clinical, nutritional and pathologic characteristics. *Journal of Health, Population, and Nutrition.* Sep 2001; 19(3):204-8.

286. Jansson UH, Kristiansson B, Albertsson-Wikland K, Bjarnason R. Short-term gluten challenge in children with coeliac disease does not impair spontaneous growth hormone secretion. *Journal of Pediatric Endocrinology and Metabolism: JPEM.* Jun 2003; 16(5):771-8.

287. Fisgin T, Yarali N, Duru F, Usta B, Kara A. Hematologic manifestation of childhood celiac disease. *Acta Haematologica.* 2004; 111(4):211-4.

288. Umarnazarova ZE. Specificity of ferrokinetics in children with enzymopathy of small intestine. *Likars'ka Sprava.* Oct-Nov 2003; (7):63-7.

289. Economou M, Karyda S, Gombakis, Tsatra J, Athanassiou-Metaxa M. Subclinical celiac disease in children: refractory iron deficiency as the sole presentation. *Journal of Pediatric Hematology/Oncology.* Mar 2004; 26(3):153-4; author reply 154.

290. Kalayci AG, Kansu A, Girgin N, Kucuk, O, Aras G. Bone mineral density and importance of a gluten-free diet in patients with celiac disease in childhood. *Pediatrics.* Nov 2001; 108(5):e89.

291. Carvalho CN, Sdepanian VL, De Morais MB, Fagundes Neto U. Celiac disease under treatment: evaluation of bone mineral density. *Jornal de Pediatria.* Jul-Aug 2003; 79(4):303-8.

292. Kavak US, Yüce A, Koçak N, et al. Bone mineral density in children with untreated and treated celiac disease. *Journal of Pediatric Gastroenterology and Nutrition.* Oct 2003; 37(4):434-6.

293. Barera G, Beccio S, Proverbio MC, Mora S. Longitudinal changes in bone metabolism and bone mineral content in children with celiac disease during consumption of a gluten-free diet. *American Journal of Clinical Nutrition.* Jan 2004; 79(1):148-54.

294. Jain V, Angitii RR, Singh S, Thapa BR, Kumar L. Proximal muscle weakness-an unusual presentation of celiac disease. *Journal of Tropical Pediatrics.* Dec 2002; 48(6):380-1.

295. Wakefield AJ, Puleston M, Montgomery SM, Anthony A, O'Leary JJ, Murch SH. Review article: the concept of entero-colonic encephalopathy, autism, and opioid receptor ligands. *Aliment Pharmacol Ther.* 2002; 16:663-674.

296. Goodwin FC, Beattie RM, Millar J, Kirkham FJ. Celiac disease and childhood stroke. *Pediatric Neurology.* Aug 2004; 31(2):139-42.

297. Suoglu OD, Emiroglu HH, Sokucu S, Cantez S, Cevikbas U, Saner G. Celiac disease and glycogenic acanthosis: a new association? *Acta Paediatrica.* Apr 2004; 93(4):568-70.

298. Stagi S, Giani T, Simonini G, Falcini F. Thyroid function, autoimmune thyroiditis and coeliac disease in juvenile idiopathic arthritis. *Rheumatology.* Apr 2005; 44(4):517-20.

299. Kolacek S, Jadresin O, Petkovic I, Misak Z, Sonicki Z, Booth IW. Gluten-free diet has a beneficial effect on chromosome instability in lymphocytes of children with coeliac disease. *Journal of Pediatric Gastroenterology and Nutrition.* Feb 2004; 38(2):177-80.

300. Loma-Sanner I, Kang E, Sepehrhad S, Goldstein S, Herman M, Accardo P, et al. A floppy child with failure to thrive. *Lancet.* Jul 2005; 366:176.

301. Kaspers S, Kordonouri O, Schober E, Grabert M, Hauffa BP, Holl RW. Anthropometry, metabolic control, and thyroid autoimmunity in type 1 diabetes with celiac disease: a multicenter survey. *Journal of Pediatrics.* Dec 2004; 145(6):790-5.

302. Peretti N, Bienvenu F, Bouvet C, et al. The temporal relationship between the onset of type 1 diabetes and celiac disease: a study based on immunoglobulin A antitransglutaminase screening. *Pediatrics.* May 2004; 113(5):E418-22.

303. Sipetic S, Vlajinac H, Kocev N, Marinkovic J, Radmanovic S, Denic L. Family history and risk of type 1 diabetes mellitus. *Acta Diabetologica.* Sep 2002; 39(3):111-5.

304. Hansen D, Brock-Jacobsen B, Lund E, et al. Clinical benefit of a gluten-free diet in Type 1 diabetic children with screening-detected celiac disease, *Diabetes Care.* 2006; 29:2452-2456.

305. Ziegler AG, Schmid S, Huber D, Hummel M, Bonifacio E. Early infant feeding and risk of developing type 1 diabetes-associated autoantibodies. *JAMA: The Journal of the American Medical Association.* Oct 1, 2003; 290(13):1721-8.

306. Högberg L, Sokolski J, Stenhammar L. Chronic bullous dermatosis of childhood associated with coeliac disease in a 6-year-old boy. *Acta Dermato-Venereologica.* 2004; 84(2):158-9.

307. Medica I, Zmak M, Persic M. Dermatitis herpetiformis in a 30-month-old child. *Minerva Pediatrica.* Apr 2003; 55(2):171-3.

308. Shamir R. Levine A. Yalon-Hacohen M, et al. Faecal occult blood in children with celiac disease. *European Journal of Pediatrics.* Nov 2000; 159(11):832-4.

309. Bolme P, Eriksson M, Stintzing G. The gastrointestinal absorption of penicillin V in children with suspected coeliac disease. *Acta Paediatrica Scandinavica.* Sep 1977; 66(5):573-8.

310. Ansaldi N, Palmas T, Corrias A, et al. Autoimmune thyroid disease and celiac disease in children. *Journal of Pediatric Gastroenterology and Nutrition.* Jul 2003; 37(1):63-6.

Index

A

Abdominal distention (#**103**), 138
    in candida albicans mucosal infection, 140
    in carbohydrate malabsorption, 139
    in collagenous colitis, 150
    in duodenal ulcerations, 148
    in gastric ulcerations, 133
    in gluten sensitive enteritis, 144
    in intestinal edema, 142
    in intestinal gas, 152
    in irritable bowel syndrome, 153
    in lactose intolerance, 146
    in lymphocytic colitis, 150
    in maltose intolerance, 147
    in sucrose intolerance, 149
    in ulcerative jejunitis, 146
    in vitamin B_3 (niacin) deficiency, 82
Abdominal pain (#**104**), 138
    bloating
        in candida albicans mucosal infection, 140
        in collagenous colitis, 150
        in Crohn's disease, 152
        in gluten sensitive enteritis, 144
        in intestinal edema from inflammation, 142
        in lymphocytic colitis, 150
    bloating and cramping
        in carbohydrate malabsorption, 139
        in constipation, 151
        in lactose intolerance, 146
        in maltose intolerance, 147
        in sucrose intolerance, 149
    cramping
        after eating fatty foods, 136
        in acute diarrhea, 140
        in small bowel intussusception, 148
    localized
        in enteropathy associated T- cell lymphoma, 184
        in postbulbar duodenal ulceration, 148
    poorly localized in vitamin B_{12} deficiency, 85
Abortion (miscarriage)
    recurrent, 101
        in antiphospholipid syndrome, 162
        in hyperprolactinemia, 101
    spontaneous (#**278**), 237
        in vitamin A deficiency, 76
        in vitamin B_9 (folic acid) deficiency, 84
Absence of volition, 207

Acidosis in acute diarrhea, 140
Addison's disease (#**132**), 154
Advocacy group, access to, 30
Allergic rhinitis (#**147**), 161
Allergy in IgA deficiency, 166
Aloofness in developmental delay, 249
Alopecia (hair loss)
    areata (sharply defined hair loss) (#**159**), 170
    diffuse (balding) (#**160**), 170
    in iron deficency anemia, 112
Alpha-linolenic acid (ALA) deficiency (#**2**), 64
Amenorrhea, secondary (#**264**), 226
    in hyperprolactinemia, 101
Amino acids, essential, deficiency of (#**15**), 75
Anemia
    in iron deficiency (#**50**), 112
        in autoimmune cholangitis, 136
        in B-cell non-Hodgkin's
            lymphoma, 183
        in copper deficiency, 69, 104
        in duodenal erosions, 142
        in H. pylori bacter infection, 135
        in pulmonary hemosiderosis, 211
        in ulcerative jejunitis, 146
        in zinc deficiency, 74, 110
        refractory in childhood (#**290**), 244
        severe in pregnancy (#**276**), 235
    in macrocytosis, 108
    in vitamin B_2 (riboflavin) deficiency, 81
    in vitamin B_6 (pyridoxine) deficiency, 83
    in vitamin B_9 (folic acid) deficiency (#**49**), 111
    in vitamin B_{12} deficiency (#**51**), 113
    in vitamin C deficiency, 86
    latent, in intestinal enzymopathies of
            small intestine (#**289**), 243
Angina pectoris (#**62**), 118
    in coronary artery disease, 120
    in iron deficiency anemia, 112
Anorexia - loss of appetite (#**71**), 123
    in Addison's disease, 154
    in cachexia, 122
    in iron deficiency, 70, 112
    in magnesium deficiency, 71, 106
    in phosphorus deficiency, 72, 107
    in potassium deficiency, 73, 105
    in primary hyperparathyroidism, 158
    in sarcoidosis, 167
    in zinc deficiency, 74, 110

Antibodies
Anti-endomysial antibody blood test (EMA), 22
Anti-endomysium (#27), 95
Anti-gliadin (#28), 95
Anti-gliadin antibody (AGA) blood test, 22
Anti-tissue transglutaminase (#29), 96
Anti-tissue transglutaminase antibody (tTG) blood test, 22
Associated autoimmune (#30), 96
Antiphospholipid syndrome (#148), 162
Anxiety
chronic maladaptive (#222), 204
in hyperthyroidism, 161
in iron deficiency, 70, 112
in magnesium deficiency, 71, 106
in potassium deficiency, 73, 105
in protein deficiency, 75, 109
in vitamin B_1 (thiamin) deficiency, 80
in vitamin B_3 (niacin) deficiency, 82
marked, in premenstrual syndrome, 229
Aortic vasculitis causing midaortic syndrome (#57), 115
Apathy (#223), 204
in autoimmune thyroiditis, 160
in copper deficiency, 69, 104
in iron deficiency, 70, 112
in protein deficiency, 75, 109
in vitamin B_1 (thiamin) deficiency, 80
in vitamin B_3 (niacin) deficiency, 82
Appetite, 34
increased (#72), 124
loss of - *see anorexia*, 123
Aphthous ulcers and non-aphthous ulcers (#73), 124
Arachidonic acid (AA) (#5), 67
Arthritis
enteropathic (#257), 222
in systemic lupus erythematosus, 168
juvenile idiopathic (#299), 251
psoriatic (#258), 222
recurrent monoarthritis (#259), 223
resembling rheumatoid arthritis in vitamin C deficiency, 86
Asthma (#149), 163
Ataxia
gait disturbance (#204), 192
gluten (#205), 193
progressive myoclonic (#206), 194
Atherosclerosis (#58), 116
in elevated homocysteine levels, 100

in omega-3 fatty acid deficiencies, 64, 65, 66
in vitamin B_6 (pyridoxine) deficiency, 83
in vitamin B_9 (folic acid) deficiency, 84, 111
in vitamin B_{12} deficiency, 85, 113
in vitamin E deficiency, 78
Attention deficit hyperactive disorder (ADHD) (#295), 249
in EPA omega-3 fatty acid deficiency, 66
Autism and learning disorders (#294), 248
in EPA omega-3 fatty acid deficiency, 66
Autoantigen in CD is tissue transglutaminase, 7
Autoimmune cholangitis (antimitochondrial antibody-negative primary biliary cirrhosis) (#99), 136
Autoimmune disorders in CD (#150), 164
Autoimmune disorders in dermatitis herpetiformis (#151), 165
Autoimmune hepatitis (#133), 154
Autoimmune polyglandular syndrome (#152), 165
Autoimmune thyroiditis (hypothyroidism) (#145), 160
Avenin in oats, 3

B

B-cell non-Hodgkin's lymphoma (#187), 183
Berberi - advanced vitamin B_1 (thiamin) deficiency, 80
Behavioral disorders in omega-3 fatty acid deficiency, 64, 66
Biopsies of small intestinal mucosa, 23
Bipolar disorder in EPA omega-3 fatty acid deficiency, 66
Bitot's spots (#238), 212
Bleeding
blood in the urine in vitamin K deficiency, 79
conjunctival hemorrhage in vitamin C deficiency, 86
easy bruising, 117
epistaxis - bright red nosebleed (#60), 117
excessive, 67, 68, 110
excessive menstrual in vitamin K deficiency, 79
from the gums, 79
in dark bluish swellings, 117
in hypoprothrombinemia, 114
in idiopathic thrombocytopenic purpura, 114
in prolonged prothrombin time, 110
increased blood clotting, 64, 65, 66
into the skin, mucous membranes and conjunctiva, 115
occult gastrointestinal bleeding (#130), 152
petechiae in vitamin C deficiency, 86
prolonged bleeding time in omega-6 fatty acid deficiencies, 67

Cardiac
  abnormalities in hyperthyroidism, 161
  disturbance in hypokalemia, 105
  dysrhythmias in magnesium deficiency, 71, 106
Cardiomegaly (#63), 119
  in vitamin B_1 (thiamin) deficiency, 80
Cardiomyopathy (#64), 119
  in selenium deficiency, 73
Carpalpedal spasms in idiopathic hypoparathyroidism, 159
Cataracts (#242), 213
  in calcium deficiency, 68, 103
  in vitamin A deficiency, 76
  in vitamin B_2 (riboflavin) deficiency, 81
Celiac disease
  associated disorders in, 20
  attributes of, 9
  atypical signs and symptoms of, 20, 27
  classic signs and symptoms of, 19
  complications of, 20
  continuous long-term follow-up by a
    multidisciplinary team in, 30
  definitive diagnosis in, 25
  diagnostic tests for, 21
  education, 29
  genetic predisposition to, 11
  genetic testing for, 24
  identification and treatment of nutritional
    deficiencies and other manifestations in, 30
  International Classification of Diseases (ICD) code
    for celiac disease, 9
  intestinal biopsy improvement in, 31
  latent, 27
  management of, 29
  manifestations of, 19
  negative antibody results for, 22
  patient classification in, 27
  phenotypes in, 27
  positive antibody results in, 22
  prevalence of, 17
  prognosis, 31
  refractory sprue, 183
  serologic antibody screening for, 21
Celiac disease-specific T-lymphocytes, 11
Celiac iceberg, 27
Cell-mediated immune response, 13
Cerebral perfusion abnormalities (#210), 197
Cheilosis (#74), 125
Chest pain

  in cancer of the esophagus, 130
  in esophageal motor abnormalities, 131
  in GERD - gastroesophageal reflux disease, 131
Cholesterol - low (#32), 98
Chorea (#207), 195
Chronic bullous dermatosis of childhood (#304), 255
Clots, abnormal in vitamin E deficiency, 78
Collagenous colitis (#123), 150
Collagenous gastritis (#95), 134
Colonic volvulus and ulcerative jejunoileitis (#122), 149
Coma in vitamin B_1 (thiamin) deficiency, 80
Common variable immunodeficiency (#153), 166
Concentration, poor in vitamin B_1 (thiamin) deficiency, 80
Confabulation in vitamin B_1 (thiamin) deficiency, 80
  in vitamin B_3 (niacin) deficiency, 82
Confusion
  in hypoglycemia - low blood sugar, 104
  in magnesium deficiency, 71, 106
  in potassium deficiency, 73, 105
  in primary hyperparathyroidism, 158
  in schizophrenia, 207
  in vitamin B_1 (thiamin) deficiency, 80
  in vitamin B_{12} deficiency, 85, 113
Congenital anomalies (#283), 240
Congenital malformations in vitamin B_9 (folic acid)
    deficiency, 84
Conjunctiva
  dryness of the bulbar (white of eyeball), 76
  inflammation of, 81
  hemorrhage in vitamin C deficiency, 86
Constipation (#126), 151
  alternating with diarrhea (#127), 151
  in hypothyroidism, 160
  in magnesium deficiency, 71, 106
  in primary hyperparathyroidism, 158
  in vitamin B_1 (thiamin) deficiency, 80
  in vitamin B_{12} deficiency, 85
Consultation with a skilled dietitian, 29
Coordination for walking - defective in vitamin D
    deficiency, 77
Copper deficiency (#8), 69
Cornea, dryness of with haziness, 76
Coronary artery disease (#65), 120
Cortical calcifying angiomatosis (#211), 197
Cough
  nocturnal in esophageal motor abnormalities, 131
  non-productive in sarcoidosis, 167
  productive in bronchopneumonia, 209

productive of purulent sputum in lung abcess, 210

Crohn's disease (#128), 152

Crypts, 10, 14

Cutaneous vasculitis (#168), 173

Cutis laxa, acquired (#169), 174

Cystic fibrosis (#285), 241

D

Dark freckles in Addison's disease, 154

Deamidation, 11, 12

Death, 76, 80

Delay in diagnosis of CD and increased risk of autoimmune
disorders, 164

Delayed puberty in boys (#308), 258

Delayed puberty in girls (#302), 253

Delirium in vitamin B_{12} deficiency, 85

Delusion - belief inconsistent with reality, 207

Dementia (#212), 198

in vitamin B_1 (thiamin) deficiency, 80

Dental enamel defects - imperfect teeth (#75), 126

Depression (#224), 205

in hyperthyroidism, 161

in magnesium deficiency, 71

in menopause, 229

in potassium deficiency, 73, 105

in vitamin B_3 (niacin) deficiency, 82

in vitamin B_6 (pyridoxine) deficiency, 83

in vitamin B_{12} deficiency, 85

in vitamin C deficiency, 86

in zinc deficiency, 74

Dermatitis herpetiformis (#170), 175

Dermatitis herpetiformis in childhood (#305), 256

Dermatitis in protein deficiency, 75, 109

Dermatomyositis (#171), 176

Developmental delay (#296), 249

Diabetes mellitus

gastrointestinal complications in type 1 (#138), 157

instability (#137), 157

juvenile type 1 (#303), 254

type 1 - insulin dependent (#136), 156

Diarrhea

acute (#108), 140

chronic (#109), 141

in carbohydrate malabsorption, 139

in collagenous colitis, 150

in Crohn's disease, 152

in enteropathy-associated T-cell lymphoma, 184

in gastric ulceration, 133

in hypokalemic rhabdomyolysis, 188

in IgA deficiency, 166

in irritable bowel syndrome, 153

in lactose intolerance, 146

in lymphocytic colitis, 150

in maltose intolerance, 147

in milk intolerance, 147

in sucrose intolerance, 149

in vitamin B_9 (folic acid) deficiency, 84, 111

intermittent in vitamin B_{12} deficiency, 85, 113

intractable in refractory sprue, 183

persistent in mesenteric lymph node cavitation, 186

serious (may be bloody) in vitamin B_3 (niacin)
deficiency, 82

with outpouring of blood in ulcerative colitis, 151

worsening of in zinc deficiency, 74, 110

Difficulty

chewing/swallowing, 167

concentrating in glucose deficiency, 63, 104

making friendships in developmental delay, 249

recalling information in vitamin B_1 (thiamin)
deficiency, 80

swallowing - see dysphagia, 130

Digestion, poor in vitamin A deficiency, 76

Disorganized speech and behavior, 207

Disorientation in vitamin B_1 (thiamin) deficiency, 80

in vitamin B_3 (niacin) deficiency, 82

Distended neck veins in vitamin B_1 (thiamin) deficiency, 80

Dizziness

in Addison's disease, 154

in hypoglycemia, 63

in hypokalemia, 105

in vitamin B_3 (niacin) deficiency, 82

Docosahexaenoic acid (DHA) deficiency (#3), 65

Down syndrome (#281), 239

Drowsiness, 73, 105

Dry eye syndrome in EPA fatty acid deficiency, 66

in vitamin A deficiency, 76

Dry mouth in vitamin A deficiency, 76

Dry skin in EPA omega-3 fatty acid deficiency, 66

Duodenal erosions in the second part of
the duodenum (#110), 142

Duodenum, 39

Dysbiosis

causing intestinal gas, 152

in constipation, 151

in diarrhea, 141

Dysgeusia - distortion/impairment of taste (#250), 216
  in Sjögren's syndrome, 167
  in vitamin B$_3$ (niacin) deficiency, 82
  in vitamin B$_{12}$ deficiency, 85, 113
  in zinc deficiency, 74, 110
Dyslexia in EPA omega-3 fatty acid deficiency, 66
Dysmenorrhea - menstrual pain (#269), 230
Dyspareunia - pain during intercourse (#270), 231
Dysphagia - difficulty swallowing (#86), 130
  in cancer of the esophagus, 130
  in cancer of the pharynx, 129
  in esophageal motor abnormalities, 131
  in esophageal small cell carcinoma, 130
  in iron deficiency, 70, 112
  in GERD - gastroesophageal reflux disease, 131
  in Plummer - Vinson syndrome, 132
  in post-cricoid carcinoma, 129
  in glycogenic acanthosis (#298), 250
Dyspraxia - movement disorder in EPA omega-3 fatty acid
  deficiency, 66

E

Ear problems in omega-3 fatty acid deficiency, 64
Early fullness after eating in delayed gastric emptying, 132
Ecchymosis (#59), 117
Eczema (#173), 177
Edema - fluid retention (#172), 176
  in infants in vitamin C deficiency, 86
  intestinal (#111), 142
  of face, legs, trunk and serous cavities in vitamin B$_1$
    (thiamin) deficiency, 80
  periorbital and facial in hypothyroidism, 160
  pulmonary and peripheral in cardiomegaly, 119
  with lung congestion in vitamin B$_1$ (thiamin)
    deficiency, 80
Eicosapentaenoic acid (EPA) deficiency (#4), 66
Emicrania - headache (#213), 198
  in anemia, 112, 113
  in chronic fatigue syndrome, 200
  in glucose deficiency, 63, 104
Encephalopathy in calcium deficiency, 68, 103
Endomysium, 11, 13, 55
Endoscopy procedure with proximal intestine biopsies, 23
  intraepithelial lymphocytosis in samples (#191), 185
  negative - poor technique, 24
Epigastric pain in gastric ulcers, 133
Epilepsy (#214), 199

occipital lobe with cerebral calcifications (#219), 201
Epistaxis, unexplained (nosebleed) (#60), 117
Epitope, 12, 55
Eructation - belching in delayed gastric emptying, 132
Erythema elevatum diutinum (EED) (#174), 177
Erythema nodosum (#175), 178
Esophageal motor abnormalities (#88), 131
Esophagus, 35
Excessive response to annoyance, 206
Eyes
  tearing, burning and itching of in vitamin B$_2$
    (riboflavin) deficiency, 81
  visual disturbances of in glucose deficiency, 63, 104
  visual impairment of in iron deficiency, 70, 112

F

Failure to gain weight in a child, 139
Failure to thrive and growth retardation (#287), 242
  in milk intolerance, 147
  severe in a child in small bowel
    intussusception (#120), 148
Faintness in glucose deficiency, 63, 104
Fatigue
  chronic / lassitude (#215), 199
  chronic fatigue syndrome (#216), 200
  in chronic ulcerative jejunitis, 146
  in hypoglycemia, 63, 104
  in iron deficiency, 70, 112
  in magnesium deficiency, 71, 106
  in Plummer-Vinson syndrome, 132
  in primary hyperparathyroidism, 158
  in protein deficiency, 75, 109
  in vitamin B$_1$ (thiamin) deficiency, 80
  in zinc deficiency, 74, 110
  progressive in primary sclerosing cholangitis, 137
Fatty liver in omega-6 fatty acid deficiency, 67
Fecal occult blood in childhood (#306), 256
Fetus
  abnormalities and malformations, 74, 110
  growth retardation in zinc deficiency, 74, 110
  perinatal deaths, 74, 110
  prematurity in zinc deficiency, 74, 110
Fluid imbalance in omega-3 fatty acid deficiency, 64
Fluid retention - see edema, 176
Follicular hyperkeratosis (#176), 178
Food Allergen Labeling and Consumer Act of 2003, 49
Food allergy, IgE and non IgE (#112), 143

G

Gall bladder motility, impaired (**#100**), 136
Gas, excessive (**#129**), 152
    in carbohydrate malabsorption, 139
    in constipation and alternating with diarrhea, 151
    in delayed gastric emptying, 132
    in diarrhea, 141
    in gluten sensitive enteritis, 144
    in irritable bowel syndrome, 153
    in lactose intolerance, 146
    in maltose intolerance, 147
    in sucrose intolerance, 149
Gastric emptying, delayed, (**#92**), 132
Gastric ulcer (**#93**), 133
Gastric ulcerations, multiple (**#94**), 133
Gastroesophageal reflux disease (GERD) (**#89**), 131
Gastrointestinal bleeding, occult (**#130**), 152
Gingival inflammation - in vitamin C deficiency, 86
Gliadin in wheat, 3, 10
Glossary, 54
Glossitis - inflammation of tongue, 70, 81, 82, 83, 84, 85
Glucose deficiency (**#1**), 63
Gluten, 3
    26-mer peptide derived from incomplete digestion of, 12
    33-mer peptide derived from incomplete digestion of, 7, 12
    anatomy of a grain of wheat, 3
    containing grains, 4
    opioid effect of, 10
    plant taxonomy, 3
    safe alternatives for, 4
    the environmental factor in CD, 11, 19
Gluten-free diet
    necessity of lifelong adherence to, 29
    "Sample of Foods Commonly Allowed and Not Allowed" - Appendix III, 49
    "Self-Management Three Step Process" - Appendix II, 45
    "Unsafe Foods and Ingredients" - Appendix I, 44
Gluten-free diet trial, 25
Gluten sensitive enteritis (**#113**), 144
Gluten sensitive enteropathy, 9
Glutenin, 3
Glycogenic acanthosis (**#298**), 250
Grave's disease (hyperthyoidism) (**#146**), 161
Gums, bleeding and/or swollen (**#76**), 127

in vitamin C deficiency, 86

H

Hair
    coiling of in skin in vitamin C deficiency, 86
    diameter lower and cuticolar scores
        higher of (**#161**), 171
    discoloration (black or brown turns reddish) of, 75
    loss of pigmentation of, 69
    thinning of, 75
Hallucinations in vitamin B_{12} deficiency, 85, 113
Hangnail (**#177**), 179
Headache - *see emicrania, also migraine*
Heart
    enlargement (cardiomegaly) and heart failure
        in vitamin B_1 (thiamin) deficiency, 80
    small size of in Addison's disease, 154
Heartburn (**#90**), 132
    in gastroesophageal reflux disease (GERD), 131
Helicobacter pylori infection (H. pylori) (**#97**), 135
Hematoma, 99
Hemochromatosis (**#52**), 113
Hemorrhage
    in idiopathic pulmonary hemosiderosis, 211
    in infants, 86
    risk for in hypoprothrombinemia, 114
    splinter-like in nails, 86
Hepatic granulomatous disease (**#135**), 155
Hepatomegaly (enlarged liver), 155
Histopathology, 14
HLA-DQ2, HLA-DQ8, 11
Hordein in barley, 3
Hunger, 34
    in hypoglycemia, 63, 104
    in obesity, 121
    in protein deficiency, 75, 109
Hyperactivity in children in vitamin B_3 (niacin) deficiency, 82
Hyperparathyroidism, primary (**#141**), 158
Hyperparathyroidism, secondary (**#142**), 159
Hyperpermeability of small intestinal lining, 9, 12
Hyperprolactinemia (**#35**), 101
Hypertension (elevated blood pressure), 68, 71, 73, 106, 161
    in aortic vasculitis, 115
    in essential fatty acid deficiency, 64, 65, 66
    intracranial, 84, 111, 197
    reversible (**#61**), 118
Hyperthyroidism - *see Grave's disease*, 161

Hypocalcemia (#37), 103
    in idiopathic hypoparathyroidism, 159
    in secondary hypoparathyroidism, 159
Hypocalciuria - low calcium excretion in urine (#260), 223
Hypochondria, in vitamin C deficiency, 86
Hypoglycemia (#39), 104
Hypogonadism in children in zinc deficiency, 74, 110
Hypogonadism, unexplained in males (#272), 232
Hypokalemic rhabdomyolysis (#195), 188
Hypoparathyroidism, idiopathic (#143), 159
Hypophosphatemia (#42), 107
    in idiopathic hypoparathyroidism, 159
    in secondary hypoparathyroidism, 159
Hypoprothrombinemia (#53), 114
Hyposplenism (#194), 187
    in lung abcess, 210
    in pneumococcal septicemia, 210
Hypotension - low blood pressure, 67, 73
Hypothyroidism - *see autoimmune thyroiditis*, 160
Hypotonia - flaccid muscles (#301), 252
Hysteria in vitamin C deficiency, 86

I

Ichthyosis, acquired (#178), 179
Idiopathic thrombocytopenic purpura (#54), 114
IgA deficiency (#154), 166
IgA nephropathy (#261), 224
Ileum, 41
Immature secondary sex characteristics
        female, 253
        male, 101, 232, 258
Immunity
        cell mediated, 13
        humoral response, 13
Immunoglobulin-A (IgA), 13
Immunoglobulin-G (IgG), 13
Impaired taste and smell in zinc deficiency, 74, 110
Impaired vibratory and sensory sensations in vitamin E
        deficiency, 78
Impotence, male (#273), 233
Inability to concentrate (#225), 206
        in depression, 205
        in DHA fatty acid deficiency, 65
Inappropriate affect in developmental delay, 249
Inattention in iron deficiency, 70, 112
Indigestion in vitamin B_1 (thiamin) deficiency, 80
        in cancer of the esophagus, 130

in esophageal small cell carcinoma, 130
Infant
    edema in vitamin C deficiency, 86
    hemorrhages in vitamin C deficiency, 86
    low birth weight in omega-6 fatty acid deficiency, 67
    reduced head circumference of in omega-6 fatty acid
        deficiency, 67
    weakness of bone, teeth, cartilage, and connective
        tissue in vitamin C deficiency, 86
Infection
    increased susceptibility to
        in iron deficiency, 70, 112, 235, 243, 244
        in zinc deficiency, 74, 110
        life-long in hyposplenism, 187
    life-threatening in transient erythroblastopenia, 115
    lowered resistance to in selenium deficiency, 73
        in protein deficiency, 75, 109
    predisposition to in neutropenia, 115
    recurrent in common variable
                immunodeficiency, 166
        in IgA deficiency, 166
    recurrent respiratory in milk intolerance, 147
    repeat and poor recovery
        in vitamin A deficiency, 76
        in zinc deficiency, 74, 110
Infertility
    both sexes
        in iron deficiency, 70, 112
        in omega-6 deficiency, 67
        in protein deficiency, 75, 109
        in vitamin B_9 (folic acid) deficiency, 84, 111
    female (#265), 227
    male (#274), 234
        in vitamin A deficiency, 76
        in vitamin D deficiency, 77
        in vitamin E deficiency, 78
        in zinc deficiency, 74, 110
Inflammation
    increased response to injury in omega-3 fatty acid
        deficiency, 64, 65, 66
    poor response to injury in omega-6 fatty acid
        deficiency, 67
Ingredient list on food packaging, 44
Insomnia (#226), 206
    in calcium deficiency, 68, 103
    in depression, 205
    in magnesium deficiency, 71, 106
    in omega-3 fatty acid deficiency, 66

in tryptophan amino acid deficiency, 75
in vitamin B_1 (thiamine) deficiency, 80
in vitamin B_6 (pyridoxine) deficiency, 83
Intellect, diminished in protein deficiency, 75
severe in brain atrophy, 196
Intercellular tight junctions (enterocytes), 11, 12
Intestinal barrier defense system, 12
Intestinal permeability, increased
(leaky gut syndrome) (#114), 145
Intrauterine growth retardation of fetus (#284), 240
in zinc deficiency, 74, 110
Iron deficiency (#9), 70
Irritability (#227), 206
in depression, 205
in magnesium deficiency, 71, 106
in premenstrual syndrome, 229
in tetany, 191
in vitamin B_1 (thiamine) deficiency, 80
in vitamin B_6 (pyridoxine) deficiency, 83
in vitamin C deficiency, 86
marked in hypoglycemia, 63, 104
Irritable bowel syndrome (#131), 153

J

Jaundice in primary sclerosing cholangitis, 137
Jejunitis, chronic ulcerative (#115), 146
Jejunum, 40
Joint pain (arthritis) in vitamin C deficiency, 86
Juvenile autoimmune thyroid disease (#309), 259
Juvenile idiopathic arthritis (#299), 251

K

Keratoconjunctivitis (#243), 214
Keratomalacia (#244), 214
Kidney stone - *see renal calculus*, 225
Koilonychia (#164), 172

L

Lack of coordination in movement and walking, 193
Lack of feeling or absence of care, 204
Lactose intolerance (#116), 146
Large intestine (colon), 42
Laryngospasm (#83), 129
Larynx, 35
Lassitude (#215), 199

in idiopathic hypoparathyroidism, 159
Leaky gut syndrome, 12
Learning
faulty in omega-6 fatty acid deficiency, 67
reduced in iron deficiency, 70, 112
Lethargy
in cachexia, 122
in calcium deficiency, 103
in rickets, 246
in vitamin C deficiency, 86
Leukopenia (low white blood cell level), 69, 104
Lightheadedness in anemia, 111, 112, 113
Linoleic acid (LA) deficiency (#6), 67
Liver enzymes, elevated, 102
in autoimmune cholangitis, 136
in hepatic granulomatous disease, 155
in non-alcoholic fatty liver disease, 155
Loss of
feeling in toes in vitamin B_1 (thiamine) deficiency, 80
power to live or go on living, 122
smell (#249), 216
speech sounds from the larynx, 80
vitality (#69), 122
in iron deficiency, 70, 112
in protein deficiency, 75, 109
in selenium deficiency, 73
Low
birth weight in intrauterine growth retardation, 240
energy in zinc deficiency, 74, 110
frustration level in attention deficit hyperactive
disorder, 249
morale in vitamin B_1 (thiamin) deficiency, 80
Lung cavities or abscesses (#232), 210
Lung failure in sarcoidosis, 167
in hypokalemia, 105
Lymphadenopathy - swollen lymph nodes (#192), 185
in B cell non-Hodgkins lymphoma, 183
in extraintestinal lymphomas, 185
Lymphocytic colitis (#124), 150
Lymphocytic gastritis (#96), 134
Lymphocytosis, 13, 185
Lymphoma
B cell non-Hodgkin (#187), 183
cryptic intestinal T-cell lymphoma
(refractory sprue) (#188), 183
enteropathy-associated T-cell lymphoma
(EATL) (#189), 184
extraintestinal (#190), 185

Lymphopenia
    in pyridoxine deficiency, 83
    in systemic lupus erythematosus, 168

M

Macroamylasemia (#43), 107
Macrocytosis (#44), 108
Macrolipasemia (#45), 108
Magnesium deficiency (#10), 71
Maltose intolerance (#117), 147
Melanoma (#179), 179
Memory
    faulty in omega-6 fatty acid deficiency, 67
    loss of immediate in vitamin B_1 (thiamin)
        deficiency, 80
        in chronic fatigue syndrome, 200
    poor in vitamin B_1 (thiamin) deficiency, 80
        in vitamin B_3 (niacin) deficiency, 82
    reduced in iron deficiency, 70, 112
Menarche, late - delayed menstruation (#266), 228
Menopause, early (#267), 229
Menstrual pain - *see dysmenorrhea*, 230
Mesenteric lymph node cavitation
        and hyposplenism (#193), 186
Migraine (#217), 200
    in cortical calcifying angiomatosis, 197
    in vitamin B_9 (folic acid) deficiency, 84, 111
Milk intolerance (bovine beta casein
        enteropathy) (#118), 147
Milk production, low in lactating women in phosphorus
        deficiency, 72, 107
Miscarriage - *see abortion*, 237
Mouth, 34
    burning sensations of, 127, 128
Mucin, 34
Mucosa
    atrophy of intestinal, 14
    complete recovery of intestinal, 31
    hypoplastic intestinal, 24
    inflamed membranes of vagina and urethra
        in vitamin B_3 (niacin) deficiency, 82
    loss of integrity in vitamin A deficiency, 76
    normal intestinal, 14
Mucous, diminished production of in vitamin A
        deficiency, 76
Multiple sclerosis (#218), 201
Muscle

atrophy of calf and thigh and tenderness
    in vitamin B_1 (thiamin) deficiency, 80
brief, rapid contraction of, 194
cramps and spasm (#197), 189
    in back and legs in calcium deficiency, 68, 103
    in idiopathic hypoparathyroidism, 159
    in potassium deficiency, 73, 105
    in tetany, especially hands and feet, 191
    in thighs in vitamin B_1 (thiamin) deficiency, 80
myoclonic jerks in potassium deficiency, 73, 105
necrosis in polymyositis, 190
pain (#196), 189
    in autoimmune thyroiditis, 160
    in chronic fatigue syndrome, 200
    in dermatomyositis, 176
poor tone in hypotonia, 252
    in protein deficiency, 75, 109
proximal weakness - upper extremities, 161, 190
stiffness in vitamin B_{12} deficiency, 85
tense calf in vitamin B_1 (thiamin) deficiency, 80
wasting (#198), 189
    in cachexia, 122
    in dermatomyositis, 176
    in polymyositis, 190
    in protein deficiency, 75, 109
    in vitamin C deficiency, 86
    of calf and thigh in vitamin B_1 (thiamin)
        deficiency, 80
weakness (#199), 189
    in chronic fatigue syndrome, 200
    in hypoglycemia, 63, 104
    in magnesium deficiency, 71, 106
    in osteomalacic myopathy, 190
    in phosphorus deficiency, 72, 107
    in primary hyperparathyroidism, 158
    in protein deficiency, 75, 109
    in selenium deficiency, 73
    in vitamin B_1 (thiamin) deficiency, 80
    in vitamin B_3 (niacin) deficiency, 82
    in vitamin D deficiency, 77
    of calf and thigh in in vitamin B_1 (thiamin)
        deficiency, 80
    sudden with inability to walk in hypokalemic
        rhabdomyolysis, 188
Myocardial ischemia in magnesium deficiency, 71, 106

N

Nails
dry and brittle nails that chip, peel, crack or break
easily (#**162**), 171
horizontal & vertical ridges in nails (#**163**), 172
koilonychia, 172
pitting in psoriasis, 181
rounded with curved ends, dark & dry (#**166**), 172
split in omega-3 fatty acid deficiency, 64
subungual splinter hemorrhages (#**165**), 172
white spots and white bands (#**167**), 173
National Institutes of Health (NIH)
panel statement on celiac disease issued August 9,
2004, xi
Nausea in delayed gastric emptying, 132
in magnesium deficiency, 71, 106
in postbulbar duodenal ulceration and stenosis, 148
in vitamin B_3 (niacin) deficiency, 82
Nerve synapses and DHA omega-3 fatty acid, 65
Nervous system disorders (#**203**), 192
Nervousness
in hypoglycemia, 63, 104
in zinc deficiency, 74, 110
Neuritis in vitamin B_3 (niacin) deficiency, 82
Neuromuscular disturbances
in magnesium deficiency, 71, 106
in phosphorus deficiency, 72, 107
Neutropenia granulocytic hypersegmentation (#**55**), 115
Nightblindness (#**245**), 214
Non-alcoholic fatty liver disease (#**134**), 155
Non-celiac gluten sensitivity reactions, 15
Non-tropical sprue, 9
Nystagmus in vitamin B_1 (thiamin) deficiency, 80

O

Oats, 3, 4, 5, 7, 30, 44
Obesity (#**66**), 121
Obstetrical complications (#**279**), 238
Occult gastrointestinal bleeding (#**130**), 152
Ocular myopathy (#**246**), 215
Ophthalmoplegia in vitamin B_1 (thiamin) deficiency, 80
Oral mucosal lesions, chronic (#**77**), 127
Osteitis fibrosa cystica (#**253**), 219
Osteomalacia (#**254**), 219
Osteomalacic myopathy (#**200**), 190
Osteonecrosis (#**255**), 220
Osteopenia in childhood (#**291**), 245

Osteoporosis (#**256**), 221
in magnesium deficiency, 71
in phosphorus deficiency, 72
in potassium deficiency, 73
in primary hyperparathyroidism, 158
in selenium deficiency, 73
in vitamin D deficiency, 77
in vitamin K deficiency, 79

P

Pallor
in chronic ulcerative jejunitis, 146
in iron deficiency, 70, 112, 244
in vitamin B_9 (folic acid) deficiency, 111
in vitamin B_{12} deficiency, 85, 113
Palpitation in hypoglycemia, 104
Palsy in hypoglycemia, 104
Pancreatic insufficiency (#**139**), 157
Paranoia in vitamin B_{12} deficiency, 85
Parathyroid hormone decreased
in magnesium deficiency, 71
Pellegra in advanced vitamin B_3 (niacin) deficiency, 82
Pelvis, flattening and narrowing of the pelvic outlet
in vitamin D deficiency, 77
Penicillin V impaired absorption in children (#**307**), 257
Peripheral neuropathy (#**229**), 208
in omega-3 fatty acid deficiency, 64
in vitamin B_6 (pyridoxine) deficiency, 83
in vitamin B_9 (folic acid) deficiency, 84
Persistent feelings of guilt or self-criticism, 205
Personality change
in hypoglycemia, 104
in magnesium deficiency, 71
in potassium deficiency, 73, 105
Pharynx, 35
Phosphorus deficiency (#**11**), 72
Photophobia
in keratoconjunctivitis sicca, 214
in vitamin B_2 (riboflavin) deficiency, 81
in zinc deficiency, 74, 110
Pityriasis rubra pilaris (#**180**), 180
Plummer-Vinson syndrome (#**91**), 132
Pneumoccocal septicemia (#**233**), 210
Polymyositis (#**201**), 190
Positivity to sugar permeability test, 145
Post-cricoid carcinoma (#**84**), 129
Post bulbar duodenal ulceration and stenosis (#**119**), 148

Potassium deficiency (#12), 73
Pregnancy
    abnormal taste sensations in zinc deficiency, 74, 110
    abnormally short or prolonged gestations, 238
    abruptio placenta in vitamin B_9 (folic acid) deficiency, 84
    atonic bleeding after delivery - uterus relaxes, 238
    complications after delivery, 238
    increased maternal morbidity (death), 238
    increased risks to fetus, 238
    inefficient labor, 238
    maternal disorders in zinc deficiency, 74, 110
    pre-eclampsia in calcium deficiency, 68, 103
    reduced rate in hyperprolactinemia, 101
    restless leg syndrome in vitamin B_9 (folic acid)
      deficiency, 84
    severe iron deficiency anemia in, 235
    toxemia of in vitamin B_9 (folic acid) deficiency, 84
    zinc-deficiency syndrome in, 74, 110
Premature ventricular and atrial contractions of the heart
    in potassium deficiency, 73
Premenstrual syndrome (PMS) (#268), 229
Primary biliary cirrhosis (#101), 137
Primary sclerosing cholangitis (#102), 137
Progressive multifocal leukoencephalopathy (#220), 202
Proinflammatory cytokines, 19
Prurigo nodularis (Hyde's prurigo) (#181), 180
Pruritic skin rash (#182), 180
Psoriasis (#183), 181
Psychiatric disorders
    in cerebral perfusion abnormalities, 197
    in vitamin B_9 (folic acid) deficiency, 84
Puerperium complicated by CD (#280), 238
Pulmonary hemosiderosis, idiopathic (#234), 211
Pulmonary permeability, increased (#235), 211
Pulse
    fast in vitamin B_1 (thiamin) deficiency, 80
    slow in hypothyroidism, 160

Q, R

Rectal bleeding in ulcerative colitis, 151
Recurring thoughts of suicide or death, 205
Reflexes
    brisk in osteomalacic myopathy, 190
    brisk in hyperthyroidism, 161
    loss of deep tendon reflexes in vitamin E deficiency, 78
    loss of knee jerk in vitamin B_1 (thiamin) deficiency, 80
Refractory sprue, 183

Renal calculus (kidney stone) (#262), 225
Restlessness in hypoglycemia, 63, 104
Retina, dysfunction of in vitamin A deficiency, 76
Retinopathy in vitamin E deficiency, 78
Rheumatic pains in legs in vitamin C deficiency, 86
Rickets (#292), 246

S

Salivary amylase, 34
Sarcoidosis (#155), 167
Schizophrenia spectrum disorders (#228), 207
    in EPA fatty acid deficiency, 66
Scleroderma (#184), 181
Scurvy - advanced vitamin C deficiency, 86
Seborrhea (#185), 182
Secalin in rye, 3
Seizures
    in cortical calcifying angiomatosis, 197
    in hypocalcemia, 103
    in magnesium deficiency, 71
    in potassium deficiency, 73, 105
Selenium deficiency (#13), 73
Semen, reduced quality of, 232
Sense of worthlessness, 205
Short duration of breast feeding (#277), 236
Short stature (#293), 247
    in omega-6 fatty acid deficiency, 67
    in zinc deficiency, 74, 110
Sjögrens syndrome (#156), 167
Skin
    cracked, itchy, pigmented red rash advancing to
      crusting in vitamin B_3 (niacin) deficiency, 82
    dry, scaly, rough with plugged hair follicles
      in vitamin A deficiency, 76
    eruptions sensitive to sunshine, 82
    extremely itchy, bullous skin rash in dermatitis
      herpetiformis, 175
    flaky in protein deficiency, 75
    itchy rash in dermatomyositis, 176
    itchy, red wet areas from chafing
      in vitamin B_3 (niacin) deficiency, 82
    lemon yellow tint of in vitamin B_{12}
      deficiency, 85, 113
    loose in copper deficiency, 69
    loss of pigmentation of in copper deficiency, 69, 104
    multiple red to brown painful nodules, 178
    raised scaly, discoid (disc-like) lesions, 168

Urticaria, chronic (hives) (**#158**), 169
Uveitis, bilateral (**#247**), 215

V

Vaginitis (**#271**), 231
Vascular membrane lipid composition, changes in, 64
Vasculitis of the central nervous system (**#221**), 203
Vasodilatation and warm extremities in thiamin deficiency, 80
Villi, intestinal, 10, 13, 14
> microscopic damage to, 14
> recovering, 31
> submicroscopic damage to, 23

Violent behavior in hypoglycemia, 63, 104
Vision
> disturbances, paroxysmal, 201
> impaired in omega-3 fatty acid deficiency, 64
> loss of visual acuity in riboflavin deficiency, 81

Vitamin A deficiency (**#16**), 76
Vitamin B$_1$ (thiamin) deficiency (**#20**), 80
Vitamin B$_2$ (riboflavin) deficiency (**#21**), 81
Vitamin B$_3$ (niacin) deficiency (**#22**), 82
Vitamin B$_6$ (pyridoxine) deficiency (**#23**), 83
Vitamin B$_9$ (folic acid) deficiency (**#24**), 84
Vitamin B$_{12}$ deficiency (**#25**), 85
Vitamin C deficiency (**#26**), 86
Vitamin D deficiency (**#17**), 77
Vitamin E deficiency (**#18**), 78
Vitamin K deficiency (**#19**), 79
Vitiligo (**#186**), 182
Vomiting (**#98**), 135
> in delayed gastric emptying, 132
> in magnesium deficiency, 71, 106
> in milk intolerance, 147
> in potassium deficiency, 73, 105
> in vitamin B$_3$ (niacin) deficiency, 82

W

Walking
> coordination for, impaired in vitamin D deficiency, 77
> delayed in children (1 to 4 year), 77
> painful with bowlegs and knock-knees in child, 77
> staggering in advanced vitamin B$_1$ (thiamin) deficiency, 80

Weakness - *see also muscle weakness*, 189
> in cachexia, 122
> in hypoglycemia, 63, 104

of extremities in peripheral neuropathy, 208
profound in neutropenia, 115
progressive in autoimmune cholangitis, 136
Weight
> gain (**#67**), 121
> loss, considerable in vitamin B$_{12}$ deficiency, 85
> loss, unexpected (**#70**), 123
>> in Addison's disease, 154
>> in B-cell non-Hodgkins lymphoma, 183
>> in cachexia, 122
>> in Crohn's disease, 152
>> in enteropathy-associated T-cell lymphoma, 184
>> in extraintestinal lymphomas, 185
>> in Grave's disease, 161
>> in mesenteric lymph node cavitation, 186
>> in phosphorus deficiency, 72, 107
>> in primary hyperparathyroidism, 158
>> in primary sclerosing cholangitis, 137
>> in protein deficiency, 75, 109
>> in refractory sprue, 183
>> in sarcoidosis, 167
>> in small bowel intussusception, 148
>> in ulcerative colitis, 151
>> in vitamin B$_1$ (thiamin) deficiency, 80

Wheat, 3, 4, 5, 7, 44
Wheezing
> in asthma, 163
> in bronchiectasis, 209
> in idiopathic hypoparathyroidism, 159

Wound healing
> impaired in vitamin C deficiency, 86
> slow in zinc deficiency, 74, 110

Writhing in chorea, 195

X

Xerophthalmia (**#248**), 215
Xerostoma - dry mouth in chronic oral mucosa lesions, 127

Y, Z

Zinc deficiency (**#14**), 74
Zonulin, 13

NOTES

NOTES

NOTES

NOTES

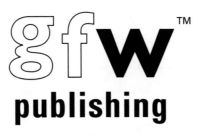

gfw™
publishing

www.glutenfreeworks.com

Gluten Free Works Publishing
Order Form

To purchase additional copies of this book for $34.95 please fill out the following form.

Fax Orders: 215-591-4566. Complete and fax this form.

Telephone Orders: 215-591-4565. We take Master Card and Visa.

Email Orders: orders@glutenfreeworks.com

Postal Orders: Gluten Free Works Publishing, PO Box 186,
                       Fort Washington, PA 19034-0186, USA.

Shipping: US: $4.00 for first book, and $2 for each additional book.
                       International: $12.00 for first book, $6.00 for each additional (estimate).

Please add 6% for products shipped to Pennsylvania addresses.

Product	Product Code	Quantity	Cost/Each	Total
1. Recognizing Celiac Disease	RCD001		$34.95	
2.				
3.				
			Subtotal:	
			Sales Tax: *(6% in PA)*	
			Shipping:	
			Total:	

Bill To:

Name _____

Address *(No P.O. Boxes)* _____

Phone _____ Email _____

Ship to: ☐ *Same as Billing*

Name _____

Address *(No P.O. Boxes)* _____

Phone _____ Email _____

Payment Method: ☐ Check   ☐ Money Order (Made payable to Gluten Free Works)
                    ☐ Visa   ☐ Master Card

Card Number _____ Expiration (MM/YY) ____

Signature _____

Please send more FREE information: ☐ Other books   ☐ Other products

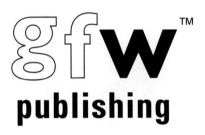

Gluten Free Works Publishing
Order Form

To purchase additional copies of this book for $34.95 please fill out the following form.

Fax Orders: 215-591-4566. Complete and fax this form.

Telephone Orders: 215-591-4565. We take Master Card and Visa.

Email Orders: orders@glutenfreeworks.com

Postal Orders: Gluten Free Works Publishing, PO Box 186,
                         Fort Washington, PA 19034-0186, USA.

Shipping: US: $4.00 for first book, and $2 for each additional book.
                         International: $12.00 for first book, $6.00 for each additional (estimate).

Please add 6% for products shipped to Pennsylvania addresses.

Product	Product Code	Quantity	Cost/Each	Total
1. Recognizing Celiac Disease	RCD001		$34.95	
2.				
3.				
			Subtotal:	
			Sales Tax: (6% in PA)	
			Shipping:	
			Total:	

Bill To:

Name _____

Address *(No P.O. Boxes)* _____

Phone _____   Email _____

Ship to: ☐ *Same as Billing*

Name _____

Address *(No P.O. Boxes)* _____

Phone _____   Email _____

Payment Method: ☐ Check   ☐ Money Order   (Made payable to Gluten Free Works)
                      ☐ Visa   ☐ Master Card

Card Number _____   Expiration (MM/YY) ____

Signature _____

Please send more FREE information: ☐ Other books   ☐ Other products